Venous Disease

Springer
London
Berlin
Heidelberg
New York
Barcelona
Budapest
Hong Kong
Milan
Paris
Santa Clara
Singapore
Tokyo

Ruckley, Fowkes and Bradbury

Venous Disease

Epidemiology, Management and Delivery of Care

Springer

Charles Vaughan Ruckley, FRCS Ed
Professor of Vascular Surgery, Vascular Surgery Office, Department of Surgery, University of Edinburgh, Royal Infirmary of Edinburgh, Edinburgh, EH3 9YW

Andrew Walter Bradbury, FRCS Ed
Senior Lecturer, Department of Surgery, University of Edinburgh, Royal Infirmary of Edinburgh, Edinburgh, EH3 9YW

Francis Gerald Reid Fowkes, FRCS Ed
Professor of Epidemiology, Wolfson Unit for Prevention of Peripheral Vascular Diseases, Department of Public Health Sciences, Teviot Place, Edinburgh, EH8 9AG

ISBN-13:978-1-4471-1212-9 Springer-Verlag London Berlin Heidelberg

British Library Cataloguing in Publication Data
Venous Disease: Epidemiology, Management and Delivery of Care
1. Veins - Diseases - Epidemiology 2. Veins - Diseases - Diagnosis 3. Veins - Diseases - Treatment
I. Ruckley, C.V. (Charles Vaughan) II. Fowkes, F.G.R.,1946 - III. Bradbury, Andrew Walter
616.1'4
ISBN-13:978-1-4471-1212-9 e-ISBN-13: 978-1-4471-0829-0
DOI: 10.1007/ 978-1-4471-0829-0

Library of Congress Cataloging-in-Publication Data
Venous Disease : Epidemiology, Management and Delivery of Care /
[Edited by] Ruckley, Fowkes and Bradbury.
p. cm.
Proceedings of a meeting sponsored by the Venous Forum of the Royal Society of Medicine, held Oct. 22-23. 1998.
Includes bibliographical references and index.
ISBN-13:978-1-4471-1212-9
1. Veins - Diseases - Congresses. I. Ruckley, C Vaughan. II. Fowkes, F.G.R., 1946 - . III. Bradbury. Andrew Walter, 1961 - . IV. Royal Society of Medicine (Great Britain). Venous Forum.
[DNLM: 1. Vascular Diseases congresses. 2.Veins Congresses. WG 600V4643 1999]
RC695.V47 1999
616.1'4-dc21
DNLM/DLC
for Library of Congress 68-35856

Softcover reprint of the hardcover 1st edition 1999

Typeset by: The Midlands Book Typesetting Company

28/3830-543210 Printed on acid-free paper

Contents

Section IV: Priorities for Treatment

Section V: Delivery of Care

Section VI: Improving Outcomes

Contributors

Dr. P.L. Allan
Senior Lecturer, Department of Medical Radiology
University of Edinburgh
Teviot Place
Edinburgh EH8 9AG

Miss M. Bello
Department of Surgery
Robert Kilpatrick Building
Leicester Royal Infirmary
Leicester LE2 7LX

Professor John J. Bergan
North Coast Surgeons
9850 Genessee Avenue
Suite 560
La Jolla
CA92037 USA

Mr D.C. Berridge
Consultant Vascular Surgeon
Departments of Vascular and Endovascular Surgery and Radiology
St James's and Seacroft University Hospitals
Beckett Street
Leeds LS9 7TF

Professor Nick Bosanquet
Professor of Health Policy
Department of Primary Care
Imperial College
Norfolk Place
London W2 1PG

Dr. Nicholas E. Bourantas
Specialist Registrar in Vascular Surgery
Cardiff Vascular Unit
University Hospital of Wales
Cardiff CF4 4XW

Mr Andrew W. Bradbury
Vascular Surgery Unit
University Department of Surgery
Royal Infirmary of Edinburgh
Edinburgh EH3 9YW

Professor K.G. Burnand
Department of Surgery
St Thomas' Hospital
Lambeth Palace Road
London SE1 7EH

Mr Michael J. Callam
Consultant Surgeon
Bedford General Hospital
Kempston Road
Bedford MK42 9DJ

Mr Philip D. Coleridge-Smith
Department of Surgery
University College London Medical School
The Middlesex Hospital
Mortimer Street
London WIN IAA

Mr. C.R.R.L. Corbett
The Princess Royal Hospital
Haywards Heath
West Sussex RH16 4EX

Mr Simon G. Darke
Royal Bournemouth Hospital
Castle Lane
East Bournemouth BH7 7DW

Dr Deborah Ellison
Research Nurse Specialist
South Manchester University Hospital
Nell Lane
West Didsbury
Manchester M20 8LR

Dr. C.J. Evans
Specialist Registrar in Public Health Medicine
Dumfries and Galloway Health Board
Grierson House
The Crichton
Bankend Road
Dumfries DG1 4ZG

Professor F.G.R. Fowkes
Professor of Epidemiology
Wolfson Unit for Prevention of Peripheral Vascular Diseases
Department of Public Health Sciences
University of Edinburgh
Teviot Place
Edinburgh EH8 9AG

Dr. Peter J. Franks
Co-director
Centre for Research & Implementation of Clinical Practice
Thames Valley University
Wolfson Institute of Health Sciences
32-38 Uxbridge Road
London W5 2BS

Dr. Tracey Gillies
Specialist Registrar in Vascular Surgery
Vascular Surgery Office
Royal Infirmary of Edinburgh
Lauriston Place EH3 9YW

Mr Ian F. Lane
Consultant Vascular Surgeon
Cardiff Vascular Unit
University Hospital of Wales
Cardiff CF4 4XW

Dr. A.J. Lee
Research Statistician
Wolfson Unit for Prevention of Peripheral Vascular Diseases
Department of Public Health Sciences
University of Edinburgh
Teviot Place
Edinburgh EH8 9AG

Dr. Gillian C. Leng
Department of Public Health Sciences
University of Edinburgh
Teviot Place
Edinburgh EH8 9AG

Professor N.J.M. London
Department of Surgery
Robert Kilpatrick Building
Leicester Royal Infirmary
Leicester LE2 7LX

Professor Gordon D.O. Lowe
Professor of Vascular Medicine
Uiversity Department of Medicine
Royal Infirmary
10 Alexandra Parade
Glasgow G31 2ER

Professor Charles N. McCollum
Professor of Sugery
University Department of Surgery
South Manchester University Hospital
Nell Lane
West Didsbury
Manchester M20 8LR

Dr. Olle Nelzén
Department of Surgery
Kärnsjukhuset
Skaraborg Hospital
S-541 33 Skövde
Sweden

Professor H.A.M. Neumann
Academisch Ziekenhuis Maastricht
Department of Dermatology
P.O. Box 5600
6200 AZ Maastricht
The Netherlands

Professor Andrew Nicolaides
Vascular Surgery Unit
St Mary's Hospital
Praed Street
Paddington
London W2 1NY

Professor H. Partsch
Dermatological Department of the Wilhelminen-Hospital
A I 1 71 Vienna
Austria

Mr A.A Quaba
Consultant Plastic Surgeon
West Lothian NHS Trust
St John's Hospital at Howden
Howden Road West
Livingston EH54 6PP

Dr. Elizabeth M. Royle
Department of Public Health Sciences
University of Edinburgh
Teviot Place
Edinburgh EH8 9AG

Professor C.Vaughan Ruckley
Professor of Vascular Surgery
Vascular Surgery Office
Royal Infirmary of Edinburgh
Lauriston Place EH3 9YW

Dr. Ann Rumley
Clinical Scientist
University Department of Medicine
Royal Infirmary
10 Alexandra Parade
Glasgow G31 2ER

Mr M. Scriven
Department of Surgery
Robert Kilpatrick Building
Leicester Royal Infirmary
Leicester LE2 7LX

Mr John H. Scurr
Consultant Surgeon
Middlesex and University College Hospital
Lister House
The Lister Hospital
Chelsea Bridge Road
London SW2W 8RE

Mr Wesley P. Stuart
Specialist Registrar
Borders General Hospital
Melrose
Roxburghshire TD6 9BS

Dr. M.J. Weston
Consultant Radiologist
Departments of Vascular and Endovascular
Surgery and Radiology
St James's and Seacroft University Hospitals
Beckett Street
Leeds LS9 7TF

Mr David D.I. Wright
Medical Director Surgicare
Dralda House
Crendon Street
High Wycombe HP13 6LS

Section I

Epidemiology and Aetiology

1 How Common Is Venous Disease in the Population?

C. J. Evans, A. J. Lee, C. V. Ruckley and F. G. R. Fowkes

Introduction

Venous disease is a common problem in the Western world. Exactly how common is difficult to determine, because relatively little epidemiological research has been conducted in this area. This is perhaps because venous conditions are rarely a cause of death and generally have a low public profile. However, venous disease causes considerable morbidity and is costly in terms of treatment, accounting for an estimated 2% of the United Kingdom's healthcare resources [1].

The term venous insufficiency covers a wide range of conditions, from asymptomatic incompetence of venous valves, through varicose veins, to chronic venous insufficiency and leg ulceration. The more severe end of the clinical spectrum will be addressed in the next chapter. The aim of this chapter is to examine how common varicose veins are in the population. Data on the incidence and prevalence of varicose veins from past studies are presented, with reference to definitions and methodologies used and populations studied. These figures are updated with results from the Edinburgh Vein Study, a recently completed cross-sectional survey of venous disease in a random population sample.

Methodological Issues

Attempts have been made recently to standardise the reporting of venous disease [2]. In addition, non-invasive methods of measurement such as Doppler and duplex ultrasound have become available and provide objective methods of assessment of venous function, acceptable for use in epidemiological studies. However, most of the studies providing data on the incidence and prevalence of varicose veins have not used such objective methods or standardised classification systems. Comparison of results from these studies is difficult due to variations in the methods and definitions used. Furthermore, many existing studies have examined selected population groups and the generalisability of results from such groups is questionable. These methodological issues will now be considered in further detail.

Definitions

Table 1.1 shows recently agreed definitions for degrees of venous dilation described by Porter, Moneta and an International Consensus Committee on Chronic Venous

Table 1.1. Definitions of venous dilation described by Porter et al. for reporting standards in venous disease [2] and definitions of varicose veins used by Widmer et al. in the Basle Study [3]

Author	Term	Definition
Porter [2]	Varicose veins	Dilated, palpable subcutaneous veins generally larger than 4 mm
	Reticular veins	Dilated, non-palpable subdermal veins 4 mm in size or less
	Telangiectases	Dilated intradermal venules less than 1 mm in size
Widmer [3]	Trunk varices	Dilated, tortuous trunks of the long or short saphenous vein and their major branches of the first or second order
	Reticular varices	Dilated, tortuous subcutaneous veins, not belonging to the main trunk or its major branches
	Hyphenwebs	Intradermal venectasis

Disease [2]. Prior to the development of these guidelines, several investigators used the definition of Arnoldi [4,5] for varicose veins: "any dilated, tortuous and elongated subcutaneous veins of the lower leg" [6–12]. In the Framingham Study [13] varicose veins were defined as "the presence of distended and tortuous veins, clearly visible in the lower limbs with the subject standing" and a similar definition was used by Abramson in a community survey in Jerusalem [14]. In the Tecumseh Community Health Study [15], the diagnosis of "any varicose veins" included "all subjects in whom prominent superficial veins were noted in the lower extremities" and was similar to definitions used in later studies in Sicily and Czechoslovakia [16,17]. In a study of hereditary factors in venous insufficiency, Gundersen and Hauge [18] used a WHO definition for varicose veins: "saccular dilation of the veins which are often tortuous". Mekky et al. [19] used the definition of Dodd and Cockett [20]: "A varicose vein is one which has permanently lost its valvular efficiency . . . As a result of continuous dilation under pressure, in the course of time a varicose vein becomes elongated, tortuous, pouched, thickened".

An important variation in definitions used is the inclusion [8,9,16,17,21] or specific exclusion [13,14,18,19,22] of abnormalities of the venules (hyphenwebs/telangiectasias) and of mild reticular varices [10,23]. This variation may have contributed to marked differences in the overall prevalence of varicose veins reported in these studies. In the Basle Study [3] varicose veins were divided into three categories, each graded 1–3 according to "the degree and extent of tortuosity and prominence" (Table 1.1). As this system was considered the best available at the time [24], it was adapted for use in the Edinburgh Vein Study [25]. Other studies have also reported different grades of severity of varices [7,10,12,15,21,26–28]. The gradings were often arbitrary and varied between studies, but reflect an attempt to distinguish between medically significant and insignificant varicose veins. In a pilot survey, Weddell defined "clinical" and "non-clinical" varicose veins by an association of signs with symptoms [29]. In the Basle Study a distinction was made between subjects with venous "disorder" and "disease", based on a statistical correlation between type and degree of varicosity and chronic venous insufficiency [3,30].

Methods of Measurement

Many studies have used both history and examination to assess the presence of varicose veins. While some studies have made use of questionnaires to standardise history-taking [10,11,15,17,19,29,31], two recent studies from England and Finland used postal questionnaires exclusively to investigate the prevalence of varicose veins in general population samples [22,32]. While being easier and cheaper to administer than physical examination of subjects, such questionnaires rely on self-reporting of varicose veins which may be unreliable. In the English study comparison of questionnaire results with examination findings for a self-selected group of subjects revealed a sensitivity of 76% and a specificity of 86% for the questionnaire [32]. In the Finnish study the sensitivity and specificity of the questionnaire was 91% and 92% respectively in women and 93% for both parameters in men. When results were compared with evaluation by a surgeon self-assessed diagnosis was shown to be less accurate in those with a familial predisposition to varicosis [33].

Sisto et al. [34] used a questionnaire to determine the prevalence of previous diagnosis of varicose veins by a physician, but no validation of this method of assessment was performed. Only 56% of women working in a department store in Czechoslovakia had themselves noticed the varicose veins which were diagnosed on examination [17]. In a study from Israel the sensitivity and specificity of interview was 47% and 95% in men and 67% and 85% in women respectively when the prevalence of varicose veins from interview data was compared with clinical examination data [14]. Hence the validity of questionnaire and interview data from different studies was variable and was affected by the characteristics of the population being assessed.

Most studies have examined subjects in a standing position. Attempts to standardise the examination technique have included an initial supervised training period for the observers [9,10], the use of only one observer [11,19] and joint classification by two observers [27]. The problems of inter-observer variability were highlighted in a study of Paris policemen. Among results from the 12 examining physicians, who each saw at least 200 men in the study, the observed prevalence of varicose veins varied from 14% to 40% [26]. In the Basle Study, in addition to physical examination of the legs, three colour photographs were taken and reclassified by one or more observers at the end of each stage of the study, to obtain a "homogeneous classification". The reproducibility of this method was shown to be between 72% and 94% for the different types of varicose veins [3].

In the Edinburgh Vein Study, several steps were taken to standardise the classification of varicose veins [25]. The two principal observers were trained together initially in the method of classification and, periodically throughout the study, all three observers independently classified the same subjects and compared results. As in the Basle Study, three colour photographs were taken of each subject. These were classified continuously throughout the study by the two members of the study team who had not examined the subject in the clinic, with periodic review of reference photographs as a reminder of the original standard. This method resulted in two independent classifications of the venous status of each subject: one based on examination in the clinic and the other on analysis of the photographic slides. There was "fair to good agreement" (kappa = 0.60) [35] between the two methods for the classification of trunk varices.

A few recent studies have used more objective methods to measure venous insufficiency. The longitudinal Bochum Study used Doppler ultrasound to detect venous reflux in schoolchildren on three occasions during their education [31]. Stvrtinova et al. [17] used Doppler ultrasound to assess patency and valvular function in the lower limbs of women working in a department store in Czechoslovakia. In the San Valentino Venous Disease Project duplex scanning is being used to evaluate patency and incompetence, and light reflection rheography to calculate the venous refilling time, in the lower limbs of the population of a village in central Italy [36]. In addition to physical examination, the study population in the Edinburgh Vein Study had eight points on the deep and superficial veins of the lower limbs assessed for the presence of venous reflux by duplex scanning [25].

Prevalence and Incidence

Table 1.2 shows the prevalence of varicose veins observed on examination of subjects in studies from various countries. As discussed above, there was no uniform definition or method of measurement used in these studies. The age and sex distribution of the populations examined also varied widely. One study sample comprised men and women randomly selected from the general population [39], while others were made up of selected occupational groups of only one sex [11,17,19,23,26] or of hospital or clinic patients [10,38]. Given these reservations, the prevalence of varicose veins in these studies varies widely from 0.1% in women from villages in rural New Guinea [12] to 60.5% in women working in a department store in Czechoslovakia [17].

In an attempt to compare more similar populations, the prevalence of varicose veins obtained from five general population surveys is shown in Table 1.3. Two of these surveys used self-administered questionnaires to assess the prevalence of varicose veins, one relying on the subject's own observation [32] and the other on the subject's report of any previous diagnosis of varicose veins made by a physician [34]. The other three studies examined subjects for the presence of varicose veins [14,15,25]. The age ranges differed among the study populations and only two of the four published studies reported age-adjusted results [14,34]. Despite this, the prevalence of varicose veins in women was similar in all five studies, ranging from 25% to 32%. However, the prevalence in men varied widely from 7% in the Finnish Study [34] to 40% in the Edinburgh Vein Study. The particularly low value in the former study was based on reported physician's diagnosis and may have been due partly to a reluctance by men to consult their doctor about varicose veins.

The classification used in the Basle Study differentiated reticular and hyphenweb varices from trunk varices (Table 1.1) [3]. When all types and severity of varices were included, 56% of men and 55% of women from the chemical industry in the Basle Study had varices. Trunk varicosity occurred in 20% of men and 11% of women, being

Table 1.2. Prevalence of varicose veins by sex, in studies from different countries

Year	[Ref]	Country	Number	Male (%)	Female (%)
1966	[37]	Bohemia	15 060	6.6	14.1
1969	[19]	Egypt	467	–	5.8
1969	[19]	England	504	–	32.1
1972	[11]	India (south)	323	25.1	–
1972	[11]	India (north)	354	6.8	–
1973	[3]	Switzerland	4 529	56.0	55.0
1973	[23]	Switzerland	610	–	29.0
1975	[6]	Cook Island (Pukapukans)	377	2.1	4.0
1975	[6]	Cook Island (Rarotongans)	417	15.6	14.9
1975	[6]	New Zealand (Maoris)	721	33.4	43.7
1975	[6]	New Zealand (Europeans)	356	19.6	37.8
1975	[6]	Tokelau Island	786	2.9	0.8
1975	[12]	New Guinea	1 457	5.1	0.1
1977	[38]	Tanzania	1 000	6.1	5.0
1981	[26]	France	7 425	26.2	–
1981	[17]	Czechoslovakia	696	–	60.5
1986	[10]	Brazil	1 755	37.9	50.9
1988	[16]	Sicily	1 122	19.3	46.2
1989	[39]	Germany	2 821	14.5	29.0
1990	[8]	Japan	541	–	45.0
1994	[9]	Turkey	850	34.5	38.3

Table 1.3. Prevalence of varicose veins in males and females from surveys of the general population

Author [Ref]	Year	Location	Age (years)	Method	Definition	Male (%)	Female (%)
Coon [15]	1973	Tecumseh, USA	> 10	Examination	Prominent superficial veins in the lower extremities	12.9	25.9
Abramson [14]	1981	Jerusalem, Israel	> 15	Examination	Distended and tortuous subcutaneous veins, excluding very small veins (venectasias)	10.4	29.5
Franks [32]	1992	London, England	35–70	Questionnaire	Asked "Have you ever had large veins or varicose veins in your legs?"	17[a]	31[a]
Sisto [34]	1995	Finland	> 30	Questionnaire	Asked whether a physician had ever made a diagnosis of varicose veins	6.8	24.6
Evans[b]	1998	Edinburgh, Scotland	18–64	Examination	Dilated, tortuous trunks of the long or short saphenous veins and their branches of first or second order	39.7	32.2

[a]Calculated from original report [32]. Figures are approximate due to unspecified missing values.
[b]Results from the Edinburgh Vein Study.

combined with hyphenweb and/or reticular varices in the majority of cases. Hyphenweb and/or reticular varices were approximately 3 and 4 times more common than trunk varices in men and women respectively, and were present in the absence of trunk varices in 36% of men and 44% of women [3]. In a study of Japanese women aged 15–90 years, reticular varices were present in 58% and hyphenweb varices in 61% of women [8]. Stvrtinova et al. [17] examined 696 women working in a department store in Czechoslovakia and found that 15.4% had reticular varices and a further 30.7% hyphenwebs, in addition to the 14.4% of women with trunk varices. The occurrence of reticular and hyphenweb varices in the Edinburgh Vein Study population is shown in Fig. 1.1. The definitions used in this study included even single hyphenweb varices and small dilated subcutaneous veins. With such a definition the presence of these varices was the norm, with each type affecting over 80% of this population. However, when further graded according to severity, the vast majority of subjects were affected only to a mild degree (Grade 1).

The prevalence of treatment for varicose veins in a population may be affected by factors such as treatment availability and perceived severity of the condition by the patient, in addition to the clinical severity of the varices. In a population survey in West London, 7% of subjects questioned said that they had used support stockings for a venous complaint [32], while 4.3% of patients attending a health centre in Brazil who had varicose veins had been operated on for the condition [10]. Results on the prevalence of treatment for varicose veins in men and women obtained in five other studies are shown in Table 1.4. Despite differences in methodology and study populations, a common finding was that treatment for varicose veins was more prevalent in women than in men. Preliminary analysis of data from the Edinburgh Vein Study data revealed that 7.8% of women had previously had operations and 5.7% injections for varicose veins compared with 5.1% and 1.4% of men respectively.

The incidence of varicose veins refers to the development of new cases over a period of time in a population initially free of disease. The longitudinal Framingham Study followed up men and women who were living in the town of Framingham, USA. Every 2 years, over a 16-year period from 1966 onwards, subjects were examined for varicose

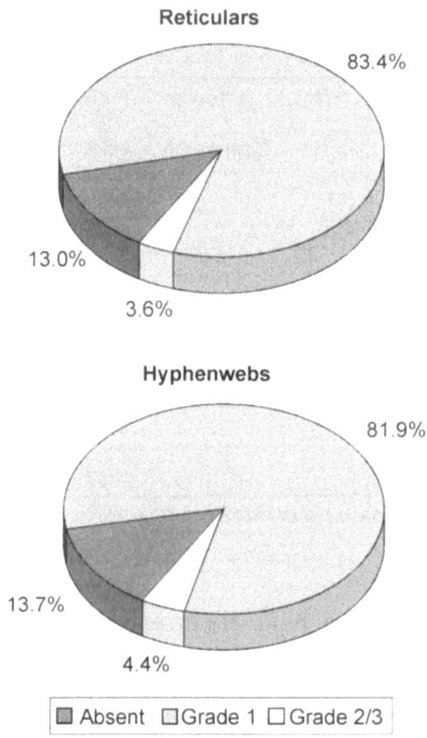

Fig. 1.1. Prevalence of hyphenweb and reticular varices in the Edinburgh Vein Study (adjusted for age and sex).

Table 1.4. Prevalence of treatment for varicose veins in different surveys

Author [Ref]	Subjects	Treatment	Male (%)	Female (%)
Widmer [3]	All subjects	Stripping/sclerotherapy	7	19
		Compression	3	8
Abramson [14]	Subjects with varices	Any treatment	15	32
Laurikka [22]	All subjects	Any treatment	5	17
	Subjects with varices		25	41
Sisto [34]	All subjects	Surgical operations	1.9	13.2
	Subjects with varices		29	53
Evans[a]	All subjects	Operation	5.1	7.8
		Injection	1.4	5.7
		Compression	2.9	9.0

[a]Results from the Edinburgh Vein Study.

veins, defined as "the presence of distended and tortuous veins, clearly visible on the lower limbs with the subject standing". Abnormalities of the venules were excluded. Over the 16-year period, 396 of 1720 men and 629 of 2102 women who were free from the condition in 1966, developed varicose veins. The 2-year incidence of varicose veins was on average 39.4 per 1000 for men and 51.9 per 1000 for women [13]. The Bochum Study examined schoolchildren on three occasions during their education. At the first examination, none of the children (aged 10–12 years) exhibited varices of the trunk veins or their tributaries, although there was already venous reflux present in the long and short saphenous veins in 2.5% of children on Doppler examination. By age 14–16 years, 1.7% of the children had trunk varices and 0.8% varices of the tributary veins while 12.3% showed saphenous reflux. These figures increased to 3.3% and 5.0% for varices of trunk and tributary veins respectively by age 18–20 years, with a prevalence of 19.8% for saphenous reflux on Doppler examination. The prevalence of reticular varices increased from 10.7% at the first examination to 35.3% by the third examination [31].

Further studies are required to determine the incidence and progression of venous disease in the general population. The San Valentino Venous Diseases Project was initiated in July 1994 with the aim of evaluating the prevalence of venous diseases in the village of San Valentino, central Italy and following progression over a period of 10 years [36]. The planned follow-up to the Edinburgh Vein Study will also provide information on the incidence and progression of venous disease in a general population sample.

Sex Differences

Most studies have found a higher prevalence of varicose veins in women compared with men (Tables 1.2, 1.3), although it has been suggested that the sex ratio decreases with increasing age [40]. Selection bias may be a problem in some of these studies, as more women than men may be aware of their varicose veins or consider them to be a problem and hence be more likely to participate in such studies. In addition, many of the results from these studies have not been adjusted for age, a factor which may contribute to the observed gender differences [38].

However, there are several studies which have not found a higher prevalence of varices in women. In the Basle Study there was little difference in prevalence between men and women, but only a relatively small proportion (17%) of the study population was female [3]. Beaglehole et al. [6] found no significant sex differences in the age-standardised prevalence rates of varices in the Cook or Tokelau Islanders from the South Pacific. In a study of villagers in New Guinea, only one woman was found to have varicose veins, resulting in a prevalence of varices of 0.1% in women compared with 5.1% in men [12]. There was no significant difference in the prevalence of varices between men (mean age 73.4 years) and women (mean age 74.2 years) examined in a Turkish study (34.5% versus 38.3% respectively) [9]. By the age of 18–20 years, the male schoolchildren examined in the Bochum Study had a higher prevalence of trunk and tributary varices and incompetent perforators than the females, while this sex difference was reversed for reticular varices and hyphenwebs. There were, however, no tests of significance reported for these results [31]. A recent study in South Wales examined more than 600 randomly selected men and women over the age of 60 years and found that gender was not a significant risk factor for varicose veins (I. Harvey, personal communication). In the Edinburgh Vein Study, the age-adjusted prevalence of trunk varices was significantly higher in men than women (40% versus 32% respectively, $p \leq 0.01$). However, there was no significant difference in the overall prevalence of hyphenweb or reticular varices between the sexes in this study (Fig. 1.2).

In addition to selection bias, methods such as self-assessment of varicose veins [32], or previous diagnosis by a physician [34], may also lead to bias in prevalence figures, as women may be more likely to report varices or to consult their doctor for this condition than men. This hypothesis is supported by findings from the Edinburgh Vein Study. Prior to examination, subjects were asked in a questionnaire whether they had

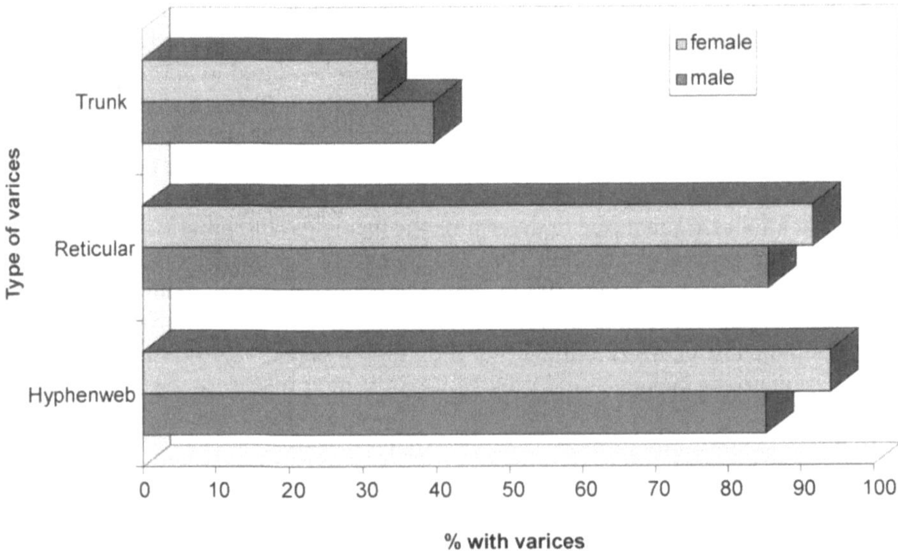

Fig. 1.2. Prevalence of varicose veins by sex in the Edinburgh Vein Study (adjusted for age).

ever been told by a doctor that they had varicose veins. Only 10% of men answered positively to this question compared with 17% of women, although men were subsequently found to have a significantly higher prevalence of trunk varices on examination (Fig. 1.2).

Effect of Age

A common finding in most studies is that the prevalence of varicose veins increases with increasing age. Figure 1.3 shows the increase in prevalence of varices with age in both males and females from general population surveys conducted in Jerusalem [14] and Edinburgh. The overall prevalence of trunk varices in the Edinburgh Vein Study increased from 11.5% in those aged 18–24 years to 55.7% in those aged 55–64 years ($p < 0.001$). In the longitudinal study of Bochum schoolchildren described above, the prevalence of both varices and venous reflux increased with age [31]. It is important, therefore, that age is taken into account when comparing the prevalence of varices between sexes, or investigating possible risk factors.

In the Framingham Study, which examined a population biannually over a 16-year period for the presence of varicose veins, the incidence of varicose veins did not increase with age [13]. The observed increase in the prevalence of varicose veins with age would therefore appear to be a result of the relatively constant development of cases as people grow older.

Geographical and Racial Differences

There is much anecdotal evidence in journal correspondence from those working in developing countries during the 1960s and 1970s to suggest that the prevalence of varicose veins is lower in those countries than in the Western world [41–44]. Barker

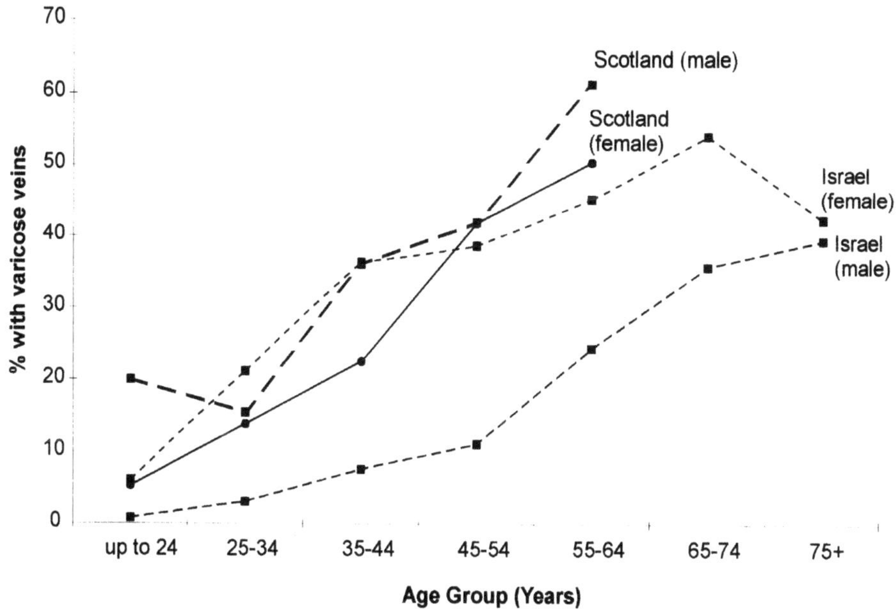

Fig. 1.3. Prevalence of varicose veins by age and sex in population surveys in Israel and Scotland. *Sources*: Abramson et al., Israel [14]: prevalence of varicose veins excluding venectasias. Evans et al., Scotland: prevalence of trunk varices in the Edinburgh Vein Study.

[45] reported only 2 cases of varicose veins out of a total of 3000 hospital patients in a Zulu area of Africa. In a letter reporting on several case series of hospital patients in India, Burkitt et al. [46] concluded that the prevalence of varicose veins in rural Indians was unlikely to exceed 2%. In Mombasa, Kenya, 294 pregnant women from different racial groups were examined for varicose veins. The prevalence of varices was 1.5% in Arab women, 3.2% in African women and 9.7% in Indian women [47]. A survey of 2084 hospital patients in Peru revealed only 3 cases of varicose veins [48], while results from a fuller report showed that 5.5% of Tanzanian outpatients had varices [38] (Table 1.2).

Although the above reports were based on hospital patients, others attempted to survey a more general population. Rougemont [49] examined all women from 10 traditional villages in the Republic of Mali using "well-standardised criteria and methods" and found an overall prevalence of 10.9% for all types of varicose veins, 4.5% of which were severe. Despite a higher than expected prevalence, none of these cases was associated with complications. Daynes and Beighton [50] examined 297 women aged 18 years and over from two adjacent villages in the Transkei, Southern Africa, and found varicosity of the main leg veins in 7.7%, the prevalence rising with age. However, none of the women complained of any associated symptoms [50]. Rivlin [51] believed that there was an equal incidence of varicose veins throughout the world but that the occurrence of symptoms and complications was virtually unknown in tropical Africa. These conflicting anecdotal accounts and the lack of well-designed epidemiological studies make it difficult to draw any conclusions about the true prevalence of varicose veins in developing countries.

Several better-documented studies have compared the prevalence of varicose veins in different racial groups. In a community study in Jerusalem, Abramson et al. [14]

found a lower prevalence of varicose veins in immigrants over 45 years of age from North Africa (men 13.2%, women 30.2%) compared with immigrants from Europe and America (men 26.9%, women 48.8%) and from other parts of Asia (men 22.4%, women 39.7%). Guberan et al. [23] found the prevalence of varices significantly lower among women from Southern Europe (Italy and Spain) than among the other women in their study from Switzerland, France and other Central European countries. In a study of cotton workers, the prevalence of varicose veins was 32% among European women compared with 6% among Egyptian women [19]. Beaglehole et al. [6] examined the prevalence of varicose veins in several contrasting South Pacific populations. There was a gradient in the prevalence of varices which followed the pattern of contact of the study populations with the Western world, being lowest in the Atoll dwellers (Tokelau Islanders and Pukapukans), intermediate in the Rarotongans and highest in the New Zealanders (European and Maori groups) (Table 1.2).

Conclusion

The prevalence of varicose veins in the general population is difficult to determine due to a lack of epidemiological data. Comparison of results from existing studies is difficult due to variations in methodologies and definitions employed and generalisability of results is further hampered by a lack of data on random population samples. Although many studies have reported a higher prevalence of varices in women than men, some of these differences may have resulted from methodological bias, and several recent studies do not support a higher prevalence in women. A common finding is that the prevalence of varices increases with age. One study examining incidence suggests that this remains relatively constant across the age ranges. Although anecdotal evidence suggests that varicose veins may be less common in developing countries, there is a general lack of epidemiological data from these countries. The recent development of guidelines for standardised reporting of venous disease should aid research in this area and the use of non-invasive techniques will allow a more objective assessment of venous function in future research studies. Longitudinal population-based epidemiological studies using such definitions and methods of measurement are required in order to increase knowledge of the incidence, prevalence and progression of venous disease in the population.

References

1. Laing W. Chronic venous diseases of the leg. London: Office of Health Economics, 1992:28.
2. Porter JM, Moneta GL and an International Consensus Committee on Chronic Venous Disease. Reporting standards in venous disease: an update. J Vasc Surg 1995;21:635–45.
3. Widmer LK, ed. Peripheral venous disorders: prevalence and socio-medical importance. Bern: Hans Huber, 1978:1–90.
4. Arnoldi CC. The aetiology of primary varicose veins. Dan Med Bull 1957;4:102–107.
5. Arnoldi CC. The heredity of venous insufficiency. Dan Med Bull 1958;5:169–176.
6. Beaglehole R, Prior IAM, Salmond CE, Davidson F. Varicose veins in the South Pacific. Int J Epidemiol 1975;4:295–299.
7. Beaglehole R, Salmond CE, Prior IAM. Varicose veins in New Zealand: prevalence and severity. N Z Med J 1976;84:396–399.
8. Hirai M, Kenichi N, Nakayama R. Prevalence and risk factors of varicose veins in Japanese women. Angiology 1990;41:228–232.

9. Komsuoglu B, Goldeli O, Kulan K, Cetinarslan B, Komsuoglu SS. Prevalence and risk factors of varicose veins in an elderly population. Gerontology 1994;40:25–31.
10. Maffei FHA, Magaldi C, Pinho SZ, et al. Varicose veins and chronic venous insufficiency in Brazil: prevalence among 1755 inhabitants of a country town. Int J Epidemiol 1986;15:210–217.
11. Malhotra SL. An epidemiological study of varicose veins in Indian railroad workers from the south and north of India, with special reference to the causation and prevention of varicose veins. Int J Epidemiol 1972;1:117–183.
12. Stanhope JM. Varicose veins in a population of New Guinea. Int J Epidemiol 1975;4:221–225.
13. Brand FN, Dannenberg AL, Abbott RD, Kannel WB. The epidemiology of varicose veins: the Framingham study. Am J Prev Med 1988;4:96–101.
14. Abramson JH, Hopp C, Epstein LM. The epidemiology of varicose veins: a survey of western Jerusalem. J Epidemiol Community Health 1981;35:213–217.
15. Coon WW, Willis PW, Keller JB. Venous thromboembolism and other venous disease in the Tecumseh Community Health Study. Circulation 1973;48:839–846.
16. Novo S, Avellone G, Pinto A, et al. Prevalence of primitive varicose veins in a randomised population sample of western Sicily. Int Angiol 1988;7:176–181.
17. Stvrtinova V, Kolesar J, Wimmer G. Prevalence of varicose veins of the lower limbs in the women working at a department store. Int Angiol 1991;10:2–5.
18. Gundersen J, Hauge M. Hereditary factors in venous insufficiency. Angiology 1969;20:346–355.
19. Mekky S, Schilling RSF, Walford J. Varicose veins in women cotton workers: an epidemiological study in England and Egypt. BMJ 1969;2:591–595.
20. Dodd H, Cockett FB. The pathology and surgery of the veins of the lower limb. Edinburgh: Livingstone, 1956:3.
21. da Silva A, Widmer LK, Martin H, Mall T, Glaus L, Schneider M. Varicose veins and chronic venous insufficiency: prevalence and risk factors in 4376 subjects in the Basle Study II. Vasa 1974;3:118–125.
22. Laurikka J, Sisto T, Auvinen O, Tarkka M, Laara E, Hakama M. Varicose veins in a Finnish population aged 40–60. J Epidemiol Community Health 1993;47:355–357.
23. Guberan E, Widmer LK, Glaus L, et al. Causative factors of varicose veins: myths and facts. Vasa 1973;2:115–120.
24. Callam MJ. Epidemiology of varicose veins. Br J Surg 1994;81:167–173.
25. Evans CJ, Fowkes FGR, Ruckley CV, et al. Edinburgh Vein Study: methods and response in a survey of venous disease in the general population. Phlebology 1998; in press.
26. Ducimetiere P, Richard JL, Pequignot G, Warnet JM. Varicose veins: a risk factor for atherosclerotic disease in middle-aged men? Int J Epidemiol 1981;10:329–335.
27. Latto C, Wilkinson RW, Gilmore OJA. Diverticular disease and varicose veins. Lancet 1973;i:1089–1090.
28. Prior IAM, Evans JG, Morrison RBI, Rose BS. The Carterton Study. 6. Patterns of vascular, respiratory, rheumatic and related abnormalities in a sample of New Zealand European adults. N Z Med J 1970;72:169–177.
29. Weddell JM. Varicose veins pilot survey, 1966. Br J Prev Soc Med 1969;23:179–186.
30. Madar G, Widmer LK, Zemp E, Maggs M. Varicose veins and chronic venous insufficiency: disorder or disease? A critical epidemiological review. Vasa 1986;15:126–134.
31. Schultz-Ehrenberg U, Weindorf N, Matthes U, Hirche H. New epidemiological findings with regard to initial stages of varicose veins (Bochum Study I–III). In: Raymond Martimbeau P, Prescott R, Zummo M, editors. Phlebologie '92. Paris: John Libbey Eurotext, 1992:234–236.
32. Franks PJ, Wright DDI, Moffatt CJ, et al. Prevalence of venous disease: a community study in West London. Eur J Surg 1992;158:143–147.
33. Laurikka J, Laara E, Sisto T, Tarkka M, Auvinen O, Hakama M. Misclassification in a questionnaire survey of varicose veins. J Clin Epidemiol 1995;48:1175–1178.
34. Sisto T, Reunanen A, Laurikka J, et al. Prevalence and risk factors of varicose veins in lower extremities: Mini-Finland Health Survey. Eur J Surg 1995;161:405–414.
35. Fleiss JL. Statistical methods for rates and proportions. 2nd ed. New York: Wiley, 1981.
36. Cesarone MR, Belcaro G, Nicolaides AN, et al. Epidemiology and costs of venous diseases in central Italy. Angiology 1997;48:583–593.
37. Bobek K, Cajzl L, Cepelak V, Slaisova V, Opatzny K, Barcal R. Etude de la fréquence des maladies phlébologiques et de l'influence de quelques facteurs étiologiques. Phlebologie 1966;19:217–230.
38. Richardson JB, Dixon M. Varicose veins in tropical Africa. Lancet 1977;i:791–792.
39. Leipnitz G, Kiesewetter P, Waldhausen P, Jung F, Witt T, Wenzel E. Prevalence of venous disease in the population: first results from a prospective study carried out in greater Aachen. In: Davy A, Stemmer R, editors. Phlebology '89. Paris: John Libbey Eurotext, 1989:169–171.
40. Beaglehole R. Epidemiology of varicose veins. World J Surg 1986;10:898–902.

41. Coles RW. Varicose veins in tropical Africa. Lancet 1974;ii:474–475.
42. Milton-Thompson DG. Varicose veins in tropical Africa. Lancet 1974;i:1174.
43. Williams EH. Varicose veins in tropical Africa. Lancet 1974;i:1291.
44. Worsfold JT. Varicose veins in tropical Africa. Lancet 1974;ii:1322–1323.
45. Barker A. Varicose veins. Lancet 1964;ii:970–971.
46. Burkitt DP, Jansen HK, Mategaonker DW, Philips C, Phuntsog YP, Sukhnandan R. Varicose veins in India. Lancet 1975;ii:765.
47. Burkitt DP, Townsend AJ, Patel K, Skaug K. Varicose veins in developing countries. Lancet 1976;ii:202–203.
48. Dalrymple J, Crofts T. Varicose veins in developing countries. Lancet 1975;i:808–809.
49. Rougemont A. Varicose veins in the tropics. BMJ 1973;2:547.
50. Daynes G, Beighton P. Prevalence of varicose veins in Africans. BMJ 1973;3:354.
51. Rivlin S. Varicose veins in tropical Africa. Lancet 1974;i:1054.

2 Leg Ulcer and Chronic Venous Insufficiency in the Community

Michael J. Callam

Introduction

Venous disease is the most common vascular condition to affect the lower limb. A knowledge of the epidemiology of venous disease is essential for a rational debate on the nature and level of resources required to provide adequate care for this widespread and costly condition.

Recently published longitudinal studies [1,2] have confirmed the clinical impression that from the initial vein valvular incompetence or deep vein thrombosis (DVT) there is a slow and often insidious development of chronic venous insufficiency and eventually venous ulceration over years or even decades. This provides an opportunity to identify people with venous disease at an early stage and to take corrective action to prevent or limit the development of ulceration. An understanding of the natural history of the condition is necessary to allow the best choice and timing of such interventions.

The data on varicose vein epidemiology are reviewed in the previous chapter and this chapter concentrates on the available evidence on chronic venous insufficiency and leg ulceration. Figure 2.1 demonstrates the inter-relationships between the total population, those with venous disease, those with chronic venous insufficiency (CVI) and those with leg ulceration. As there have now been a large number of studies on the prevalence of leg ulceration and several on CVI it might be expected that the

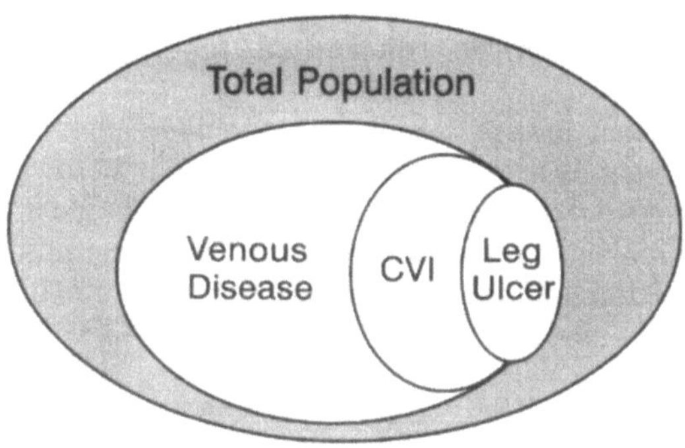

Fig. 2.1. Association between venous disease and leg ulceration.

percentage of the population in each group would be known. However, the variations between definitions and methodology employed in the different studies make it difficult to obtain a clear picture [3]. Any analysis of these studies must allow for the variations in definitions and methodology and these are outlined in the next section.

Definition and Methodological Variation

What Is Chronic Venous Insufficiency?

There has been no internationally accepted classification of CVI and so it is not surprising that different criteria were used. The classification devised by Widmer in the Basle Studies (Table 2.1) [4] seems to have been most widely utilised but in many studies the exact criteria used are not specified. No epidemiological studies using the recently proposed CEAP classification [5] appear to have been published yet.

What Is a Chronic Leg Ulcer?

Although any break in the skin anywhere on the leg or foot could be classified as a leg ulcer, different studies of prevalence of leg ulceration have limited the definition by duration, site or aetiology. Many have only included ulceration of more than 4–6 weeks' duration, some have excluded ulcers on the forefoot and some have only included ulcers thought to be of venous origin. Some studies have only included people with open active ulcers and others have included everyone who had ever suffered from ulceration even if the ulcer was healed at the time of the survey. These limitations will clearly have marked effects on the overall results, with the narrower definitions resulting in lower prevalences.

What Is Prevalence?

Point prevalence is the number of patients with a condition at one point in time, whereas period prevalence is the number of patients presenting with the condition over a specified period of time. Chronic venous ulceration is both chronic and prone to recurrence and therefore there may be a marked difference between point and period prevalence.

It should be noted that any prevalence study of a population only gives an indication of the level and severity of venous disease at that point in time. Some of the study population will go on to develop venous disease subsequently and in others the severity of the venous disease will increase over time. It is only longitudinal studies such as the Bochum [1] and Edinburgh studies (C. Evans, personal communication) which will

Table 2.1. Widmer classification of chronic venous insufficiency

Grade	Description
CVI I	Corona Phlebectatica (venous flare)
CVI II	Hyper-depigmented areas
CVI III	Open/healed ulcer

provide definitive information on progression of venous disease in the general population.

What Population Was Assessed?

The size and selection of the sample population and the completeness of the survey are crucial to the accuracy of prevalence data. For example, some studies have looked at clinic attendees [6,7], where the level of venous disease would be expected to be higher than the normal population. Others have looked at factory populations [4,8], where the prevalence might be lower than normal. The larger and more random the sample selected the more truly representative the findings. Accuracy of prevalence will, however, decrease if the proportion of the sample population assessed, i.e. response rate, is low [9].

When Was the Study Carried Out?

It is possible that the prevalence of CVI and leg ulceration might have altered over time. The widespread use of DVT prophylaxis and heparin in the treatment of DVT, for example, might have had some effect on the prevalence between the early studies in the 1960s and those published in the 1990s. However, analysis of the data does not suggest any significant drop (or increase) in the prevalence, so this factor can perhaps be discounted. A reduction in post-thrombotic ulcers could be masked by an increase in other types of ulcer.

What Method of Assessment Was Used?

The assessment method used has varied between studies, from a questionnaire only, through simple clinical examination, to complex vascular laboratory tests such as plethysmography or even colour duplex ultrasound scanning. Questionnaires are known to give rise to substantial false positive and false negative results [10], which usually result in an overestimate of the prevalence. The use of duplex assessment will also give a high figure for the prevalence of venous abnormalities as it will detect asymptomatic venous valvular incompetence which may give rise to venous insufficiency in the future.

Prevalence Study Data

Prevalence studies of CVI and leg ulcer can be split up into three groups (Tables 2.2–2.4). Group 1 consists of studies in which the authors have contacted health care workers in a defined geographic area, to identify all patients undergoing treatment for leg ulceration in the population. Most of the group 1 studies have also examined a subset of the identified patients to obtain detailed information on the natural history of leg ulceration. Group 2 consists of direct questionnaire studies of a selected sample of the population to identify those with leg ulceration. In some group 2 studies positive responders have been examined to confirm the diagnosis and in one study a sample of negative responders were also seen to assess the false negative rate [10]. Group 3 consists of true epidemiological studies, which have examined population samples in detail for evidence of CVI and leg ulceration.

Table 2.2. Group 1 studies

Study[a] [Ref.]	Year	Population	Ulcer No.	Ulcer %	% Venous leg ulceration
Lothian & Forth, Scotland [11]	1981	1 000 000	1477	0.15	0.1(0.08)
Harrow, U.K. [12]	1981/2	200 000	357	0.21	0.12
Skaraborg, Sweden [8]	1988	270 800	827	0.31	0.22
Perth, Australia [13]	1989	238 000	259	0.11	0.06
Malmö, Sweden [14]	1990	232 908	275	0.12	0.07
Newcastle, UK [19]	1991	240 000	206	0.08	N/K
Stockholm, Sweden [15]	1993	241 804	294	0.12	0.06
Stockport, UK [16]	1993	540 000	587	0.11	0.07

N/K, not known.
[a]The study from Gothenberg [17] has been excluded because it was a retrospective review of case records and the figure published was an estimate only.

Table 2.3. Group 2 studies

Study[a] [Ref.]	Year	No. (Ages, years)	Response rate (%)	False +ve	False −ve	Prevalence of open and healed ulcers
Klatov, Czechoslovakia [18]	1961	16 781 (15–89)	89.3%	N/R	N/R	1%
Stockbridge, UK [10]	1981	760 (65–81)	77%	40%	5%	3.6%
Malmö, Sweden [8]	1990	12 000 (50–89)	90%	43%	N/R	2.1%
Skvolde, Sweden [8]	1996	2785 (30–65)	87%	64%	N/R	1.7%
Skaraborg, Sweden [19]	1977	8000 (>5)	70%	0%*	N/R	1.1%

N/R, not recorded.
[a]The Dublin study [20] was excluded as it was based on households not individuals and so the sample size could not be ascertained.
[b]All responders checked by nurse.

Group 1 studies cover large populations and will therefore provide the best estimate of the current workload in the treatment of leg ulceration. Group 3 studies, although only assessing relatively small populations in detail, will provide the best estimates of the prevalence of CVI, which is found commonly, but may be less accurate for leg ulceration, which will be found rarely in small samples. Group 2 studies tend to have larger populations than group 3 studies. They are less accurate but can bridge the gap between the other two groups. Data from these studies, making allowances for the variations in definition and methods, are summarised in the following section as representing the best available estimates of prevalence of CVI and leg ulceration.

What Is the Prevalence of Leg Ulceration?

A combination of the group 1 health worker studies covers a population of just under 3 million people in Scandanavia, the United Kingdom and Australia and indicates a point prevalence of active ulceration requiring treatment of 1.5 per 1000 of the adult population. However, this does not allow for any of the variables (see below) and is perhaps unduly influenced by the large number of ulcers found in the Skaraborg study [8].

Table 2.4. Group 3 studies

Study [Ref.]	Year	No. (Ages, years)	Population	Comments
Tecumseh, USA [21]	1962/5	9226 (> 0)	Population sample	Town population
Basle, Switzerland [4]	1978	4529 (25–74)	Factory workers	Mostly men
Munich, Germany [6]	1984	1000 (> 18)	Clinic attenders	? Selection bias
Botucatu, Brazil [7]	1986	1755 (> 15)	Clinic attenders	? Selection bias
Amsterdam, Netherlands [22]	1997	387 (15–65)	Working males	Standing occupation
San Valentino, Italy [23]	1997	746 (8–94)	Population sample	Village population
Edinburgh, Scotland	1998	1566 (18–64)	Population sample	City population

Table 2.5. Group 3 study results by class of CVI

Study [Ref.]	CVI I	CVI II	CVI III Ulcer O & H	Comments
Tecumseh, USA (All) [24]		3.3%	0.2%	
Men	N/R	3.7%	0.1%	
Women		3.0%	0.3%	
Klatov, Czechoslovakia (All) [18]*		2.8%	1%	Only +ve
Men	N/R	1.9%	0.8%	responders
Women		3.4%	1.2%	seen
Basle, Switzerland [4]	8%	6%	1%	
Munich, Germany [6]	N/R	7%	4%	
Botucatu, Brazil [7]	N/R	2.3%	3.7%	
Amsterdam, Netherlands [22]	18%	11%		No open ulcers
SanValentino, Italy [23]	N/R	0.5% @ 20–30 9% @ 90–100	1% @ 30–40 11% @ 90–100	Total not given
Edinburgh, Scotland				
Men	6.9%	1.3%	1.0%	
Women	5.3%	1.1%	0.2%	

N/R, not recorded.

Leg Ulcer and Age

It is clear that one of the most important of the variables is age. The group 2 studies which included both open and healed ulcers demonstrated that the older the population studied the higher the detected prevalence, ranging from 1% for all adults [10] to 3.6% for people over 65 years [18]. Figure 2.2 shows the prevalence data for the group 1 studies where population corrected age-specific data were available. All the values fell between the upper and lower limits shown. A log scale has been used to demonstrate the steady rise of prevalence with age although it minimises the variation between studies in the values in the older age groups which are revealed with a linear scale (Fig. 2.3). Studies which gave values towards the upper limit tended to include both leg and foot ulcers and to be the figures for the female population only, while those towards the lower limit represent studies excluding toe and forefoot lesions and comprising male populations only. Correction for sex and inclusion of foot lesions would narrow the range of possible prevalence values which, if applied

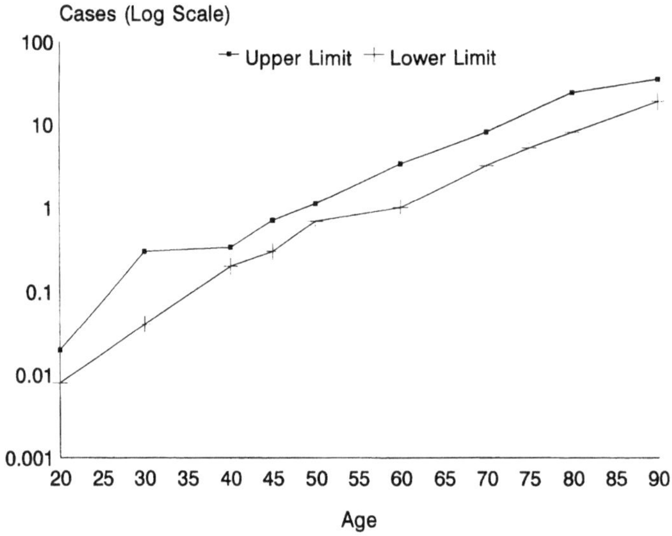

Fig. 2.2. Number of leg ulcer cases per 1000 population: log scale.

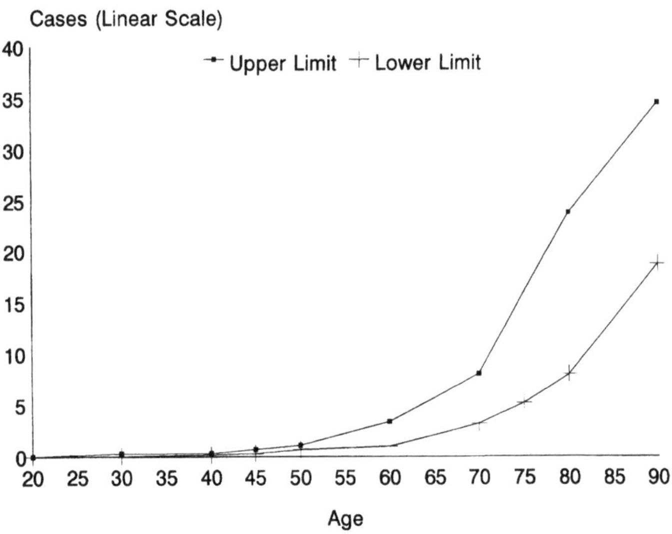

Fig. 2.3. Number of leg ulcer cases per 1000 population: linear scale.

to a population with a known age/sex distribution, could be used to estimate the ulcer case workload.

Leg Ulcer and Sex

It is widely believed that leg ulceration is more common in women because almost all the group 1 studies identifying treated leg ulcer patients in the community have shown a marked predominance of females (1:2–3) [3]. However the group 3 studies have suggested a more equal distribution and in the Edinburgh study even a male predominance of open or healed ulcers. There are two possible explanations to account for these seemingly incompatible results. Firstly Nelzen [8] has argued that women are more likely to seek treatment and has produced evidence that men are more likely to be self-caring, particularly when of working age. However, the data to show that the ulcers in these younger males who treat themselves are similar in aetiology and outcome to the professionally treated ulcers are not available. It is possible that these self-treated ulcers are simply traumatic, reflecting a factory working environment. Secondly it could be expected that, with greater lifespan in females and the rapid increase in the rate of ulceration in the later decades, a female predominance would be found. The predominance is primarily age-related rather than sex-related. However, there still appears to be a slight female predominance overall but much less than had previously been estimated.

Leg Ulcer and Venous Aetiology

The percentage of leg ulcers which are of venous aetiology depends on whether the sample included forefoot ulcers and what definition and method of assessment were used to diagnose the venous disease. The final column of the group 1 studies (Table 2.2) shows the prevalence of active venous leg ulceration which, with the exception of the Skaraborg study, gives a range of 0.06–0.12%. The figure in parentheses for the Lothian & Forth Valley study represents the percentage of patients in whom venous disease was thought to be the main or only cause. These results demonstrate that by including only venous disease the variation between the studies is markedly reduced despite the varying methods of assessment used. The prevalence of active venous ulceration being treated is therefore estimated to be 0.8–1 per 1000. Unfortunately too few studies provide sufficient information on the relationship between age and venous aetiology to allow an equivalent age curve for venous ulcers similar to that drawn for all ulcers in Fig. 2.2. However, analysis of the data available raises the interesting possibility that the percentage of ulcers where venous disease is thought to be the main aetiological factor falls in the older age groups.

Prevalence of Chronic Venous Insufficiency

The only studies which cast any light on the prevalence of CVI are the group 3 studies which were set up to assess the full spectrum of venous disease in selected populations. Although the numbers are relatively small, this is compensated for by the fact that the lesser degrees of venous disease are common and the sample populations were assessed in detail. Figure 2.4 shows the results from these studies for all grades of CVI plotted against age. It is quite clear that the prevalence increases with age, but there is a huge variation in the values in the later decades making meaningful interpretation difficult. Table 2.5 shows the data by class of CVI for the group 3 studies. The Munich and Botucatu studies were of clinic attendees and did not represent the prevalence in a general population and so should be discarded.

There are three studies where the CVI I prevalence is recorded separately and there is good agreement between the Basle and the Edinburgh studies, which showed prevalences of about 7%. The Basle study includes a slightly higher age group, which might account for the small difference in prevalence found. The Amsterdam study showed a much higher percentage of CVI I (18%), which may represent a true increase in people of standing occupation or different assessment criteria. This trend is also

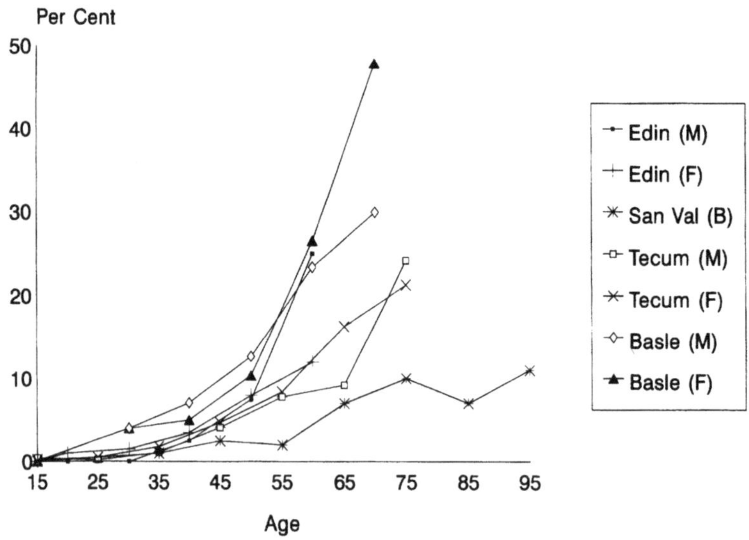

Fig. 2.4. Percentage of population with chronic venous insufficiency.

noticed in the results for CVI II, as both the Amsterdam study and the Basle study (factory workers) give higher figures for the prevalence compared with the other studies which have included the general population. A reasonable estimate for the prevalence of CVI II is 1–3%.

There is even better agreement for CVI III (open and healed ulceration). A figure of 1% for the whole adult population is a reasonable estimate.

Future Trends

There is clear evidence that the prevalence of both CVI and venous ulceration increases with age. Therefore as the number of elderly in the population increases, a commensurate increase in the number of cases of CVI can be expected. Support for the view that this is already occurring comes from data on Scottish hospital admissions for leg ulceration where the annual admission rate for leg ulceration has increased sharply from 15 to 25 per 100 000 population since 1990 (C. V. Ruckley, personal communication). However, this increase is not necessarily inevitable as the progression towards CVI and ulceration is slow and there is evidence that there are a number of interventions which can be effective.

Figure 2.5 outlines the pathways which can lead to CVI and ulceration and the points at which intervention has been shown to affect the natural history. The first opportunity is DVT prevention. A recent meta-analysis showed that the routine use of prophylaxis with heparin, graduated compression stockings and intermittent pneumatic sleeves can reduce the incidence of peri-operative thrombosis; compression alone reduces the incidence from 27% to 11% [27]. The treatment of DVT also offers opportunities for the reduction of CVI. There is evidence which has demonstrated a fall in the development of the post-thrombotic syndrome with the routine use of heparin in the treatment of DVT, although much of the data depends on historical controls [11]. More recent studies have demonstrated that there appears to be a benefit in selected cases in reducing the frequency

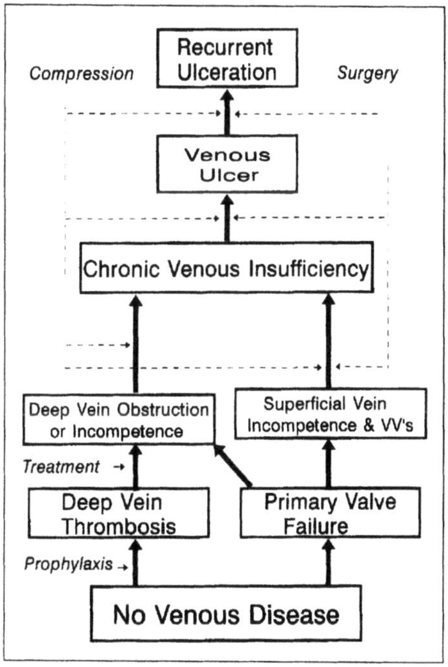

Fig. 2.5. Venous pathological pathways and prevention points. VV's, varicose veins.

with which the post-thrombotic syndrome develops by means of thrombectomy [24] and thrombolysis [25], although trial numbers are still small.

The efficacy of graduated elastic compression in limiting the development of CVI after a DVT has been demonstrated in at least one controlled study, with a 50% reduction in the CVI rate at 5-year follow-up [28]. The benefits of graduated elastic compression in preventing patients with CVI from going on to ulceration and preventing recurrence of ulceration [26] have also been demonstrated.

It is interesting to note that the evidence from controlled trials that surgery is of benefit in preventing the development of CVI and ulcers in patients with varicose veins and superficial venous insufficiency is more difficult to obtain, although most clinicians would accept that it is indeed the case. There is, however, evidence that treatment of superficial venous disease will reduce recurrence of ulceration significantly in the absence of post-phlebitic deep venous disease [29].

The extent to which these interventions have already affected the incidence of CVI is not known, but there is certainly no evidence of a decrease in the prevalence as yet.

Much of the available evidence will be covered in subsequent chapters, but a great deal of research remains to be done to confirm the size of each group in the venous pathway (Fig. 2.5) and to clarify the extent of benefit from particular interventions at each point in the pathway so that cost-benefit analysis can be applied.

Conclusions

Any discussion of prevalence of leg ulceration and CVI must take account of the definition and methodological differences discussed in the Introduction. The influence of the age of the population under consideration is the most important factor in view of the progressive rise in prevalence with age for all grades of CVI and leg ulceration.

On the currently available evidence, the best estimates for the whole adult population are a point prevalence for open leg ulceration of 0.15% with an open venous leg ulcer rate of 0.08–0.1% (excluding toe and forefoot lesions). However, the use of the age prevalence curve will give a more accurate estimate for a target population. Although many more women than men present for treatment, this is at least in part due to their greater lifespan, and the sex difference in prevalence has previously been overstated.

The prevalence of CVI is less certain. There is such variation between the study methodology and results that interpretation is more speculative. However, using the available data we can estimate that for the whole adult population the overall prevalence of CVI I is 7–8%, CVI II is 1–3% and CVI III is 1%. The percentages are very much lower than this in the early decades of life but increase sharply with age, so that they are considerably higher in old age.

References

1. Schultz-Ehrenberg U, Weindorf N, Matthes U, Hirche H. Etude épidémiologique sur la pathogenèse des varices. Etude de Bochum I–III. Phlebologie 1992;45:497–500.
2. Van Haarst EP, Liasis N, Van Ramshorst B, Moll FL. The development of valvular incompetence after deep vein thrombosis: A 7 year follow-up study. Eur J Vasc Surg 1996;12:295–299.
3. Callam MJ. Prevalence of chronic leg ulceration and severe chronic venous disease in Western countries. Phlebology 1992;7 (Suppl 1):6–12.
4. Widmer LK. Peripheral venous disorders: Basle III. Bern: Hans Huber, 1978.
5. Beebe HG, Bergan JJ, Berqvist D, et al. Classification and grading of chronic venous disease in the lower limbs: a consensus statement. Eur J Vasc Endovasc Surg 1996;12:487–492.
6. Eberth-Willershausen W, Marshall W. Prevalenz, Risikofaktoren und Komplikationen peripherer Venenerkrankungen in der Münchner Bevolkerung. Hautarzt 1984;35:68–77.
7. Maffei FHA, Magaldi C, Pinho SZ, et al. Varicose veins and chronic venous insufficiency in Brazil: prevalence among 1755 inhabitants of a country town. Int J Epidemiol 1986;15:210–217.
8. Nelzen O. Patients with chronic leg ulcer: aspects on epidemiology, aetiology, clinical history, prognosis and choice of treatment. Uppsala University Dissertation 1997. Stockholm: Almquist & Wiksell, (distributor).
9. Lees TA, Lambert D. Prevalence of lower limb ulceration in an urban health district. Br J Surg 1992;79:1032–1034.
10. Dale JJ, Callam MJ, Ruckley CV, Harper DR, Berrey PN. Chronic ulcer of the leg: a study of prevalence in a Scottish community. Health Bull 1983;41:310–314.
11. Callam MJ. Chronic leg ulceration: the Lothian & Forth Valley survey. Ch.M. thesis, University of Dundee, 1989.
12. Cornwall JV, Dore CJ, Lewis JD. Leg ulcers: epidemiology and aetiology. Br J Surg 1986;73:693–696.
13. Baker SR, Stacey MC, Jopp-McKay AG, Hoskin SE, Thompson PJ. Epidemiology of chronic venous ulcers. Br J Surg 1991;78:864–867.
14. Lindholm CA, Bjellerup M, Christensen OB, Zederfeldt B. A demographic survey of leg and foot ulcer patients in a defined population. Acta Derm Venereol (Stockh) 1992;72:227–230.
15. Ebbeskog B, Lindholm C, Ohman S. Leg and foot ulcer patients: epidemiology and nursing care in an urban population in South Stockholm, Sweden. Scand J Primary Health Care 1996;14:239–243.
16. Simon DA, Freak L, Kinsella A, Walsh J, Lane C, Groake L, McCollum C. Community leg ulcer clinics: a comparative study in two health authorities. BMJ 1996;312:1648–1651.
17. Andersson E, Hansson C, Swanbeck G. Leg and foot ulcers: an epidemiological survey. Acta Derm Venereol (Stockh) 1984;64:227–232.
18. Bobek K, Cajzl L, Cepelak V, Slaisova V, Opatzny K, Barcal R. Etude de la fréquence des maladies phlébologiques et de l'influence de quelques facteurs étiologiques. Phlebologie 1966;19:217–230.
19. Hallbrook T. Leg ulcer epidemiology. Acta Chir Scand 1988; Suppl 544:17–20.
20. Henry M. Incidence of varicose ulcers in Ireland. Irish Med J 1986;79:65–67.
21. Coon WW, Willis PW, Keller JB. Venous thrombo-embolism and other venous disease in the Tecumseh Community Health Study. Circulation 1973;98:839–846.

22. Krijnen RMA, De Boer EM, Ader HJ, Bruynzeel DP. Venous insufficiency in male workers with a standing profession. Dermatology 1997;194:111–120.
23. Cesarone MR, Belcaro G, Nicolaides AN, et al. Epidemiology and costs of venous diseases in central Italy. The San Valentino Venous Disease Project. Angiology 1997;7:583–593.
24. Plate G, Eklof B, Norgren L, Ohlin P, Dalstrom JA. Venous thrombectomy for iliofemoral vein thrombosis: 10 year results of a prospective randomised study. Eur J Vasc Endovasc Surg 1997;14:367–374.
25. Barras JP, Widmer MT, Zemp E, Voilin R, Widmer LK. Sequelles de la thrombose veineuse. J Mal Vasc 1991;16:115–118.
26. Dinn E, Henry M. The effectiveness of graduated compression stockings with regular follow up in prevention of venous ulcer recurrence. Swiss Med 1988;10:127–128.
27. Colditz GA, Tuden RL, Oster G. Rates of venous thrombosis after general surgery: combined results of clinical trials. Lancet 1986; 2:143–146.
28. Brandjes DP, Buller HR, Heijboer H, Huisman MV, et al. Randomised trial of effect of compression stockings in patients with symptomatic proximal vein thrombosis. Lancet 1997;349:759–762.
29. Burnand K, Lea Thomas M, O'Donnell T, Browse NL. Relation between post-phlebitic changes in the deep veins and results of surgical treatment of venous ulcers. Lancet 1976;I:936–938.

3 What Are the Risks of Thrombophilia?

Gordon D. O. Lowe and Ann Rumley

Introduction

Deep vein thrombosis of the leg (DVT), whether symptomatic or asymptomatic, is a common cause of venous insufficiency (calf pump failure syndrome): when there is evidence of previous DVT from the history or at venography the term "post- thrombotic syndrome" is used [1]. The incidences of the post-thrombotic syndrome, and of recurrent DVT, in a large, prospective observational study were recently reported [2]. The cumulative incidence of recurrence following conventional treatment of acute DVT with heparin followed by 3 months of warfarin was 17.5% after 2 years, 25% after 5 years and 30% after 8 years. The cumulative incidence of the post-thrombotic leg syndrome was 23%, 28% and 29% respectively, and was strongly associated with ipsilateral recurrent DVT. Recurrence was associated positively with thrombophilias and with malignant disease, and negatively with DVT following recent trauma, fracture or surgery [2].

Because both initial and recurrent DVT are major causes of venous insufficiency, it is important to identify persons at increased risk of DVT and of recurrent DVT, in order to institute appropriate prophylaxis of both the post-thrombotic leg syndrome and pulmonary thromboembolism (PTE). Figure 3.1 illustrates the concept of a "multiple hit model" for the pathogenesis of DVT [3]. As with arterial and cardiac thromboembolism, the incidence of venous thromboembolism increases exponentially with age.

Genetic abnormalities in the haemostatic system (inherited thrombophilias) increase the risk from birth, especially if multiple [4]. Acquired risk situations (oestrogen therapy, pregnancy and puerperium, trauma, surgery, medical illnesses and immobilisation) also increase the risk. The risk is higher in women (partly due to the effects of endogenous and exogenous oestrogens), in obesity, and in the presence of malignant disease (especially pelvic, abdominal, metastatic, primary proliferative polycythaemia or malignant paraproteinaemias) (Fig. 3.1; Tables 3.1, 3.2).

The poor prognosis in many patients with malignant disease and DVT means that relatively few will live long enough to develop the post-thrombotic syndrome; however, prolonged anticoagulation in such patients may be considered to reduce the risks of recurrent, symptomatic DVT or PTE, especially in the presence of chemotherapy, central venous catheters or tamoxifen prophylaxis in breast cancer. Prevention of post-thrombotic syndrome may therefore best be focused on identification of thrombophilia, which may be defined as changes in the blood (increased or acquired) that increase the risk of DVT, whether primary episodes or recurrences.

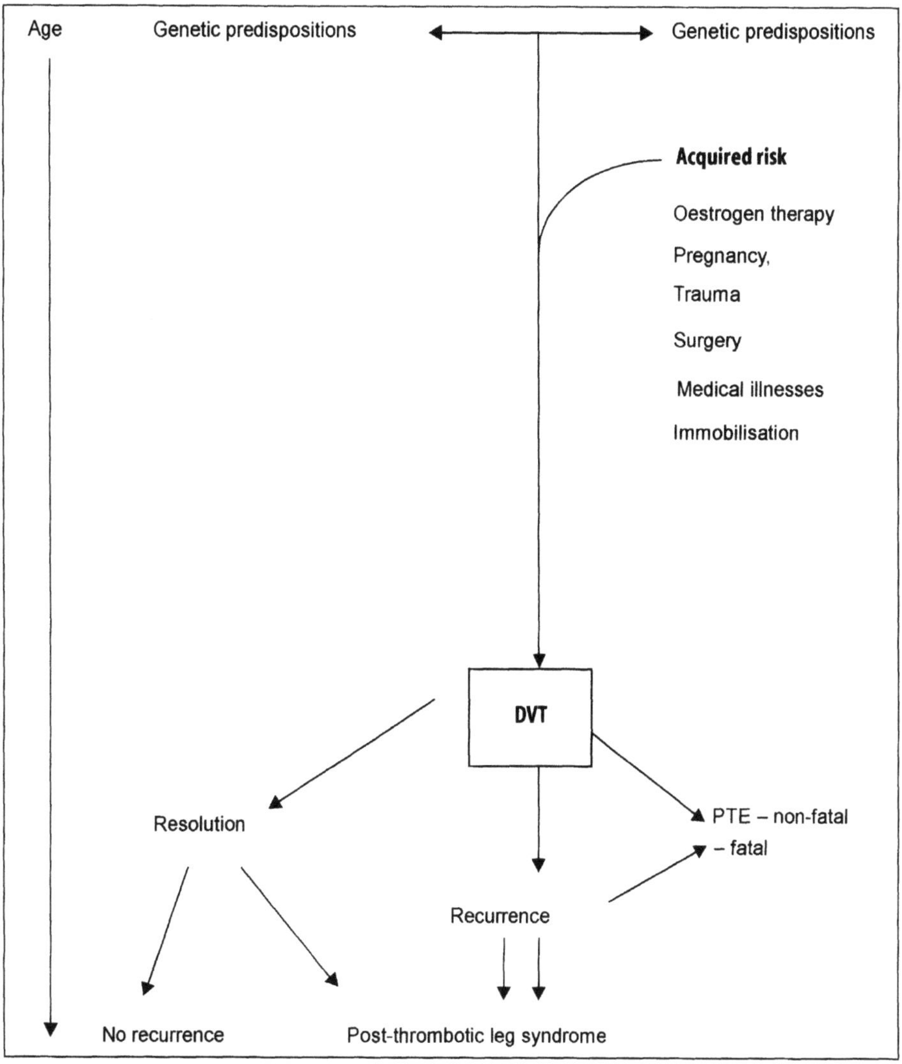

Fig. 3.1. Multiple hit model for deep vein thrombosis (DVT). PTE, pulmonary thromboembolism. From [3].

Genetic Thrombophilias

Genetic thrombophilias should be suspected clinically if there is a past history, or a family history in blood relatives, of "premature" (e.g. onset before 40–45 years) DVT, PTE or recurrent fetal loss (spontaneous abortion or stillbirth); if there is recurrent venous thromboembolism or thrombophlebitis; or if thromboembolism occurs at an unusual site (upper limb veins, retina, cerebral venous sinuses, mesenteric, portal or hepatic veins) [5]. Protein C or protein S deficiency may also present with coumarin-induced skin necrosis [4,5]. Congenital deficiencies of the three coagulation inhibitors (antithrombin, protein C or protein S) are usually due to heterozygosity for autosomal dominant gene defects. In the population-based Leiden study of 474 persons with a first, objectively confirmed DVT (excluding patients over 70 years with

Table 3.1. Risk factors for deep vein thrombosis

Patient factors	Disease or surgical procedure
Age	Trauma or surgery, especially of pelvis, hip, lower limb
Obesity	Malignancy, especially pelvic, abdominal, metastatic
Varicose veins	Heart failure
Immobility (bed rest of > 4 days)	Recent myocardial infarction
Pregnancy	Paralysis of lower limb (e.g. stroke)
Puerperium	Infection
Oestrogen therapy	Inflammatory bowel disease
Previous deep vein thrombosis or pulmonary embolism	Nephrotic syndrome
Thrombophilias	Polycythaemia
Activated protein C resistance	Paraproteinaemia
Factor V Leiden	Paroxysmal nocturnal haemoglobinuria
Other	Behçet's disease
Increased factor VIII or fibrinogen	
Deficiency of antithrombin, protein C or protein S	
Antiphospholipid antibodies ± lupus anticoagulant	
Homocystinaemia	

From [3].

Table 3.2. Risk factors for deep vein thrombosis: Leiden Thrombophilia Study

Risk factor	Cases (%) ($n = 474$)	Controls (%) ($n = 474$)	Odds ratio[a] (95% confidence intervals)
Acquired risk situations			
Surgery	18	3.6	6 (4–10)
Hospitalisation without surgery	12	1.3	12 (6–24)
Prolonged immobilisation at home	3.6	0.2	16 (3–72)
Pregnancy	5.0	1.3	4 (1–17)
Puerperium	8.2	0.6	14 (2–107)
Total	33	5.9	11 (6.2–19)
Thrombophilias			
Factor V Leiden	19	3.0 8 (4–15)	
High factor VIII (150 IU/dl or over)	24	10	3 (2–4.5)
Antithrombin or protein C deficiency	8	3	2.5 (1.5–4.5)
Population attributable risks			
Acquired risk situation	0.30		
Factor V Leiden	0.17		
High factor VIII	0.16		
Antithrombin or protein C deficiency	0.05		
Total	0.55		

Data from [3] and [6].
[a]Adjusted for age and sex.

malignancy) and 474 controls aged 16–73 years (mean 47 years) such functional deficiencies were found in 8% of patients and 3% of controls: the population attributable risk was 0.05 (Table 3.2). In other words, about 5% of DVT in the population is attributable to the presence of these "classical thrombophilias" [6]. The prevalence of a recently described mutation in coagulation factor V (factor V Leiden, which confers resistance to its inactivation by activated protein C [4]) was 19% in patients and 3% in controls: the population attributable risk was 0.17 (Table 3.2). The low prevalence of this mutation in non-Western countries may explain their low incidence of DVT and PTE [4]. The combination of the factor V Leiden mutation with a deficiency of antithrombin, protein C or protein S increases the risk of thrombosis [4]. Unlike other thrombophilias, the impact of the factor V Leiden mutation on risk of DVT appears to *increase* with age [7].

DVT in the population is also associated with increased plasma levels of fibrinogen and coagulation factor VIII [6], which are also risk factors for arterial thrombosis (ischaemic heart disease). The population attributable risk for high factor VIII (≥ 150 IU/dl) was 0.16 (Table 3.2). The associations with fibrinogen appear partly genetic in origin; the inter-relationships between factor VIII, ABO blood group and thrombosis await clarification [6].

Homozygous homocystinuria has long been recognised as a risk factor for premature arterial and venous thrombosis. More recently, hyperhomocysteinaemia has also been associated with increased risk of both venous and arterial thrombosis: this is partly due to heterozygosity for cystein synthase or methylene-tetrahydrofolate reductase (MTHRF) deficiency (whose cumulative prevalence in the general population is 0.4–1.5%) and partly due to deficiencies of vitamins (folate, cobalamine and pyridoxine), especially in the elderly [4]. Drugs interfering with metabolism of folate (methotrexate, anticonvulsants), cobalamine (nitrous oxide) or pyridoxine (theophylline) can also cause moderate homocysteinaemia. There is much current interest in the possibility that dietary supplementation of these vitamins could have a major impact on venous as well as arterial thrombosis, especially in the elderly: however, randomised trials are required.

Acquired Risk Factors

As noted above, increasing age, and (potentially) vitamin deficiencies, increase the risk of DVT. Obesity (body mass index of 30 kg/m^2 or over) also increases the risk of DVT and PTE, especially in women [8], possibly due to concomitant changes in coagulation factors or activated protein C resistance [9,10]. Smoking has no effect on risk of DVT or PTE [8]. Varicose veins increase the risk of post-operative DVT [11], possibly because they may be a marker of previous (often asymptomatic) DVT in older persons. The increased risks of DVT and PTE with increased oestrogens – in pregnancy and the puerperium [11], combined oral contraceptives [11] that interact with the factor V Leiden mutation [12] and most recently hormone replacement therapy [13] – suggest a common mechanism, such as low protein S activity, high factor VIII activity or activated protein C resistance [9,10].

The population-based Leiden study investigated the impact of acquired risk situations on a first, objectively confirmed DVT in persons aged under 70 years and without malignancy. These situations included pregnancy at time of DVT; puerperium (within 30 days of DVT); or surgery, hospitalisation without surgery or prolonged (≥ 2 weeks) immobilisation at home (including plaster casts) within the year preceding the DVT (Table 3.2). An acquired risk situation was recorded in 33% of cases and 6% of controls, and the population attributable risk was 0.30 [6] (Table 3.2). When these acquired risk situations were combined with thrombophilias (antithrombin or protein C deficiency, factor V Leiden, high factor VIII) the combined population attributable risk was 0.55 [6] (Table 3.2).

Immobilisation (at home or in hospital) and surgery are usually due to trauma or illness (e.g. infection, malignancy, heart failure, myocardial infarction, stroke). The cumulative risk of DVT and PTE increases with the duration of immobility, suggesting a role for venous stasis in the inactive leg in the pathogenesis of DVT [11]. Venous stasis also increases in patients with paralysed legs, heart failure or polycythaemia, which are also risk factors for DVT [11]. Activation of blood coagulation also occurs following trauma, surgery and immobilising illnesses including infection, malignancy, infarction and haemorrhage. The hypothesis that the combination of immobility and coagulation activation predisposes to DVT formation is supported by the prophylactic efficacy of both mechanical measures that increase leg vein blood flow and anti-thrombotic drugs especially anticoagulants, and by the increased efficacy of combinations of mechanical and anticoagulant prophylaxis [11].

Relevance of Thrombophilias to Recurrent Thrombosis and the Post-thrombotic Leg Syndrome

Both genetic thrombophilias and continued acquired risk factors (e.g. malignancy and lupus anticoagulants) increase the risk of recurrent DVT, and hence the risk of developing the post-thrombotic leg syndrome [2]. However, at present these risks remain poorly defined, and require clarification in large, prospective studies.

While thrombophilias such as factor V Leiden [7] or congenital thrombophilias or lupus anticoagulants [2] increase the risk of recurrent DVT, two recent calculations of benefit–risk ratios for prolonged oral anticoagulant therapy for the commonest thrombophilia (factor V Leiden) do not support its use [14,15]. Hence, further prospective studies are required to determine the optimal therapeutic strategies for prevention of recurrent DVT and of the post-thrombotic leg syndrome in patients with thrombophilias.

Blood Abnormalities in the Post-thrombotic Leg Syndrome

A complementary approach to investigating the relationships of blood abnormalities to post-thrombotic leg syndrome is to measure haemostatic variables in patients with this syndrome compared with controls. Browse and colleagues [1] have performed a series of studies showing high levels of plasma fibrinogen and decreased fibrinolytic activity in such patients, which may be relevant to their histological findings of a fibrin "cuff" around skin venules/capillaries. This group hypothesised that such a cuff may promote skin hypoxia and ulceration, and showed that stimulation of endogenous fibrinolytic activity with the anabolic steroid, stanozolol, was associated with some therapeutic effect [1]. However, the adverse hormonal (and other) effects of anabolic steroids limit their clinical application in this situation.

A recent randomised trial has shown that compression stockings should be prescribed routinely to be worn on the affected legs during the day long-term, to reduce the risk of the post-thrombotic leg syndrome [16]. The role of venotropic drugs such as hydroxyethylrutosides is less well established [17]. Interestingly, use of either compression stockings or venotropic drugs was associated in a cross-sectional study with decreased red cell aggregability [18]. Increased red cell aggregability (partly due to increased plasma fibrinogen levels) has been associated with the severity of venous insufficiency [19].

In the Edinburgh Vein Study, we are currently studying the relationships of blood abnormalities with venous abnormalities in a random sample of the general population. Preliminary findings will be presented at the symposium upon which this book is based.

References

1. Browse NL, Burnand KG, Lea Thomas M. Diseases of the veins: pathology, diagnosis and treatment. London: Edward Arnold, 1988.
2. Prandoni P, Lensing AWA, Cogo A, et al. The long-term clinical course of acute deep venous thrombosis. Ann Intern Med 1996;125:1–7.
3. Lowe GDO. Venous thromboembolism. In: Pathy MSJ, editor. Principles and practice of geriatric medicine. Chichester: Wiley, 1998.
4. Lane DA, Mannucci PM, Bauer KA, et al. Inherited thrombophilia. Thromb Haemost 1996;76:651–662, 824–834.
5. British Committee for Standards in Haematology. Guidelines on the investigation and management of thrombophilia. J Clin Pathol 1990;43:703–709.
6. Koster T. Deep-vein thrombosis. A population-based case–control study: Leiden Thrombophilia Study. MD Thesis, University of Leiden, 1995.
7. Ridker PM, Glynn RJ, Miletich JP, Goldhaber SZ, Stampfer MJ, Hennekens CH. Age-specific incidence rates of venous thromboembolism among heterozygous carriers of Factor V Leiden mutation. Ann Intern Med 1997;126:528–531.
8. Goldhaber SZ, Savage DD, Garrison RJ, et al. Risk factors for pulmonary embolism: the Framingham Study. Am J Med 1983;74:1023– .
9. Woodward M, Lowe GDO, Rumley A, et al. Epidemiology of coagulation factors, inhibitors and activation markers: the Third Glasgow MONICA Survey. II. Relationships to cardiovascular risk factors and prevalent cardiovascular disease. Br J Haematol 1997;97:785–797.
10. Lowe GDO, Rumley A, Woodward M, Reid E. Oral contraceptives and venous thromboembolism. Lancet 1997;349:1623.
11. Thromboembolic Risk Factors (THRIFT) Consensus Group. Risk of and prophylaxis for venous thromboembolism in hospital patients. BMJ 1992;305:567–574.
12. Vandenbroucke JP, Rosendaal FR. End of the line for "third-generation" pill controversy? Lancet 1997;349:1113–1114.
13. Vandenbroucke JP, Helmerhorst FM. Risk of venous thrombosis with hormone-replacement therapy. Lancet 1996;348:972.
14. Baglin C, Brown K, Luddington R, Baglin T. Risk of recurrent venous thromboembolism in patients with the factor V Leiden (FVR506Q) mutation: effects of warfarin and prediction by predisposing factors. Br J Haematol 1998;100:764–768.
15. Sarasin FP, Bounameaux H. Decision analysis model of prolonged anticoagulant treatment in factor V Leiden carriers with first episode of deep vein thrombosis. BMJ 1998;316:95–9.
16. Brandjes DP, Buller HR, Heijboer H, Huisman MV, de Rijk M, Jagt H, ten Cate JW. Randomised trial of effect of compression stockings in patients with symptomatic proximal-vein thrombosis. Lancet 1997;349:759–762.
17. Wadworth AN, Faulds D. Hydroxyethylrutosides: a review of its pharmacology, and therapeutic efficacy in venous insufficiency and related disorders. Drugs 1992;44:1013–1032.
18. Chabanel A, Horellou MH, Conard J, Samama MM. Red blood cell aggregability in patients with a history of leg vein thrombosis: influences of post-thrombotic treatment. Br J Haematol 1994;88:174–179.
19. Chabanel A, Zuccarelli F, Samama MM. Red cell aggregability increases with the severity of venous insufficiency. Int Angiol 1995;14:69–73.

4 Does Lifestyle Really Affect Venous Disease?

A. J. Lee, C. J. Evans, C. V. Ruckley and F. G. R. Fowkes

Introduction

Venous disease is common in the Western world, resulting in considerable morbidity and a heavy burden on national healthcare resources [1]. In the last two decades a number of reviews on the epidemiology of venous disease have been published [2–6]. However, the question as to whether varicose veins are due to an inherited defect or to some environmental influence remains unanswered. The aims of this chapter are to review the evidence relating lifestyle factors to venous disease and to update this evidence using data from the recently completed Edinburgh Vein Study. The Edinburgh Vein Study is a cross-sectional survey of 1566 men and women aged 18–64 years resident in Edinburgh. Full details of its methodology and response rates are given elsewhere [7]. It is beyond the scope of this chapter to discuss the underlying pathophysiological mechanisms that may cause varicose veins, but there is evidence to suggest that some or all of the following lifestyle factors may have an effect.

Social Class and Socio-economic Factors

There have been inconsistent findings on the relationship between venous disease and social class. One study noted a higher proportion of people in the lower social classes with venous disease [8], whilst others have shown no effect of occupation [9, 10]. Figure 4.1 shows that, in the Edinburgh Vein Study, there was no obvious relationship between social class and the prevalence of trunk varices. The age- and sex-adjusted prevalence of trunk varices was higher in manual workers (social classes IIIM–V) than non-manual workers (social classes I–IIIN), although the difference did not reach statistical significance. Venous disease has been related to other measures of socio-economic status such as estimated family income and level of education [9, 11]. Preliminary analysis of data from the Edinburgh Vein Study suggests that the prevalence of trunk varices was significantly lower among those who reported either a university or college degree or a professional qualification (29.8%) compared with those who said that they had been educated to secondary school level only (41.7%).

Standing, Lifting and Physical Exercise

There is widespread belief that certain occupations, particularly those involving prolonged standing and/or heavy lifting, are associated with the development of varicose

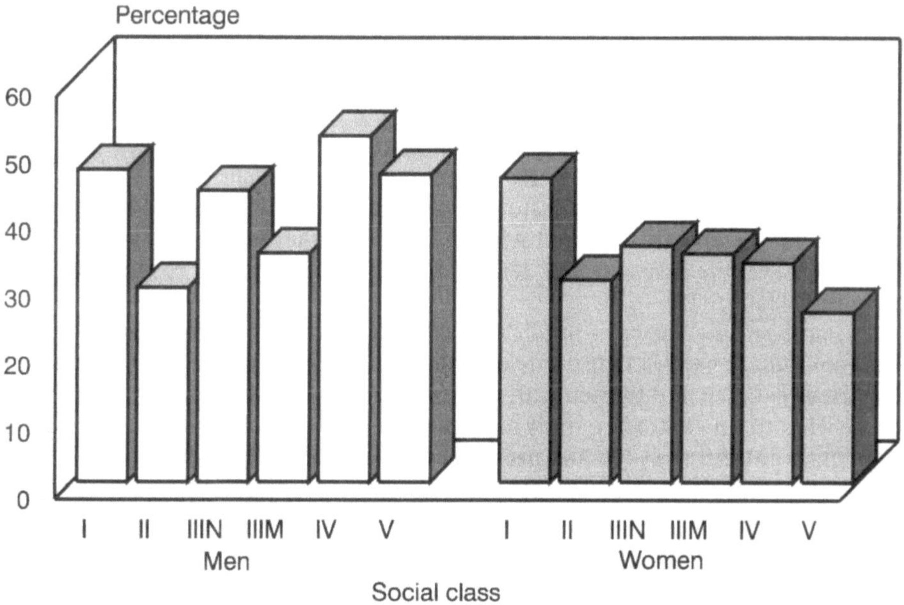

Fig. 4.1. Prevalence of trunk varices in the Edinburgh Vein Study in relation to social class.

veins. Studies that have reported such data are summarised in Table 4.1. Care must be taken in drawing conclusions from these studies because of the difficulties in measuring levels of posture, particularly over a subject's lifetime. In general, however, these studies

Table 4.1. Summary of those studies which have examined the association between mobility at work and varicose veins

Reference	Subjects	Type and place of study	Measure of mobility
Some association found			
Abramson et al. [9]	2245 M, 2557 F Aged 15–75+	Population, W. Jerusalem	Standing
Kakande [12]	64 M, 36 F Aged 10–70+	Clinic, Nairobi	Standing
Brand et al. [13]	396 M, 629 F Aged 40–89	Population, Framingham	Standing/sitting
Sadick [14]	1000 F Aged 18–74	Clinic, New York	Standing
Pinto et al. [15]	48 M, 152 F Aged 15–50+	Outpatients, Italy	Standing
Sisto et al. [10]	3322 M, 3895 F Aged 30–75+	Population, Finland	Standing (F only)
Edinburgh Vein Study (unpublished)	699 M, 867 F Aged 18–64	Population, Edinburgh	Standing, sitting, walking, heavy lifting (all F only)
No association found			
Maffei et al. [16]	443 M, 1312 F Aged 15+	Attendees of health centre, Brazil	Standing, sitting, walking
Stvrtinova et al. [17]	696 F Aged <19–60+	Store workers, Czechoslovakia	Standing, sitting
Scott et al. [11]	23 M, 106 F Aged 43.7 ± 1.3	Case–control, Boston	Standing

M, = male; F, = female.

suggest that subjects who are involved in occupations which require long periods of standing have an increased incidence of varicose veins [9, 10, 12–15], although a lack of association has been reported by others [11, 16, 17]. Figure 4.2 shows the relationship between the prevalence of trunk varices and the amount of time women from the Edinburgh Vein Study reported sitting and standing at work. A clear inverse trend in prevalence is seen with increasing amount of work time spent sitting, whilst the opposite effect is seen for the amount of time spent standing. Although standing may be an aggravating factor for varicose veins, it is unlikely to be a primary cause. There is no evidence that Africans, for example, stand for less time than Europeans, yet the prevalence of venous disease in the former is considerably less than in the latter [18].

Physical activity has been implicated as a risk factor for venous disease due to the functional changes that occur during exercise. The Framingham Study [13] reported that men and women with varicose veins were less physically active than those without. In contrast, a study of women working in a department store found no significant difference in the prevalence of varicose veins between those who reported no physical activity compared with those who were active at least once a week [17]. Conversely, a recent American study found that those with varicose veins reported the highest frequency of exercise compared with a control group [11]. Care must be taken when interpreting studies which have examined physical activity and posture as risk factors of venous disease since the presence of distended and often painful veins may bias the type of occupation and level of activity chosen by the individual.

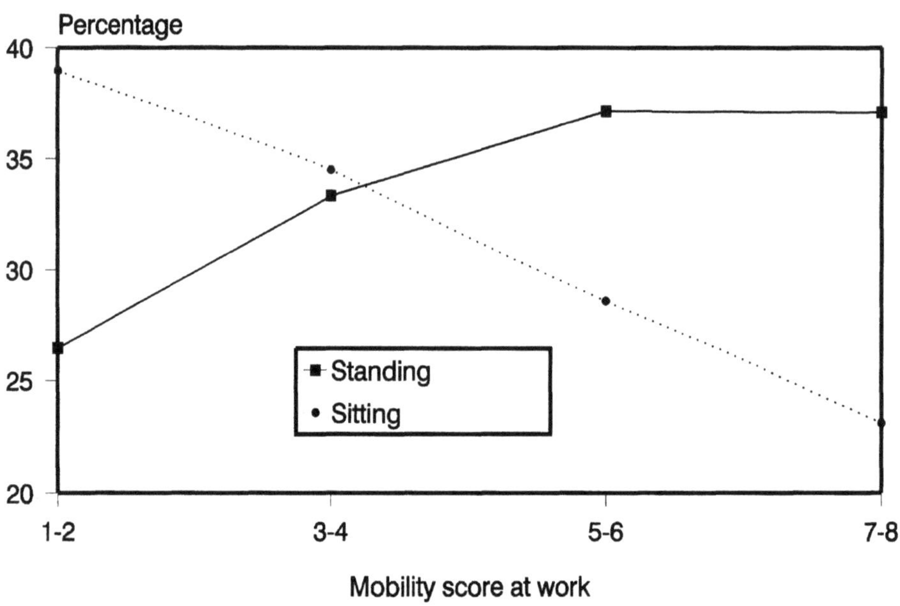

Fig. 4.2. Prevalence of trunk varices in women from the Edinburgh Vein Study in relation to amount of time spent standing and sitting at work. Mobility was calculated from the position of the subject's cross on a scale which ran from "never" to "all of the time". This scale was subsequently divided into eight sections and the cross given a score from 1 to 8. A score of 1 corresponded to the subject never doing this activity during working hours and a score of 8 to them doing this activity all of their working time.

Height, Weight and Obesity

Very few studies have examined height as a risk factor for varicose veins. Discriminant analysis of data from New Zealand found it to be positively associated with risk in male and female Maoris and in male Pakehas [19]. In a study from Jerusalem, patients with venous disease were 1.4 cm taller, on average, than patients without venous disease, although this association became non-significant when weight was controlled for [9]. A recent cross-sectional study from Finland reported that height was only slightly associated with varicose veins in men, whilst women showed a smoothly graded increase in prevalence with increasing height which remained independent on multivariate analyses [10]. In contrast, no association between height and prevalence of varicose veins was observed in the Basle Study II [20], among men from New Guinea [21], in Japanese women [22] or in elderly Turks [23]. Men and women in the Edinburgh Vein Study who were identified as having trunk varices were not significantly taller than those who had no evidence of trunk varices (Table 4.2).

Although some surgeons might remark that the majority of patients who present with varicose veins tend to be overweight, whether obesity is a primary risk factor or merely acts as a promoter for venous disease is open to debate. Obesity has been found to be significantly more common in selective subgroups with varicose veins; for example, in young Israeli men and in Israeli women of all ages [9], in Maori men [19], in American clinic patients [11], in French policemen [8], in Sicilian villagers [24], in a German cohort study [25] and in women of varying nationalities [10, 14, 17, 26]. Other reports have shown no association between obesity and an increased prevalence of varicose veins [12, 21–23, 27, 28]. Controversy between the sexes concerning the importance of obesity as a risk factor seems to exist. In keeping with findings from the Basle [29] and Framingham studies [13], preliminary analyses of the Edinburgh Vein Study data suggest a significant association of trunk varices and both weight and body mass index in women, but no comparable effect in men. Furthermore, this relationship is maintained across increasing grades of severity of trunk varices in women (Table 4.2). Since it is unlikely that obesity is a risk factor for one sex and not the other, it may be that being overweight merely accentuates the development of varicose veins in those already susceptible to the condition.

Table 4.2. Association between trunk varices and each of height, weight and body mass index in the Edinburgh Vein Study

Trunk varices	Height (m)	Weight (kg)	Body mass index (kg/m^2)
Men			
None	1.75 (0.01)	79.18 (0.65)	25.79 (0.19)
Grade 1	1.75 (0.01)	77.49 (0.77)	25.29 (0.25)
Grade 2	1.75 (0.01)	83.71 (2.11)	27.34 (0.73)
Grade 3	1.73 (0.03)	79.60 (5.82)	26.43 (1.41)
p value for trend	NS	NS	NS
Women			
None	1.62 (0.01)	65.72 (0.49)	25.06 (0.19)
Grade 1	1.62 (0.01)	68.40 (0.89)	26.25 (0.35)
Grade 2	1.64 (0.01)	73.30 (2.14)	27.44 (0.82)
Grade 3	1.61 (0.06)	74.00 (11.82)	28.09 (3.23)
p value for trend	NS	≤0.0001	≤0.0001

Values are mean (SE); NS, = not significant.
Grades are based on the Basle classification (Widmer).

Diet and Bowel Habit

It has been postulated that diets deficient in fibre-rich plant foods are a fundamental cause of varicose veins. There is a direct relationship between the amount of dietary fibre eaten by a group of people and both the intestinal transit time and stool weight, bulk and consistency. Cleave [30] hypothesised that varicose veins developed as a result of constipation within the loaded caecum causing compression of the iliac veins and a resultant small pressure increase which then obstructs venous return from the legs. An alternative hypothesis proposed by Burkitt [31, 32] is that constipation and the resultant straining causes an inherent increase in intra-abdominal pressure which, over a period of time, leads to dilatation or other changes in both the superficial and the deep venous system of the leg.

There are very few studies which have examined the dietary habits of subjects with varicose veins. Most are of limited use since they often make no allowance for confounding factors. In the Paris Prospective Study [8], a significantly higher total calorie intake was seen among men with varicose veins, but there was no difference in the distribution of various nutrients (including proteins, lipids and carbohydrates), nor in the consumption of fruit and vegetables. However, estimates of the amount of dietary fibre were not made and since the dietary analysis was done only on a small subsample (497 of 7432 subjects), large individual variation was apparent. Figure 4.3 shows the relationship between stool weight and prevalence of varicose veins in three communities eating different diets, the results being consistent with a dietary hypothesis. A study of Tanzanians, who ate a diet intermediate between a rural African diet and a typically Westernised diet, showed an intermediate prevalence of varicose veins [33].

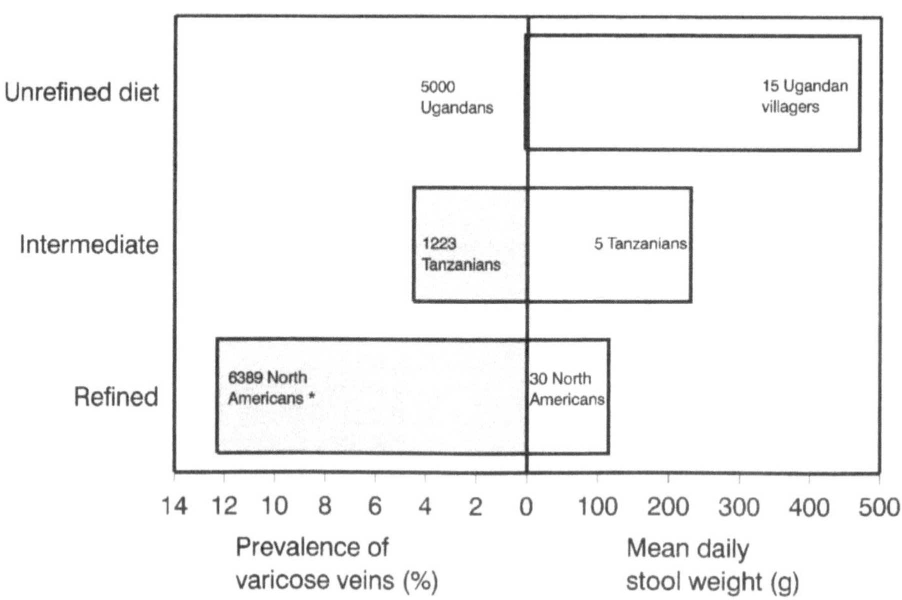

Fig. 4.3. Mean daily stool weights and prevalence of varicose veins in communities eating different diets. Prevalence in North America is age- and sex-adjusted to the Tanzanian population. (After [3]. Reproduced with permission of the editor, *Lancet*.)

A later African study of 100 people with varicose veins reported a typical, unrefined, high residue diet and a related low sufferance of chronic constipation [12]. Constipation was found to be a positive risk factor among a study of Sicilian people [24]. However, in a group of Israelis, constipation was shown to have only a weak association with varicose veins in women and none in men [9]. Given the proposed hypotheses, a direct effect of constipation might, for anatomical reasons, be expected to involve predominantly the veins of the left leg, yet varicose veins appear to occur equally on both sides [9, 16, 29]. A dietary history which estimated vegetable and cereal fibre intake, together with questions concerning bowel habit, was taken as part of the Edinburgh Vein Study. Subsequent analysis should clarify the roles of diet and constipation as risk factors for varicose veins in a Westernised population. In general, studies to date which have looked at the role of diet and constipation in venous disease have been far from conclusive.

Squatting

Squatting to defecate may provide mechanical protection for the leg veins by preventing the rise in mechanical pressure being transmitted down the legs [34]. With the adoption of raised toilets, flexion of the thighs is minimised and the valves of the leg veins are exposed to this pressure. However, an early study from Tanzania [33] found that almost all (97%) of those people with varicose veins reported that they had always squatted to defecate. A later population study from Brazil [16] reported no significant difference in the age-adjusted prevalence of varicose veins among those people who squatted to defecate compared with those who had always used a pedestal water closet. It appears that squatting does not guarantee protection against the development of varicose veins.

Pregnancy, Menopause and Oral Contraception

Many women attribute the onset of varicose veins to pregnancy and it is commonly accepted that there is some association between the two. An editorial in the *British Medical Journal* in 1965 estimated that between 8% and 20% of women develop varicosities during pregnancy [35]. The Basle Study demonstrated a significantly higher age-adjusted prevalence of trunk varices and of combined reticular and hyphenweb varices in parous women compared with childless women [29]. This has been confirmed by others [9, 12, 17, 23, 24, 36], although the effect was only significant among young women in one study [22], and it disappeared after age adjustment in another [28]. A positive relationship between prevalence and an increasing number of pregnancies has been well reported [10, 14, 16, 19, 23, 24], although in only a few studies was the effect independent of age [10, 16, 36]. Figure 4.4 shows the clear correlation between prevalence of varicose veins and number of pregnancies in a group of Brazilian women [16]. In contrast, the Tecumseh Community Health Study [37], most age groups of the Jerusalem community survey [9], the Framingham Study [13], a Japanese study [22] and a recent American case–control study [11] failed to show any association between prevalence of varicose veins and the number of pregnancies.

Although varicose veins are more frequently observed in pregnant women, the belief that the pressure of the pregnant uterus obstructs venous return from the legs is debatable [38]. Varicose veins often develop during the first trimester of pregnancy (before

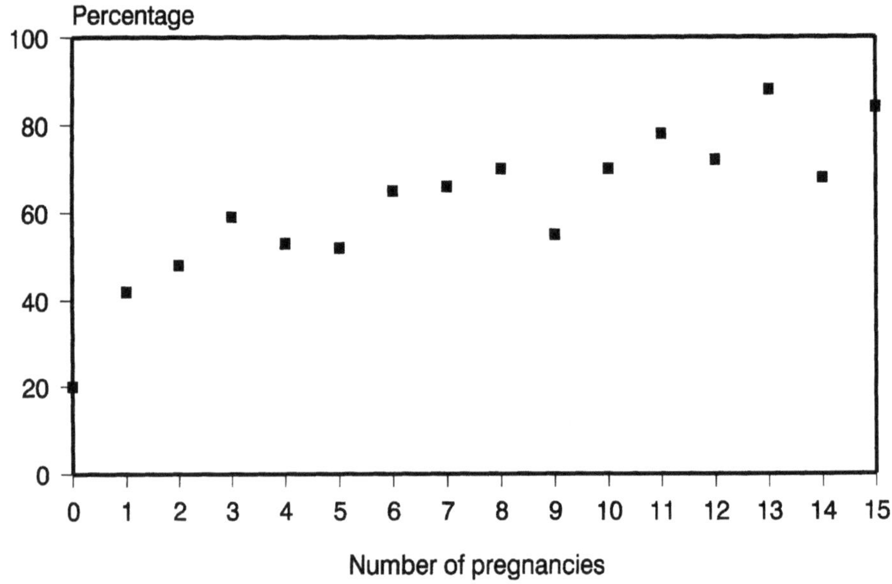

Fig. 4.4. Prevalence of varicose veins in 1312 Brazilian women aged 15 years and over in relation to the number of pregnancies. (After [16]. Reproduced with permission of the editor, *International Journal of Epidemiology*.)

significant uterine enlargement), and can disappear after birth. In addition, women have more pregnancies in developing countries than in Westernised ones, yet the prevalence of varicose veins is much lower in the former. The evidence relating pregnancy to varicose veins is slightly inconsistent and may be biased in the early studies which have not accounted for age. It is still unclear whether the mechanisms by which pregnancy has its effect are direct or merely act as accelerators in susceptible individuals.

Increasing age at menopause has been associated with an increase in risk of varicose veins [13, 38]. However, no independent relationship was reported by others [9] and preliminary analysis of data from the Edinburgh Vein Study appears to support this lack of association.

Very few studies have investigated the use of oral contraceptives and risk of varicose veins. Women with telangiectatic or varicose veins showed an increased incidence of oral contraceptive usage compared with a control group in one study [14]. In contrast, the Basle Study [29], the Mini-Finland Health Survey [10] and a North American case–control study [11] all reported no relationship between varicose veins and oral contraceptive use. However, in the Basle Study, the exposure period was short since the pill was only introduced in Switzerland 4 years before the study took place. In addition, there may be selection bias in such studies because of the known association of oral contraceptives and other venous disorders such as deep vein thrombosis.

Tight Undergarments

Mekky et al. [39] reported that tight undergarments in British women workers in the textile industry was the most important cause of varicose veins, after allowing for the effects of age, weight, parity and working posture. Similarly, a higher prevalence of varicose veins was noted among those Jewish women who habitually wore stockings or corsets [9]. Such findings support the theory of an aetiological role of raised intra-abdominal pressure. However, none of those with varicose veins in a study of Northern and Southern Indian railroad workers wore tight underwear [27] and there was no association of corset wearing with varicose veins in Swiss women after adjustment for age [28]. With fashion now moving away from corsets and restrictive clothing, the incrimination of such items in the aetiology of varicose veins has dwindled.

Smoking

Despite the obvious relationship between smoking and atherosclerosis, very few studies have examined the association between smoking and venous disease. The Framingham Study noted a relationship in men, but not in women [13]. Similarly, a study on French male employees [8], a German cohort study [25] and an American case–control study [11] all reported a positive association. A cross-sectional study from Finland noted that female smokers showed a significantly *lower* prevalence of varicose veins than those who had never smoked, whilst no effect was apparent in men. Furthermore, the association remained after controlling for obesity [10]. In contrast, other studies, including preliminary analysis from the Edinburgh Vein Study, have shown no effect of smoking [9, 22, 23, 40]. Possible mechanisms for a positive relationship between smoking and venous disease may include a decrease in fibrinolytic activity – a plausible hypothesis which is supported by two studies. In a study of Indian railway workers, a significantly lower clot lysis time was found among those with varicose veins compared with age-matched controls [27]. A later British study reported that subjects with severe varicose veins associated with liposclerosis exhibited reduced venous wall fibrinolytic activity (measured by dilute blood clot lysis time and fibrin plate lysis area) compared with healthy subjects [41].

Other Factors

Alexander [42] proposed the "chair sitting" hypothesis, which relies on the fact that chair sitting may have a substantial effect on childhood leg vein stress and calibre resulting in a vein which shows an acceleration of the normal dilatation with age and a hypersensitivity to other factors such as erect posture or pregnancy. Chair sitting is a recently acquired habit of Westernised societies. Some support for the hypothesis came from a study in New Guinea, where it was found that the male villagers (who sit on stools, squat or sit on benches) suffered from varicose veins whilst the women (who sit cross-legged on the ground) did not [21]. However, there seems to be no reliable direct evidence to link chair sitting to clinical varicose veins.

The treatment of varicose veins places a major burden on the healthcare resources in a community. The primary cause of varicose veins is still unknown and evidence for a genetic predisposition will be discussed in the next chapter. While much research has been done on therapeutic procedures, little consideration has been given to possible prevention. Since the prevalence of varicose veins is rare in developing countries, emphasis has tended to be placed on environmental factors associated with Westernised living. After reviewing those epidemiological studies which have examined lifestyle factors, a definitive answer to whether there is any causal association remains elusive.

The process of Westernisation involves a multifactorial lifestyle and factors which have been implicated including pregnancy, prolonged standing, heavy lifting and obesity may be only accelerating causes in those already susceptible to the condition. Based on the epidemiological evidence, the hypothesis incriminating a fibre-deficient diet is the most consistent and would appear to offer the best prospect for any intervention aimed at reducing the prevalence of varicose veins.

References

1. Laing W. Chronic venous diseases of the leg. London: Office of Health Economics, 1992:28:1–44.
2. Burkitt DP. Varicose veins: fact and fantasy. Arch Surg 1976;111:1327–1332.
3. Beaglehole R. Epidemiology of varicose veins. World J Surg 1986;10:898–902.
4. Madar G, Widmer LK, Zemp E, Maggs M. Varicose veins and chronic venous insufficiency disorder or disease? A critical epidemiological review. Vasa 1986;15:126–134.
5. Franks PJ, Wright DDI, McCollum CN. Epidemiology of venous disease: a review. Phlebology 1989;4:143–151.
6. Evans CJ, Fowkes FGR, Hajivassiliou CA, Harper DR, Ruckley CV. Epidemiology of varicose veins: a review. Int Angiol 1994;13:263–270.
7. Evans CJ, Fowkes FGR, Ruckley CV, et al. Edinburgh Vein Study: methods and response in a survey of venous disease in the general population. Phlebology 1998; in press.
8. Dulcimetiere P, Richard JL, Pequignot G, Warnet JM. Varicose veins: a risk factor for atherosclerotic disease in middle-aged men? Int J Epidemiol 1981;10:329–335.
9. Abramson JH, Hopp C, Epstein LM. The epidemiology of varicose veins: a survey in Western Jerusalem. J Epidemiol Community Health 1981;35:213–217.
10. Sisto T, Reunanen A, Laurikka J, et al. Prevalence and risk factors of varicose veins in lower extremities: Mini-Finland Health Survey. Eur J Surg 1995;161:405–414.
11. Scott TE, LaMorte WW, Gorin DR, Menzoian JO. Risk factors for chronic venous insufficiency: a dual case-control study. J Vasc Surg 1995;22:622–628.
12. Kakande I. Varicose veins in Africans as seen at Kenyatta National Hospital, Nairobi. East African Med J 1981;58:667–676.
13. Brand FN, Dannenberg AL, Abbott RD, Kannel WB. The epidemiology of varicose veins: the Framingham Study. Am J Prev Med 1988;4:96–101.
14. Sadick NS. Predisposing factors of varicose and telangiectatic leg veins. J Dermatol Surg Oncol 1992;18:883–886.
15. Pinto A, Galati D, Corrao S, et al. Clinical-anamnestic and instrumental data in outpatients suffering from venous disease. Int Angiol 1995;14:400–403.
16. Maffei FHA, Magaldi C, Pinho SZ, et al. Varicose veins and chronic venous insufficiency in Brazil: prevalence among 1755 inhabitants of a country town. Int J Epidemiol 1986;15:210–217.
17. Stvrtinova V, Kolesar J, Wimmer G. Prevalence of varicose veins of the lower limbs in the women working at a department store. Int Angiol 1991;10:2–5.
18. Geelhoed GW, Burkitt DP. Varicose veins: a reappraisal from a global perspective. Southern Med J 1991;84:1131–1134.
19. Beaglehole R, Prior IAM, Salmond CE, Davidson F. Varicose veins in the South Pacific. Int J Epidemiol 1975;4:295–299.
20. Da Silva A, Widmer LK, Martin H, Mall T, Glaus L, Schneider M. Varicose veins and chronic venous insufficiency: prevalence and risk factors in 4376 subjects of the Basle study II. Vasa 1974;3:118–125.
21. Stanhope JM. Varicose veins in a population of lowland New Guinea. Int J Epidemiol 1975;4: 221–225.
22. Hirai M, Naiki K, Nakayama R. Prevalence and risk factors of varicose veins in Japanese women. Angiology 1990;41:228–232.
23. Komsuoglu B, Göldeli O, Kulan K, Cetinarslan B, Komsuoglu SS. Prevalence and risk factors of varicose veins in an elderly population. Gerontology 1994;40:25–31.
24. Novo S, Avellone G, Pinto A, et al. Prevalence of primitive varicose veins of the lower limbs in a randomised population sample of Western Sicily. Int Angiol 1988;7:176–181.
25. Leipnitz G, Kiesewetter H, Waldhausen P, Jung F, Witt R, Wenzel E. Prevalence of venous disease in the population: first results from a prospective study carried out in Greater Aachen. In: Davy A, Stemmer R, editors. Phlebologie '89. Paris: John Libbey Eurotext, 1989:169–171.
26. Seidell JC, de Groot LCPGM, van Sonsbeek JLA, Deurenberg P, Hautvast JGAJ. Associations of moderate

and severe overweight with self-reported illness and medical care in Dutch adults. Am J Public Health 1986;76:264–269.
27. Malhotra SL. An epidemiological study of varicose veins in Indian railroad workers from the South and North of India, with special reference to the causation and prevention of varicose veins. Int J Epidemiol 1972;1:177–183.
28. Guberan E, Widmer LK, Glaus L, et al. Causative factors of varicose veins: myths and facts. Vasa 1973;2:115–120.
29. Widmer LK, Käch K, Madar G, Kamber V. Risk factors for varicosity. In: Widmer LK, editor. Peripheral venous disorders. Bern: Hans Huber, 1978:58–66.
30. Cleave TL. Varicose veins: nature's error or man's? Lancet 1959;ii:172–175.
31. Burkitt DP, Walker ARP, Painter NS. Dietary fibre and disease. JAMA 1972;229:1068–1074.
32. Burkitt DP. Varicose veins, deep vein thrombosis and haemorrhoids: epidemiology and suggested aetiology. BMJ 1972;2:556–561.
33. Richardson JB, Dixon M. Varicose veins in tropical Africa. Lancet 1977;i:791–792.
34. Burkitt DP. Haemorrhoids, varicose veins and deep vein thrombosis: epidemiologic features and suggested causative factors. Can J Surg 1975;18:483–488.
35. Editorial. Varicose veins in pregnancy. BMJ 1965;ii:3.
36. Dindelli M, Parazzini F, Basellini A, Rabaiotti E, Corsi G, Ferrari A. Risk factors for varicose disease before and during pregnancy. Angiology 1993;44:361–367.
37. Coon WW, Willis PW, Keller JB. Venous thromboembolism and other venous disease in the Tecumseh Community Health Survey. Circulation 1973;48:839–846.
38. Arnoldi CC. The aetiology of primary varicose veins. Dan Med Bull 1957;4:102–107.
39. Mekky S, Schilling RSF, Walford J. Varicose veins in women cotton workers: an epidemiological study in England and Egypt. BMJ 1969;2:591–595.
40. Franks PJ, Wright DDI, Moffatt CJ, et al. Prevalence of venous disease: a community study in West London. Eur J Surg 1992;158:143–147.
41. Browse NL, Gray L, Jarrett PEM, Morland M. Blood and vein wall fibrinolytic activity in health and vascular disease. BMJ 1977;1:478–481.
42. Alexander CJ. In-vivo estimation of vein-wall tension and hoop stress. Med J Aust 1972;1:311–313.

5 What Makes Veins Varicose?

K. Burnand

Introduction

Varicose veins are probably the commonest disorder presenting to general surgeons [1]. There is, however, no precise definition of what constitutes a varicose vein. The World Health Organisation defines varicose veins as "saccular dilatation of the veins which are often tortuous" [2]. This and other descriptive definitions are imprecise [3], but are easier to apply clinically than functional definitions [4]. The exact prevalence of varicose veins in a population depends on the diagnostic criteria used [5]. National surveys in Europe [6,7] and North America [8,9] estimate the prevalence at around 2%. Other local studies have suggested that the prevalence could be as high as 40% in some sub-groups [10]. Whatever their true prevalence, varicose veins appear in the limbs of a large proportion of the population of both genders. Varicose veins may arise without an obvious cause, when they are called "primary", or they may be secondary to another pathological process. Primary varicose veins have some recognised predisposing factors, and structural abnormalities and their development may be influenced by abnormal haemodynamic effects [5].

Predisposing Factors

Several conditions may predispose to the development of primary varicose veins and these are summarised in Table 5.1.

Table 5.1. Predisposing factors for the development of primary varicose veins

Age	Height
Gender	Weight
Pregnancy	Posture
Heredity	Occupation
Race	Clothing
Diet	Alcohol
Bowel habit	smoking

Adapted from [5]

Age

Many reports suggest that the prevalence of varicose veins increases with age [11–15]. Prospective, longitudinal surveillance of a cohort of German school children, the Bochum studies I–III [16,17], found that the children did not develop varicose veins until they became teenagers. In 1974, da Silva and Widmer's group showed a peak frequency of varicose veins in the sixtieth decade [18]. This may reflect the fact that elderly patients are rarely referred for varicose vein surgery, and a census of the over-sixties attending two hospitals in Turkey demonstrated a rise in prevalence with increasing age [19]. Further follow-up of the Bochum children may help to elucidate the exact role of age and tissue degeneration in the development of varicose veins.

Gender

Most studies show a female-to-male preponderance of between 2:1 and 4:1 for the prevalence of varicose veins [12–14 and others]. The Basle study [11], however, shows an almost equal sex distribution (the population survey was, however, on steel-workers!) and in New Guinea [20], Kenya [21] and Hong Kong [22] many more men than women reported varicose veins, although the overall incidence in these countries was low. It has been postulated that the female-to-male predominance in most Western surveys may be attributable to women's concerns about cosmesis [23,24], although the Bochum children's studies have also shown a female preponderance [16,17]. This suggests that hormonal or other gender differences may be involved in the development of varicose veins.

Pregnancy

Many authors have reported an increased incidence of varicose veins in parous women [25,26 and others]. This might be thought to explain the observed differences in gender incidence. In 1942, Lake and co-workers examined the prevalence of varicose veins in a group of 536 employees in a New York department store [27]. They found an increased incidence in the parous compared to the nulliparous women, and even when a correction was made for gender, the effect of pregnancy persisted. This suggests that pregnancy and gender influence the development of varicose veins independently. There also appears to be a greater incidence with increasing numbers of pregnancies, even correcting for advancing age [14], although these findings have not been confirmed in all studies [12,13]. The relative risk of developing varicose veins during pregnancy has been investigated prospectively and found to be between 1.2 and 3.8, increasing with both age and number of births [28]. Other workers have examined lower limb veins in women pre- and post-partum with duplex ultrasonography, occlusion plethysmography and light reflection rheography and found that all veins were more distensible after birth although other functional measures were unchanged [29]. The same group compared primipara with multipara and found a slight increase in vein wall distensibility only, suggesting that the first pregnancy had a greater effect than subsequent ones [30].

Heredity and Race

Virchow first proposed in 1860 that heredity influenced the development of varicose veins in [31]. The exact role of genetic predisposition is not known as most studies have relied on patient reporting, which may be highly inaccurate [32]. In one study, Belcaro used [33] Doppler ultrasonography to assess saphenofemoral incompetence in parents and offspring and found a positive association, although the sample size was small. A higher incidence of blood group A has also been reported in patients with varicose veins [34]. It has been suggested that twin studies might be helpful in elucidating the role of genetics in the development of varicose veins [5].

Post-mortem examination of black Africans has shown them to have more venous valves than Caucasians [35], suggesting a protective role for heredity. Black Africans have few varicose veins but the prevalence is equal among black and white Americans [36]. In Brazil, however, there are different prevalence rates in the white and the native populations [14], as there are in the Siberian and Mongolian peoples of Siberia [37]. There does appear to be a genetic predisposition to the development of varicose veins, but its exact nature is still to be determined.

Diet and Bowel Habit

It is difficult to disentangle the influences of heredity and environmental factors. Many surveys have found a lower prevalence of varicose veins in less industrialised regions [20,21,38] – a trend that is often reversed when these populations move to Westernised area [36,38]. This may reflect a greater concern about varicose veins in Western cultures, and also perhaps a higher reporting rate. In 1960, Cleave [39] proposed that lack of dietary fibre causes "faecal arrest" which results in compression of the iliac veins by the distended caecum and sigmoid colon. Burkitt [40] claimed that lack of dietary fibre combined with straining at defaecation on Western-style lavatory seats raised venous pressure. This was refuted by two investigators who measured venous pressures in the sitting and squatting positions during straining and found that there was no difference in the transmission of intra-abdominal pressure to the leg veins [41]. Diverticular disease is another pathology that is often blamed on a constipating diet and patients with this condition do have a higher incidence of varicose veins when compared with controls [42]. This might reflect a predisposing defect in connective tissue, however, rather than a common cause.

Height and Weight

There is a significant correlation between the height of an individual and the resting venous pressure in their legs [43]. In 1913, Miyauchi [44] suggested that the higher prevalence of varicose veins observed in German compared with Japanese soldiers was attributable to their greater height. The excessively tall Zulus have a very low reported incidence of varicose veins [38] however, and Widmer found a similar incidence in very tall and very short people [11].

The role of obesity in the development of varicose veins is also contentious. In Israel, obesity was found to be significantly more common in younger men and women with varicose veins [12]; Widmer only showed an increased incidence in obese women and then this was only for dilated intradermal venules not actual varicosities [11]. A retrospective study of English males showed no association with weight or body mass [45], although there was a positive association found in Maori men [10]. There does appear to be an association between superficial thrombophlebitis and concurrent hyperlipidaemia [46]; but as the premorbid lipid status of the subjects was unknown it is unclear whether this is cause or effect.

Posture, Occupation and Clothing

In the 1942 New York department store study, 74% of standing employees had varicose veins compared with 57% of those who sat [27]. Other surveys have also shown a higher prevalence in people who stood still at work [12,25 and others]. This has not been confirmed in every census however [14,32]. A 1969 audit of English and Egyptian cotton workers found that prevalence of varicose veins was significantly related to age, parity, weight, tight corsetry and standing at work [47]. A correlation between tight corsetry and varicose vein prevalence was also found in the Israeli study [12], but this may not be independent of increasing age. Prolonged sitting at work has also been proposed as a risk factor for the development of varicose veins [48]. On balance, the evidence is probably slightly in favour of an association between prolonged standing and varicose veins.

Conclusion

There appear to be associations between increasing age, female gender, pregnancy and heredity and the development of varicose veins. Other putative risk factors have yet to be determined.

Structural Factors

Structural factors in the development of varicose veins can be divided into valvular deficiency and vein wall abnormalities.

Valvular Deficiency

Peripheral venous valves normally prevent the reflux of blood. Their function is thought to be to protect the capillaries and venules from sudden excessive rises in pressure during muscular exercise [5]. This idea is supported by the fact that normal veins can withstand retrograde pressure in excess of 200 mmHg [49] and the physiological venous dilatation in these associated with exercise or reactive hyperaemia does not induce reflux [50].

Trendelenburg introduced the concept of descending valvular incompetence as the main cause of varicose veins. He suggested that a venous valve protects the vein wall below it from the pressure in the vein above it, and that varicose veins begin when the highest valve in the long saphenous vein becomes incompetent. He therefore introduced high saphenous ligation, proposing that this would prevent retrograde flow, allowing the saphenous vein to regain its former dimensions and thus causing the varicosities in the tributaries to regress [51]. This theory was supported by Ludbrook [52], who found that the reduction of venous pressure on exercise was equally poor in patients with mild and severe varicose veins and thus he thought that incompetence of the long saphenous vein preceded the development of distal varicosities. No attempt was made to exclude the presence of long saphenous incompetence in patients with mild disease, however, and the pressure falls found in patients with long saphenous incompetence were significantly worse than those found in patients with mild disease. Ludbrook was unable to prove that long saphenous valvular incompetence simply developed as a result of venous dilatation. It has never been shown that long saphenous ligation reverses the dilation of existing tributary varicose veins or prevents the development of new ones.

In 1951, Moore [53] suggested that almost half the patients with varicose veins had defective deep venous valves, but the technique used to demonstrate this was disputed [54], and descending phlebography and duplex scanning in patients with varicose veins do not confirm Moore's findings [5]. Valves in varicose veins are certainly stretched and become atrophic [55] and the valve cusps may even calcify in grossly dilated varices [56], but these phenomena are probably secondary to the disease process. This is supported by the finding that there are no differences in the number of saphenous valves or their degree of atrophy in varicose as compared with non-varicose cadavers [57] and 20–40% of normal individuals have an absent valve in and above the femoral vein without necessarily having long saphenous incompetence [58]. Others have used scanning electron microscopy to examine long saphenous veins excised from patients undergoing varicose vein surgery and found no structural abnormalities [59].

There are a few individuals with a congenital valvular aplasia syndrome [60,61]. These patients have an absence of all venous valves and often develop severe varicose veins [5]. Despite the fact that some animals have venous valves and some do not, however, Foote [23] could find no evidence of varicose veins in any creature other than humans except one poor donkey! At present, there seems little evidence overall to suggest a role for an inherent valvular abnormality as the main cause of primary varicose veins.

Vein Wall Abnormalities

There are a number of studies which support the hypothesis that valvular incompetence follows rather than precedes a change in the vein wall. In 1950, King [62] noted that varicose veins initially dilate distal and not proximal to valves. This was confirmed by Cotton in 1961 [55]. Cotton also noticed that this dilatation was always eccentric, whereas valve cusps are concentric, and so was not caused by regurgitant blood impinging on the vein wall below an incompetent valve. Valve cusps have twice the tensile strength of the vein wall suggesting that valves are less likely than the vein wall to yield under pressure [63]. Clinical observations also uphold the vein wall theory: normal veins function well when used as arterial substitutes in bypass surgery, even when they are reversed and their valves are destroyed, but varicose veins invariably dilate or develop localised aneurysms [64].

In 1963, Svejcar and Prerovsky's group [65] found that the collagen content in both varicose and normal veins in patients with varicose veins was significantly lower than in veins from unaffected patients, suggesting that affected individuals might have abnormal collagen metabolism. These findings have been disputed ever since. Even in the 1990s, some biochemical and histological analyses have supported this idea [66] whereas others have not [67]. Changes in the elastin content have been detected by some groups [66]. It has also been proposed that an increase in smooth muscle rather than a change in collagen or elastin might be responsible for the development of varicose veins [67]. This change in smooth muscle, if confirmed, is likely to be quantitative not qualitative as the reaction to distension of smooth muscle from normal and varicose veins shows no significant differences [68]. Whatever the mechanisms, various studies have found a significantly reduced vein wall elasticity in affected patients [69] and this may represent the final pathway in the development of varicose veins.

Haemodynamic Effects

Haemodynamic effects can be divided into venous flow effects and microcirculatory factors.

Venous Flow Effects

The concept that increased blood flow causes turbulence and thus venous dilatation in susceptible individuals is attractive. Varicose veins certainly develop upstream of an arteriovenous fistula [70]. Some workers have consistently proposed that arteriovenous fistulae are important aetiological factors in the development of varicose veins [71], but the methods used to demonstrate these communications have been challenged. Raised oxygen tensions have been found in blood taken from varicose veins compared with arm veins in the same patients [72]. This could be caused by arteriovenous shunting, although samples drawn from saphenous varicosities show a lower oxygen content than popliteal artery specimens [73]. A role for arteriovenous fistulae in the development of primary varicose veins, therefore, has yet to be established.

It has been suggested that retrograde flow occurring through incompetent valves in communicating veins causes turbulent flow in the superficial system [74]. An asymmetrical fine jet of high-velocity retrograde flow might affect the overlying vein wall, but there is no clinical or experimental evidence to support this hypothesis.

Microcirculatory Factors

Several microcirculatory factors have been suggested in the pathogenesis of varicose veins. Venous stasis might obstruct the vasa vasorum leading to endothelial hypoxia and the resultant release of inflammatory mediators that could ultimately cause venous wall damage [75]. It has also been postulated that increased circulating or endogenous vasa vasorum derived noradrenaline might cause localised dilatation, and this has been demonstrated experimentally in dogs [76,77]. Microcirculation white cell trapping has been proposed as another causative factor; the leucocytes obstructing the vasa venorum, and so inducing hypoxia, or the white cells releasing potent enzymes which destroy the post-capillary vein wall [50]. Others have noted increased mast cell infiltration in stripped varicose veins compared with controls, and have as a consequence suggested that mast cells may be involved in their development [78]. Clearly further studies are required to define any microcirculatory factors involved in the development of varicose veins.

Secondary Varicose Veins

Secondary varicose veins arise as a result of other pathologies such as post-thrombotic damage, pelvic tumours (including pregnancy), arteriovenous fistulae and congenital abnormalities such as Klippel-Trenaunay and Parkes-Weber syndromes. Most, if not all, of these disorders cause venous hypertension. Interestingly, not all individuals with these conditions develop varicosities and if they do the degree of severity is very variable [5]. These observations also refute the idea that haemodynamic factors alone lead to the development of varicose veins.

Summary

Varicose veins are a very common problem. The precise aetiology of primary varicose veins remains unclear. It seems likely from the available evidence that inherited structural weakness combined with haemodynamic or microcirculatory abnormalities eventually lead to reduced vein wall elasticity, dilatation and the formation of varicosities. Increasing age, female gender, parity and occupation may all promote the development of varicose veins in susceptible individuals. Further clinical and experimental studies are necessary if the relative contribution of each of these factors is to be fully elucidated.

References

1. Editorial. The treatment of varicose veins. Lancet 1975;ii:311.
2. Prerovsky I. Diseases of the veins. World Health Organisation, internal communication, MHO-PA 10964.
3. Weddell JM. Varicose veins: pilot study. Br J Surg 1969;23:179–186.
4. Hobsley M. Pathways in surgical management. 2nd ed. London: Edward Arnold, 1986.
5. Browse NL, Burnand KG, Lea Thomas M. Diseases of the veins. London: Edward Arnold, 1988.
6. Logan WPD, Brooke EM. The survey of sickness. Studies on medical and population subjects no. 12. London: General Register Office, 1957.
7. The committee on the Danish national morbidity survey. The sickness survey of Denmark. Copenhagen, 1960.
8. US Department of Health. Education and welfare: national health survey 1935–1936. Washington, DC, 1938.
9. The Department of National Health and Welfare and the Dominion Bureau of Statistics. Illness and health care in Canada. Canadian Sickness Survey 1950–1951. Ottawa, 1960.
10. Beaglehole R, Salmond CE, Prior IAM. Varicose veins in New Zealand: prevalence and severity. NZ Med J 1976;84:396–399.
11. Widmer LK. Peripheral venous disorders. Prevalence and socio-medical importance. Observations in 4529 apparently healthy persons. Basle III study. Bern: Hans Huber, 1978.
12. Abramson JH, Hopp C, Epstein LM. The epidemiology of varicose veins: a survey of western Jerusalem. J Epidemiol Community Health 1981;35:213–217.
13. Coon WW, Willis PW, Keller JB. Venous thromboembolism and other venous disease: the Tecumseh Community Study. Circulation 1973;48:839–846.
14. Maffei FHA. Varicose veins and chronic venous insufficiency in Brazil: prevalence among 1755 inhabitants of a country town. Int J Epidemiol 1986;15:210–217.
15. Hirai M. Prevalence and risk factors of varicose veins in Japanese women. Angiology 1990;3:228–232.
16. Schultz Ehrenburg U, Weindorf N, Vonuslar D, Hirche H. Prospective epidemiological investigations in early and preclinical stages of varicosis. In: Davy A, Stemmer R, editors. Phlebology, 89. Paris: Eurotext, John Libbey, 1989: 163–165.
17. Schultz Ehrenburg U, Weindorf N, Matthes U, Hirche H. Etude épidémiologique sur la pathogenèse des varices. Etude de Bochum I–III. Phlebologie 1992;45:497–500.
18. da Silva A, Widmer LK, Martin H, Mall TH, Glaus L, Schneider M. Varicose veins and chronic venous insufficiency. Vasa 1974;3:118–125.
19. Komsuoglu B, Goldeli O, Kulan K, Cetinarslan B, Komsuoglu SS. Prevalence and risk factors of varicose veins in an elderly population. Gerontology 1994;40:25–31.
20. Stanhope JM. Varicose veins in a population of New Guinea. Int J Epidemiol 1975;4:221–225.
21. Kakande I. Varicose veins in Africans as seen at Kenyatta National Hospital, Nairobi. East African Med J 1981;58:667–676.
22. Alexander CJ. The epidemiology of varicose veins. Med J Aust 1972;1:215–218.
23. Foote RR. Varicose veins. London: Butterworth, 1954.
24. Burkitt DP. Varicose veins: facts and fantasy. Arch Surg 1976;111:1327–1332.
25. Strvtinova V, Kolesar J, Wimmer G. Prevalence of varicose veins of the lower limbs in the women working at a department store. Int Angiol 1991;10:2–5.
26. Novo S, Avellone G, Pinto A, et al. Prevalence of primitive varicose veins in a randomised population sample of western Sicily. Int Angiol 1988;7:176–181.

27. Lake M, Pratt GH, Wright IS. Arteriosclerosis and varicose veins: occupational activities and other factors. JAMA 1942;119:696–701.
28. Dindelli M, Parazzini F, Basellini A, Rabiotti E, Corsi G, Ferrari A. Risk factors for varicose disease before and during pregnancy. Angiology 1993;44:361–367.
29. Sohn C, Stolz W, von Fournier D, Bastert G. Einfluss der Schwangerschaft und der Parität auf das Beinvenensystem. Zentralbl Gynakol 1991;113:829–839.
30. Karl C, Sohn C. Einfluss der Parität auf das Beinvenensystem. Geburtshilfe Frauenheilk 1989;49:49–52.
31. Virchow R. Cellular pathology. London: Churchill, 1860.
32. Weddell JM. Varicose veins: pilot survey. Br J Prev Soc Med 1966;23:179–186.
33. Belcaro GV. Sapheno-femoral incompetence in young asymptomatic subjects with a family history of varices of the lower limbs. In: Negus D, Jantet G, editors. Phlebology '85. Paris: John Libbey, 1985: 30–32.
34. Cornu-Thenard A, Dab W, de Vinconzi I, Valty J. Relationship between blood groups (ABO) and varicose veins: a case control study. Phlebology 1989;4:37–40.
35. Banjo AO. Comparative study of the distribution of venous valves in the lower extremities of black Africans and Caucasians: pathogenetic correlates of the prevalence of primary varicose veins in the two races. Anat Rec 1987;217:407–412.
36. Cleave TL. The saccharine disease. Bristol: John Wright, 1974: 44–65.
37. Listsyn KM. Epidemiology of diseases of the veins of the lower extremities in various climato-geographic conditions. Vestn Khir 1986;137:71–72.
38. Dodd HJ. The cause, prevention and arrest of varicose veins. Lancet 1964;ii:2:809–811.
39. Cleave TL. On the causation of varicose veins and their prevention and arrest by natural means. Bristol John Wright, 1960.
40. Burkitt DP. Varicose veins, deep vein thrombosis, and haemorrhoids: epidemiology and suggested aetiology. BmJ 1972;ii:556–561.
41. Martin A, Odling-Smee W. Pressure changes in varicose veins. Lancet 1976;I:768–770.
42. Latto C, Wilkinson RW, Gilmore OJA. Diverticular disease and varicose veins. Lancet 1973;i:1089–1090.
43. Burnand KG. Studies on the causes of venous ulceration. MS thesis, University of London, 1981.
44. Miyauchi K. Die Haufigkeit der varizen am Unterschenkel bei Japanem und der Erfolg einiger operativ beihandelter Falle. Arch Klin Chir 1913;100:1079–1085.
45. Stewart AM, Webb AJ, Hewitt D. Social medicine studies based on Civilian Medical Board records. II. Physical and occupational characteristics of men with varicose conditions. Br J Prev Soc Med 1955;9:26–32.
46. Albitskii AV, Lakunin KIU, Petukhov VA. Rol' giperlipidemii v patogeneze ostrogo tromboflebita poverkhnostnykh ven nizhnikh konechnostei (English abstract). Grudnaia i Serdechno-Sosudistaia Khirurgiia 1993;6:53–54.
47. Mekky S, Schilling RSF, Walford J. Varicose veins in women cotton workers: an epidemiological study in England and Egypt. BmJ 1969;ii:591–595.
48. Brand FN, Dannenberg AL, Abbott RD, Kannel WB. The epidemiology of varicose veins: the Framingham study. Am J Prev Med 1988;4:96–101.
49. Thuselius O, Gjöres JE. Functional study of isolated venous valves, with special comments on the etiology of varicose veins. Am Eur Symp Venous Dis, Montreux 1974: 74–76.
50. Thulesius O. The venous wall and valvular function in chronic venous insufficiency. Int Angiol 1996;15:114–118.
51. Trendelenburg F. Über die Unterbindung der Vena Saphena Magna bei unterschenkel Varicen. Beitr Klin Chir 1891;7:195–210.
52. Ludbrook J. Valvular defect in primary varicose veins: cause or effect? Lancet 1964;ii:2:1289.
53. Moore HD. Deep venous valves in the aetiology of varicose veins. Lancet 1951;ii:7–10.
54. Murley RS. Deep venous valves in the aetiology of varicose veins. Lancet 1951;i:176.
55. Cotton L. Varicose veins: gross anatomy and development. Br J Surg 1961;48:589–598.
56. Obitsu Y, Ishimaru S, Furukawa K, Yoshihama I. Histopathological studies of the valves of varicose veins. Phlebology 1990;5:245–254.
57. Ortega Santana F, Anitua Solano M, Guijarro de Pablos J, Centol Ramirez A, Lopez Calbet JA, Gonzales Sequeros O. Role of venous valves in the etiology of essential varices (English abstract). Angiologia 1991;43:153–157.
58. Basmajian JV. The distribution of valves in the femoral, external iliac and common iliac veins and their relationship to varicose veins. Surg Gynecol Obstet 1952;95:537–542.
59. Mashiah A, Rose SS, Hod I. The scanning electron microscope in the pathology of varicose veins. Israel J Med Sci 1991;27:202–206.
60. Lodin A, Lindvall N, Gentele H. Congenital absence of venous valves as a cause of leg ulcers. Acta Chir Scand 1959;116:256.
61. Lindvall N, Lodin A. A congenital absence of venous valves. Acta Chir Scand 1962;124:310–319.

62. King ESJ. The genesis of varicose veins. Aust NZ J Surg 1950;20:126.
63. Ackroyd JS, Pattison M, Browse NL. A study of the mechanical properties of fresh and preserved human femoral vein wall and valve cusps. Br J Surg 1985;72:117–119.
64. Rose SS, Ahmed A. Some thoughts on the aetiology of varicose veins. J Cardiovasc Surg 1986;27:534–543.
65. Svejcar J, Prerovsky I, Linhart J, Kruml J. Content of collagen, elastin, and water of the internal saphenous vein in man. Circ Res 1962;11:296.
66. Chello M, Mastroroberto P, Romano R, Crillo F, Cusano T, Marchese AR. Alteration in collagen and elastin content in varicose veins. J Vasc Surg 1994;28:23–27.
67. Travers JP, Dalton CM, Baker DM, Makin GS. Biochemical and histological analysis of collagen and elastin content and smooth muscle density in normal and varicose veins. Phlebology 1992;7:97–100.
68. Thulesius O, Gjöres JE. Reactions of venous smooth muscle in normal men and patients with varicose veins. Angiology 1974;25:145–154.
69. Clarke GH, Vasdekis SN, Hobbs, Nicolaides AN. Venous wall function in the pathogenesis of varicose veins. Surgery 1992;111:402–408.
70. Holman EF. The development of arterial aneurysms. Surg Gynecol Obstet 1955;100:599.
71. Schalin L. Role of arteriovenous shunting in the development of varicose veins. In: Ecklof B, Gjöres JE, Thulesius O, Berqvist D, editors. Controversies in the management of venous disorders. London: Butterworth, 1989:182–192.
72. Brewer AC. Arteriovenous shunts. BMJ 1950;ii:270.
73. Reikeras O, Sorlie D. The significance of arteriovenous shunting for the development of varicose veins. Acta Chir Scand 1983;149:479.
74. Fegan WG, Kline AL. The cause of varicosity in superficial veins of the lower limb. Br J Surg 1972;59:798–801.
75. Michiels C, Arnould T, Janssens D, Bajou K, Geron I, Remacle J. Interactions between endothelial cells and smooth muscle cells after their activation by hypoxia: a possible aetiology for venous disease. Int Angiol 1996;15:124–130.
76. Crotty TP. Is circulating noradrenaline the cause of varicose veins? Med Hypoth 1991;34:243–251.
77. Crotty TP. The role of turbulence and vasa vasorum in the aetiology of varicose veins. Med Hypoth 1991;34:41–48.
78. Yamada T, Tomita S, Mori M, Sasatomi E, Suenaga E, Itoh T. Increased mast cell infiltration in varicose veins of the lower limbs: a possible role in the development of varices. Surgery 1996;119:494–497.

6 How Does a Leg Ulcerate?

Philip D. Coleridge-Smith

Introduction

Varicose veins have been recognised since the time of the Papyrus of Ebers (*c.* 3500 BC) and venous ulceration from the works of Hippocrates, and yet the pathogenesis of these conditions is incompletely understood. Many factors are involved in the development of venous ulceration. These probably include those which also cause varicose veins and involve both inherited and environmental components. Inherited factors have been shown to be important in the pathogenesis of varicose veins [1], but a detailed analysis of genetic factors in patients with leg ulcers has not been published. Recently an association has been shown between factor V Leiden gene defect and venous ulceration [2]. This may simply reflect the increased likelihood of deep vein thrombosis (DVT) in patients with this gene defect, or may be related in a more complex way to the development of venous ulceration.

Factors Leading to Venous Ulceration

There is reasonable evidence that DVT is a risk factor for the skin changes and oedema that may precede ulceration in the lower limbs [3,4]. In a study of chronic venous ulcers in Perth, Western Australia, 17% of patients reported a history of DVT and a large number had a history of conditions that might predispose to DVT [5]. No control group was reported with which to compare these data. In a population-based study of 3600 people in Copenhagen, Denmark, history of DVT or pulmonary embolism was related to the occurrence of venous disease independently of age, sex and other possible risk factors [3]. The incidence of ulcers has been identified in follow-up studies of patients having a diagnosis of DVT [4,6]. Follow-up of 61 patients for an average of 39 months revealed the development of three ulcers (5%). These studies suggest that the annual incidence of ulceration in individuals who have had a DVT is around 1–2% per annum, but relate to series collected over 10 years ago. More recent data suggest that prompt diagnosis and treatment of venous thrombosis leads to even less likelihood of ulceration [7].

Arterial disease alone may result in lower limb ulceration, but patients with venous disease often have associated arterial disease, which is common in the age group of patients affected by leg ulceration. Some studies have reported a relatively high prevalence of arterial disease in leg ulcer patients [8,9]. However, in a recent case-control comparison in Edinburgh, Scotland, arterial disease (angina, intermittent claudication, hypertension, and low ankle brachial pressure index) did not occur more commonly in 331 leg ulcer patients compared with an equal number of age- and sex-matched population controls [10].

Venous ulceration occurs when the muscle pumping mechanisms of the leg are impaired due to disease in the superficial or deep venous systems [11]. This may be simply a consequence of varicose veins, which account for 20–50% of venous leg ulcers [12,13] or arise from incompetence of the valves of the deep veins. This may result from a previous DVT or be due to primary valve failure, in a manner similar to that which results in incompetence of the superficial veins in patients with varicose veins [14]. The consequence of incompetent lower limb vein valves is that the pumping mechanism no longer reduces the pressure in the veins to low levels during walking. A cannula placed in the dorsal foot vein usually shows a reduction of the resting pressure from 80–100 mmHg to 10–20 mmHg in a fit person. Patients with severe calf muscle pump impairment may not be able to reduce the foot vein pressure below the resting level [15] (Fig. 6.1).

The severity of venous incompetence, as indicated by the ambulatory venous pressure in the foot, may be related to the risk of ulceration. In one study of 220 unselected patients with venous problems, no ulceration occurred in limbs with ambulatory venous pressure < 30 mmHg [16]. With higher ambulatory venous pressures there was a greater risk of ulceration, ranging from 14% in limbs with pressure between 31 and 40 mmHg to 100% in limbs with a pressure of > 90 mmHg. This relationship occurred in both those with superficial venous reflux and those with deep venous reflux with or without venous occlusion. However, there tends to be considerable overlap in venous pressure measurements between patient groups (varicose veins, skin changes, ulceration), suggesting that several additional factors are also involved in the development of venous ulceration. Another way of looking at these data is to say that there is considerable variability between patients in their susceptibility to venous hypertension.

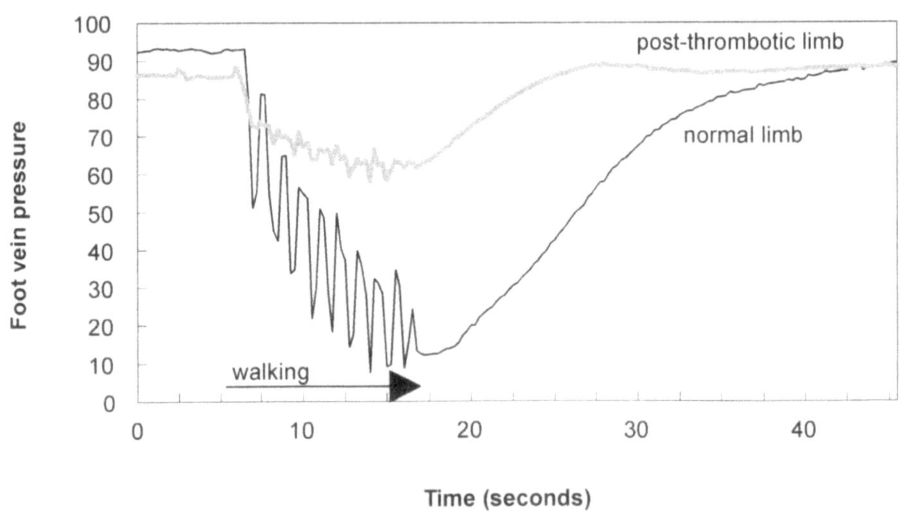

Fig. 6.1. Ambulatory venous hypertension: a recording showing traces from a patient who had suffered a previous venous thrombosis in one limb. The ambulatory venous pressure is high and the refilling time short in the affected limb.

Several other factors may contribute to the development of venous ulceration. These include minor trauma, oedema (not necessarily related to venous insufficiency), obesity, and co-existing conditions such as arthritis or neuropathies. However, the relative importance of these factors is not well established.

Mechanisms of Ulceration

Homans [17] suggested that ulceration of the skin overlying large varicosities was caused by low oxygen levels in the stagnant blood of the varicosities causing hypoxia of the skin. The oxygenation of blood in varicose veins has been the subject of several studies since that time [18,19]. It is now clear that with the patient lying supine the haemoglobin saturation with oxygen of blood in varicose veins is greater than in the veins of normal limbs. When the patient stands, there is no difference between normal subjects and patients with varicose veins. So even if venous blood was responsible for nutrition of the skin, there would be no difference between normal subjects and those with varicose veins [20]. The raised blood oxygen tension in veins of patients with venous disease led to the suggestion by some that arteriovenous fistulae were present, which might deprive the skin of oxygen [21,22]. Research using microspheres and macroaggregates has failed to demonstrate an increase in arteriovenous shunting in the skin of patients with venous disease [23].

Fibrin Cuffs

In 1982 Browse and Burnand [24] proposed that oxygen diffusion into the tissues of the skin was restricted by a pericapillary fibrin cuff that they had observed histologically. They suggested that increased capillary pressure as a consequence of the raised venous pressure results in an increased loss of plasma proteins through the capillary wall. This includes fibrinogen, which polymerises to provide the "fibrin cuff" that may be seen around capillaries in the skin, using both histochemical and immunohistochemical methods. Measurements of protein loss from capillaries showed that fibrinogen was quantitatively the most important plasma protein leaking into the tissues in patients with venous disease. Measurements of fibrinolysis have shown that patients with venous disease have reduced fibrinolytic activity in the blood and veins, perhaps explaining why the fibrin cuff persists [25].

This theory considers that venous ulceration occurs when the tissues are deprived of oxygen. Surprisingly, it is difficult to find reliable evidence that the skin and subcutaneous tissues are hypoxic in liposclerotic skin. There is no published evidence to prove that fibrin provides a barrier to oxygen diffusion. It seems probable from the composition of other human connective tissues that a fibrin gel would comprise much water with a small amount of fibrin. Diffusion of small molecules through such a cuff might be expected to be very similar to diffusion through water and other human tissues. If the assumption is made that the fibrin layer contains 0.5% fibrin, similar to that of a fibrin blood clot, calculations reveal no impairment of oxygen delivery to the tissues [26]. Even a cuff consisting of 100 times more fibrin that this would result in a reduction of oxygen delivery of only 50%. The results of these calculations have not been confirmed by measurement.

The evidence that is adduced to support the assumption that the skin is hypoxic in chronic venous insufficiency (CVI) was obtained by transcutaneous oximetry [27,28]. A Clark-type electrode equipped with an integral heater is applied to the skin in order to register the oxygen availability at the skin surface. These devices were originally devised for neonatal monitoring, and skin heating was used to produce maximal vasodilatation to ensure that the measurement accurately reflects the arterial oxygen tension. In venous disease, different findings have been obtained depending on whether the transducer is heated to 43 °C or 37 °C. At the higher temperature, used by most authors, it has been found that patients with venous disease tend to have lower $tcPO_2$ readings than normal subjects [27,28] (Fig. 6.2). Measurements made with an electrode temperature of 37 °C are paradoxical [29]. Under these circumstances, the oxygenation of the skin is greater in patients with venous disease than in normal subjects! This technique has a number of limitations and transcutaneous oxygen tensions may be influenced by many factors other than skin oxygenation. Subsequently direct needle electrode measurements have been made in liposclerotic skin, and these show a moderate reduction in tissue oxygenation, but insufficient to result in skin necrosis [30].

Less invasive methods have also been used to study skin oxygenation. Hopkins et al. [31] used positron emission tomography techniques to assess blood flow and oxygen extraction in the skin and subcutaneous tissues of patients with venous disease. They showed that the oxygen extraction ratio was reduced in such tissues, but that skin flow was increased by a substantial amount, so it is unclear from these measurements whether oxygen delivery was increased or decreased.

I have measured the clearance of xenon-133 from the skin as an assessment of the efficiency of the microcirculation in handling a molecule of similar size to oxygen. Xenon has a molecular weight 4 times that of oxygen, so its diffusion rate would be half that of oxygen, assuming similar solubility for oxygen and xenon in body fluids (water). Sjerson's technique [32] was used in which the xenon gas is applied topically to the skin and readily reaches the dermis and subcutaneous fat by diffusing through the skin. This avoids direct intradermal injection of solutions of xenon, which might

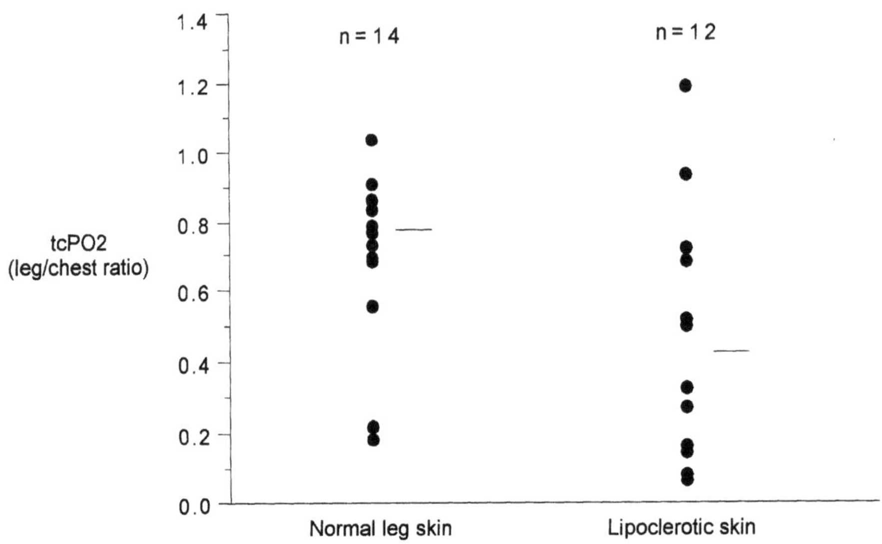

Fig. 6.2. Reduced $tcPO_2$ of the leg skin in venous disease (from measurements made at the Middlesex Hospital Vascular Laboratory). The results are expressed as the ratio of leg $tcPO_2$ to the chest wall $tcPO_2$.

alter blood flow in the skin. Measurements were made in the liposclerotic skin of patients with venous disease, and compared with values in control subjects under conditions of reactive hyperaemia after 5 min of cuff-occlusion of the arterial supply to the leg. No difference in xenon clearance was found between patients with venous disease and control subjects [33]. This was a considerable surprise and led me to assess further measures of gas exchange with the skin.

The rate of recovery of the $tcPO_2$ after a period in which arterial blood supply has been interrupted is a way of determining whether a diffusion barrier exists to delivery of oxygen to the skin. I measured the time taken for re-oxygenation of the skin after a period of ischaemia produced by inflating a cuff on the leg above systolic arterial pressure for 5 min. No difference was found between control and venous disease groups [34]. These results led me to conclude that in patients with CVI it is unlikely that there is a substantial abnormality in the delivery of oxygen to the skin causing skin damage. There remains the possibility that some elements in the skin may receive insufficient nutrition and that this renders them susceptible to injury by mechanical or other factors.

The "White Cell Trapping" Hypothesis

White cell margination is a normal event in the microcirculation, occurring most frequently in the post-capillary venules. This phenomenon is thought to be important in the mechanism that results in tissue injury following ischaemia. White blood cells are substantially larger than red cells and are responsible for many of the rheological properties of blood. White cells take 1000 times longer than red cells to deform on entering a capillary bed, and are responsible for about half the peripheral vascular resistance despite their small numbers in the circulation compared with red cells [35]. In myocardial infarction they cause capillary occlusion, which can be prevented in experimental animals by rendering the animal leucopoenic [36,37]. White blood cells have been implicated as the mediators of ischaemia in many tissues including myocardium, brain, lung and kidneys [38–41]. Polymorphonuclear leucocytes, particularly those attached to capillary endothelium, may become "activated", meaning that cytoplasmic granules containing proteolytic enzymes are released [42]. In addition a non-mitochondrial "respiratory burst" permits these cells to release free radicals, including the superoxide radical, which have non-specific destructive effects on lipid membranes, proteins and many connective tissue compounds [43]. Leucotactic factors are also released, attracting more polymorphonuclear cells.

The search for alternative mechanisms of skin damage in venous disease has resulted in investigation of the role of leucocytes in the events which follow venous hypertension. Moyses et al. [44] studied the limbs of normal subjects in response to raised venous pressure, and measured haematological parameters to assess the effect of venous hypertension. Their subjects sat on a bicycle saddle with the limbs dependent for a period of 40 min without moving. Blood samples were taken from the long saphenous vein at the ankle. They found that the haematocrit and red cell count increased in parallel as would be expected. They noticed that the white cell count remained unchanged, despite the increased haematocrit. White cells were being "lost" from the circulation, which after 40 min amounted to a 25% change. Thomas et al. [45] performed a similar study in which they compared patients with normal lower limbs with patients with venous disease resulting in lipodermatosclerosis and ulceration. Their patients were permitted to sit with their legs dependent, a less stringent requirement than that of Moyses et al. Blood sampling was again from the long saphenous vein at the ankle. After 60 min patients with venous disease were "trapping" 30% of the white cells and control subjects were trapping 7% (Fig. 6.3). This led me to examine the microcirculation using capillary microscopy. I found that venous hypertension appeared to reduce the number of visible capillary loops in patients with venous disease, but not in control subjects [46], suggesting that capillary damage may be occurring during venous hypertension.

Bollinger et al. [47] have investigated the events in venous disease using fluorescence video capillary microscopy. They measured the rate of diffusion of fluorescein out of capillaries after an intravenous injection. They showed that capillaries in venous disease are much more permeable than normal to this molecule, contrary to the suggestions made in the "fibrin cuff" hypothesis. Using simultaneous fluorescence and light capillary microscopy Franzeck et al. [48] have described the appearances of capillary loops which are filled with red blood cells but did not appear to be perfused. They suggested that this may be due to capillary "thrombosis".

I published a hypothesis suggesting that white cell trapping resulted in neutrophil activation, causing damage to the tissues [49] (Fig. 6.4). Based on the literature on myocardial ischaemia, I proposed that white cells caused occlusion of capillaries, a suggestion originally made by Moyses et al. [44]. If some of the capillaries were occluded this might result in heterogeneous perfusion and therefore tissue hypoxia and ischaemia. This seemed a reasonable suggestion at the time, since it pre-dated our attempts to measure the severity of the "diffusion block", and I included this to explain the "hypoxia" observed by transcutaneous oximetry. My conclusion from the data presented above is that tissue hypoxia is not the main cause of venous ulceration. In fact, I have specifically investigated the response of the microcirculation to venous hypertension to see whether this causes degradation of microcirculatory function. Using laser Doppler fluxmetry and transcutaneous oximetry to assess the skin microcirculation during a 30-min period of experimental venous hypertension produced by standing, I could show no progressive microcirculatory deficit to suggest occlusion of large numbers of capillaries [46]. Subsequently I have applied a more severe venous hypertensive insult

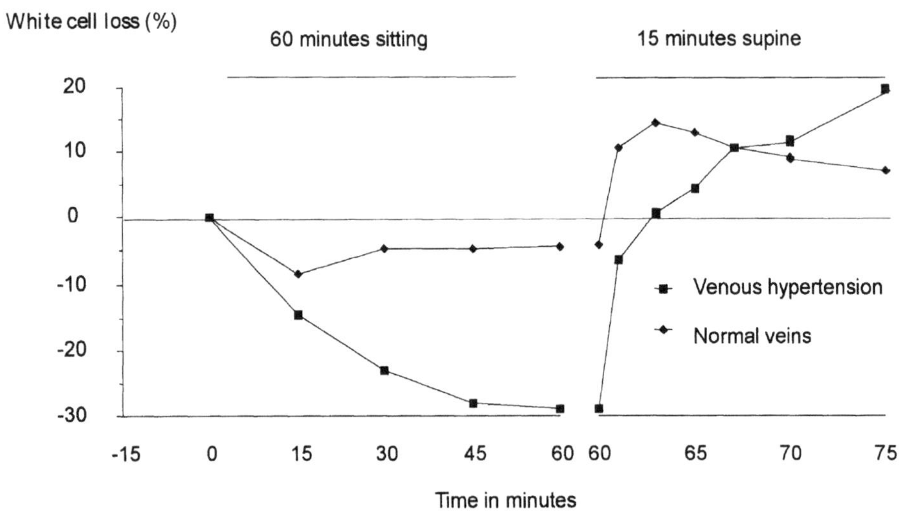

Fig. 6.3. "White cell trapping" in patients compared with controls. (Re-drawn from [45].)

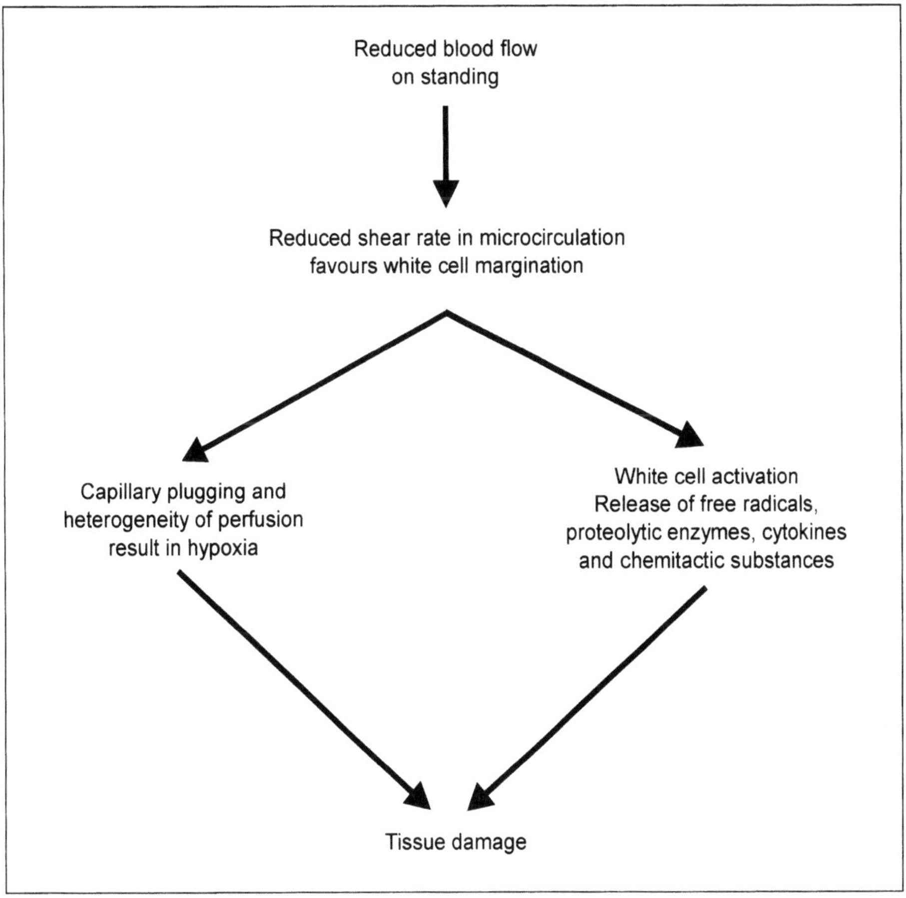

Fig. 6.4. "White cell trapping" hypothesis, derived from [49]. As indicated in the text, we now believe that if white cells cause occlusion of capillaries, they probably do not cause local hypoxia. It seems that the toxic products released by white cells may be more likely candidates for the mediators of tissue injury.

to the normal circulation, by inflating a cuff around the leg to 80 mmHg for 15 min and measuring the hyperaemic response. I found a small reduction in microcirculatory function by this means, which suggests that microcirculatory injury may be produced in the short term (15 min) by raised venous pressure in the leg. Although white cell trapping occurs in the lower limb this does not cause capillary occlusion to the extent that perfusion of the skin is impaired and this part of my original hypothesis was incorrect.

Histological Studies

The involvement of leucocytes in the processes that lead to leg ulceration has been investigated in a number of ways. The microcirculation of the skin has been investigated by histology [50] and by capillary microscopy [51]. Both methods demonstrate capillary proliferation in patients with CVI – vastly more capillaries are visible by both techniques. However, capillary microscopy shows that these probably arise from a single capillary loop and appear like a glomerulus, rather than an increase in the numbers of capillaries. Recent immunohistochemical investigations have shown that the peri-capillary cuff contains far more than fibrin. The capillary endothelium is perturbed, expressing increased amounts of factor VIII related antigen [52,53], and adhesion molecules, especially ICAM-1. ELAM-1 may be slightly upregulated but VCAM appears to be normal in patients without venous ulceration. Perturbed endothelium is more likely to attract the adhesion of leucocytes. The presence of the peri-capillary fibrin cuff has been confirmed, but it also contains collagen IV, laminin, fibronectin and tenascin [54]. A strong leucocyte infiltration has been measured in patients with venous disease [55]. These cells are macrophages and T lymphocytes [52]. The cytokines involved include the interleukins IL-1α and IL-1β; tumour necrosis factor alpha (TNFα) was not detected in these histological sections. The presence of the perivascular "fibrin cuff" (with other components) is a reflection of the inflammatory process and is seen in other chronic inflammatory conditions. In patients with venous disease increased plasma D-dimer levels have been observed suggesting enhanced deposition of fibrin [56]. The perturbed state of the endothelium allows the passage of large molecules though the endothelium, permitting their perivascular accumulation, and explains the presence of the "fibrin cuff".

Leucocyte Activation

The effect of venous hypertension on leucocyte activation has been studied in my laboratory using a series of plasma and cellular markers. Control subjects exposed to lower limb venous hypertension produced by standing were studied by taking blood samples from the hand and the leg veins. Degranulation of neutrophils was studied by measuring plasma levels of neutrophil elastase (a primary neutrophil granule enzyme) and lactoferrin (a secondary neutrophil granule enzyme). After a 30-min period of experimental venous hypertension, a rise in plasma lactoferrin concentration was observed in the blood taken both from the foot and from the arm [57]. When venous hypertension was produced by inflation of a cuff around one lower limb, a rise in lactoferrin was observed only in that limb. Subsequently expression of the surface neutrophil ligand, CD11b, has been investigated as a marker of neutrophil activation. The experiment was repeated as before on control subjects. Blood was taken from a dorsal foot vein. CD11b expression was assessed by fluorescent-labelled monoclonal antibody used to label neutrophils in whole blood which were counted using flow cytometry. During the period of ambulatory venous hypertension in control subjects no rise in CD11b expression was seen in the lower limb blood [58]. Following return to the supine position, when neutrophils might be expected to leave the lower limb, according to the studies of Thomas et al. [45], increased levels of CD11b were observed (Fig. 6.5). This indicates that neutrophils were upregulated by their period of adhesion to normal endothelium. An increased white cell:red cell ratio was also observed during this phase confirming white cell egress from the lower limb.

This study has also been conducted in patients with venous disease, including only subjects with un-ulcerated skin to avoid the possibility that the inflammatory processes involved in the ulcer may result in up-regulation of inflammatory mediators in a way unrelated to the development of the ulcer. Two groups of patients were studied: one group with uncomplicated varicose veins and one with skin changes (lipodermatosclerosis) attributable to venous disease. The adhesion of neutrophils and monocytes to endothelium was investigated (Fig. 6.6). This is a two-stage process. Initially these cells roll along the endothelium, binding in a loose manner using a

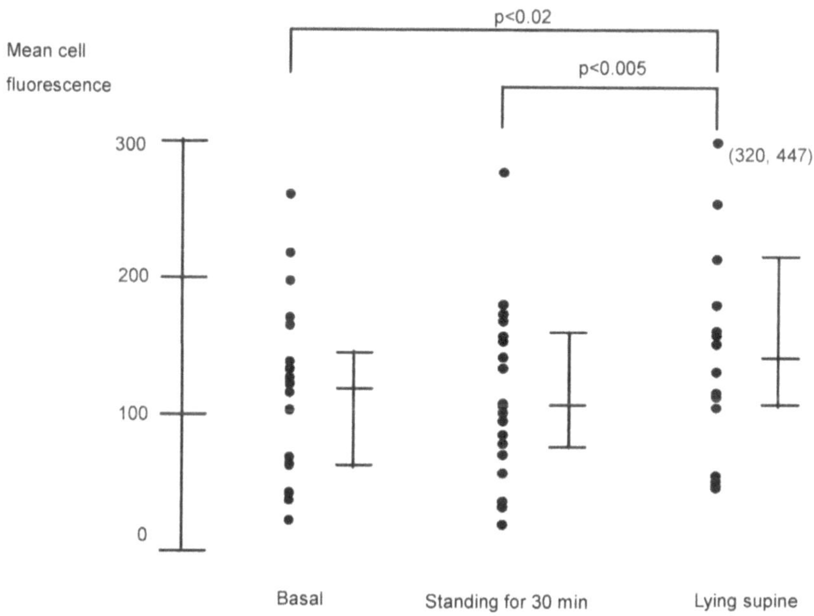

Fig. 6.5. Neutrophil CD11b expression measured by flow cytometry in volunteers before and 10 min after a period of ambulatory venous hypertension produced by standing. Increased CD11b expression is noted on return to the supine position during the period of leucocyte efflux. Error bars show the median and interquartile range of data. Statistical significance was tested by the Mann–Whitney *U*-test

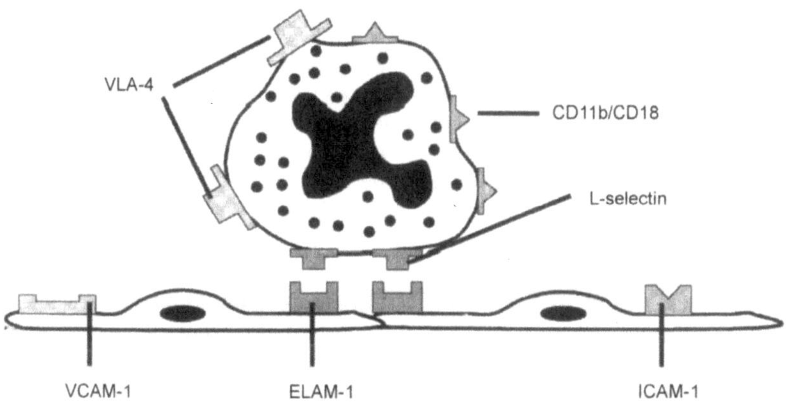

Fig. 6.6. Surface ligands of neutrophils and monocytes (CD11b/CD18, L-selectin, VLA-4) and the endothelial adhesion molecules with which they interact (ICAM-1, ELAM-1, VCAM-1).

ligand on the leucocytes known as CD62L or L-selectin (Fig. 6.7a). When binding occurs a fragment of L-selectin is released into the plasma (soluble L-selectin) and can be detected by an ELISA. It was found that the concentration of soluble L-selectin rose during venous hypertension, confirming that endothelial:leucocyte binding had occurred [59]. There was no major difference in magnitude between the two groups of patients.

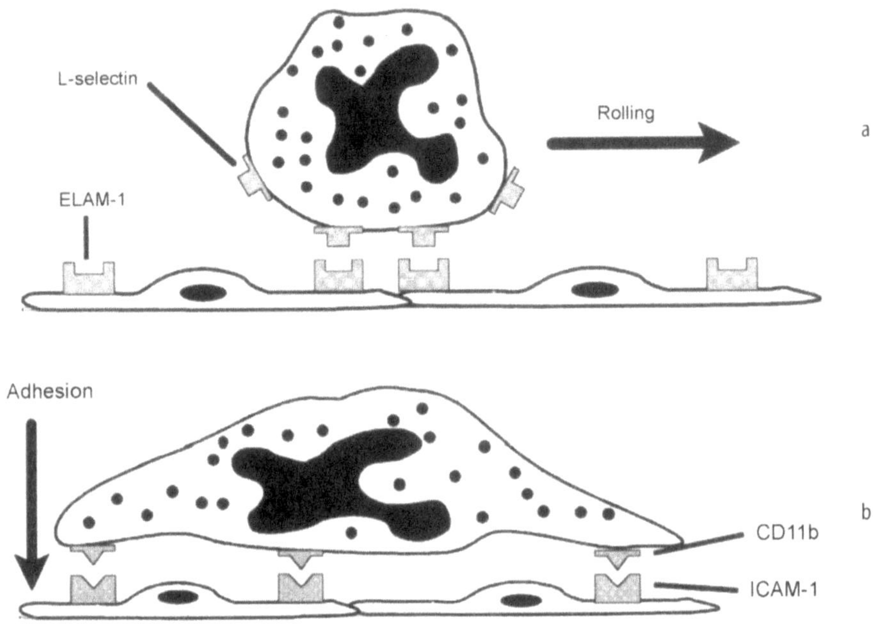

Fig. 6.7a The leucocyte ligand L-selectin mediates the initial "rolling" interaction between neutrophils or monocytes and the endothelium. **b.** Subsequently CD11b/CD18 mediates firm adhesion of leucocytes to the endothelium.

Subsequently, firm binding of neutrophils and monocytes occurs using CD11b/CD18 ligands which link to endothelial ICAM (Fig. 6.7b). This is reflected in the peripheral blood by a fall in the cells expressing most CD11b. Just such a fall was seen in the blood taken from the leg in both groups of patients. On return to the supine position I had expected to see an egress of leucocytes expressing more CD11b in these patients, but this was not observed, in contrast to the studies on control subjects. In the time-scale of this experiment (up to 10 min following venous hypertension), the more activated neutrophils and monocytes remained bound to the endothelium of the lower limb.

Plasma lactoferrin and elastase have been assessed in groups of patients with active venous disease. Blood was taken from the arm veins (not the lower limb veins) of patients with varicose veins, liposclerotic skin change and active venous ulceration [60,61]. In all samples, the levels of lactoferrin and elastase were higher in the patients than the age- and sex-matched control groups (Fig. 6.8, 6.9). However, it was found that the highest levels of plasma lactoferrin were present in patients with active varicose veins. Subsequently blood was taken from the arms of patients for measurement of neutrophil CD11b expression. This was elevated in patients with varicose veins, but depressed in patients with lipodermatosclerosis [62]. The explanation may be that the more active leucocytes are attracted to the region of the inflammatory process and do not circulate in the peripheral blood. Alternatively, such patients may have high circulating levels of neutrophil inhibitors.

In recent studies undertaken in the Department of Surgery, University College London, measurements of plasma levels of endothelial adhesion molecules have been performed along with von Willebrand factor. These may reflect endothelial injury in the microcirculation. Patients with chronic venous disease (a group with uncomplicated varicose veins and

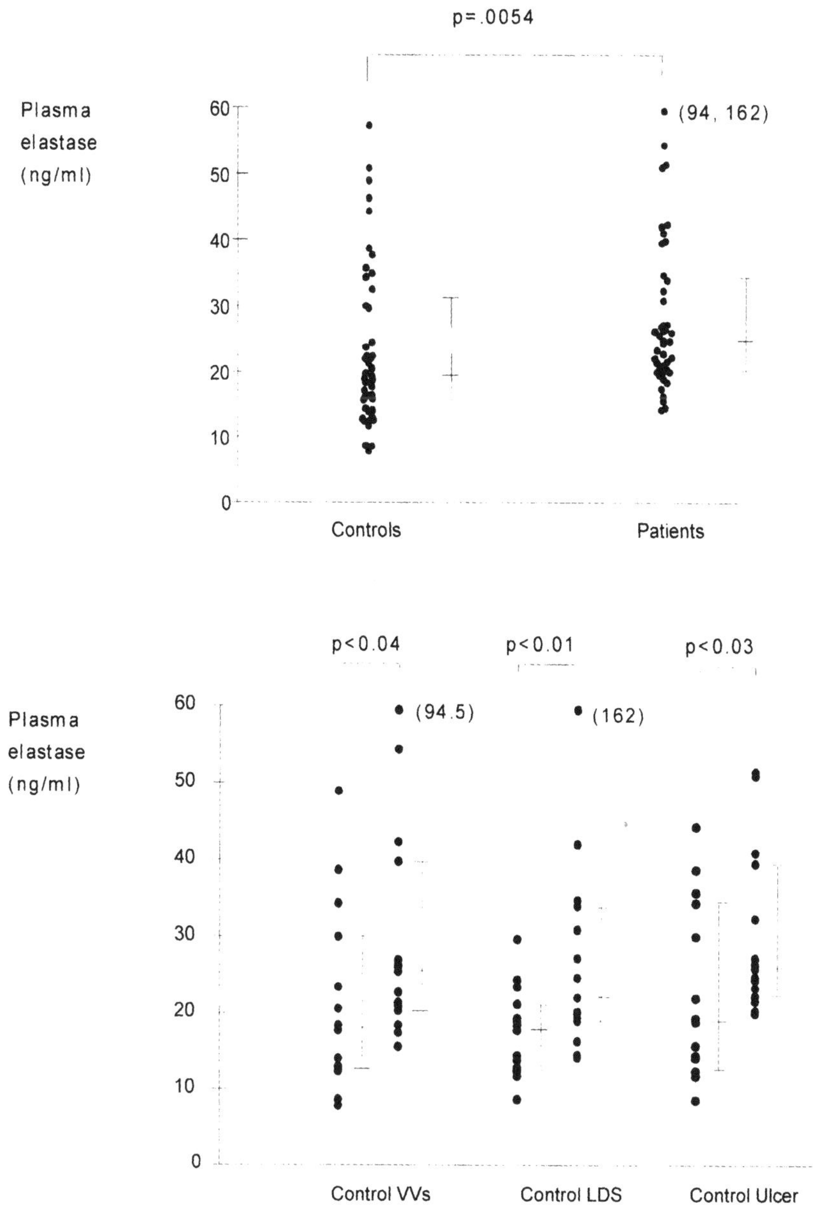

Fig. 6.8. Results of plasma neutrophil elastase measurements in patients and control subjects. Error bars show the median and interquartile range of data. Statistical significance was tested by the Mann–Whitney *U*-test. *Vvs*, varicose veins; *LDS*, lipodermatosclerosis.

a group with skin changes) were again studied and compared with normal controls. The concentration of soluble VCAM (vascular endothelial adhesion molecule) was elevated in both patient groups compared with control subjects, and was highest in the group with skin changes. Smaller elevations of von Willebrand factor, soluble ICAM and E-selectin were also observed (Fig. 6.10, 6.11). All subjects were then exposed to venous hypertension for 30 min using the protocol described in earlier sections. Further rises of soluble

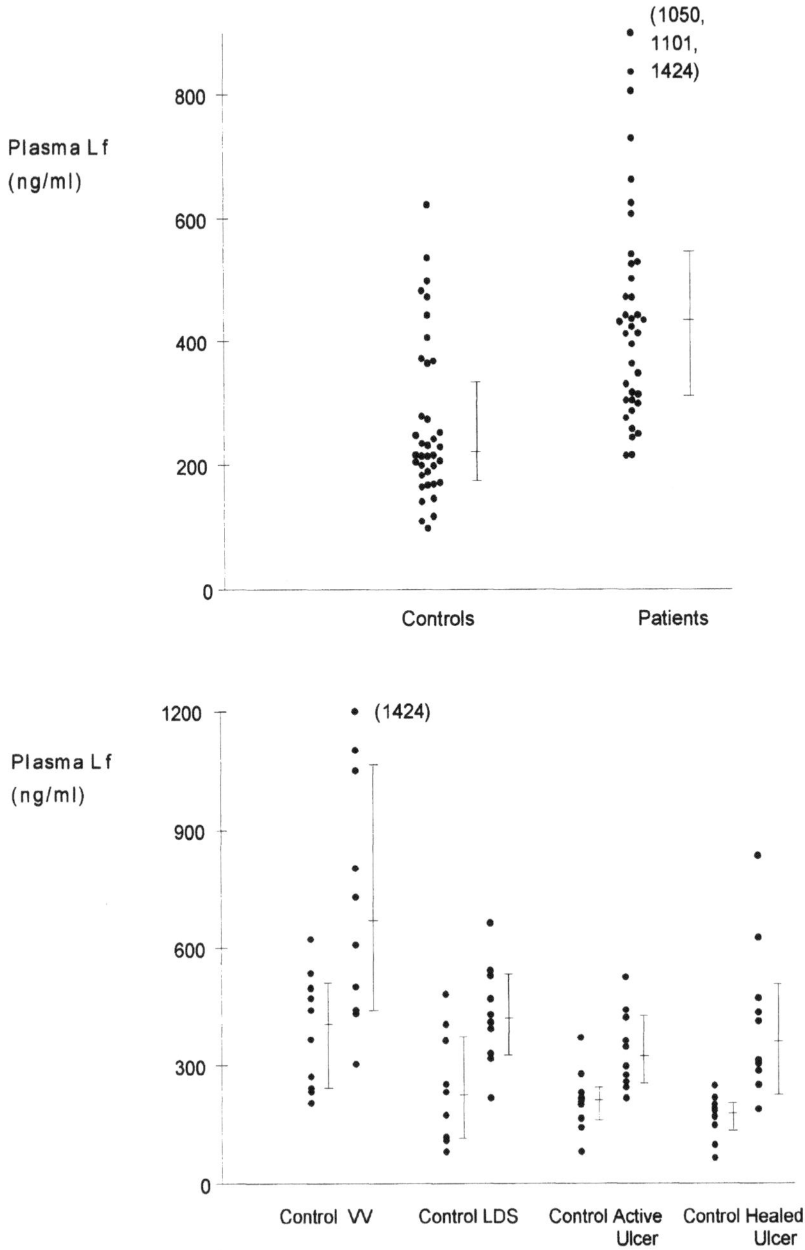

Fig. 6.9. Results of plasma neutrophil lactoferrin (*Lf*) measurements in patients and control subjects. Error bars show the median and interquartile range of data. *VV*, varicose veins; *LDS*, lipodermatosclerosis.

adhesion molecules were noted, of which the rise in soluble VCAM was the most marked, and was greatest in the patients with skin changes attributable to venous disease. These elevations of soluble endothelial adhesion molecules probably reflect endothelial injury in response to short-term experimental venous hypertension, which occurs both in control subjects and patients with venous disease.

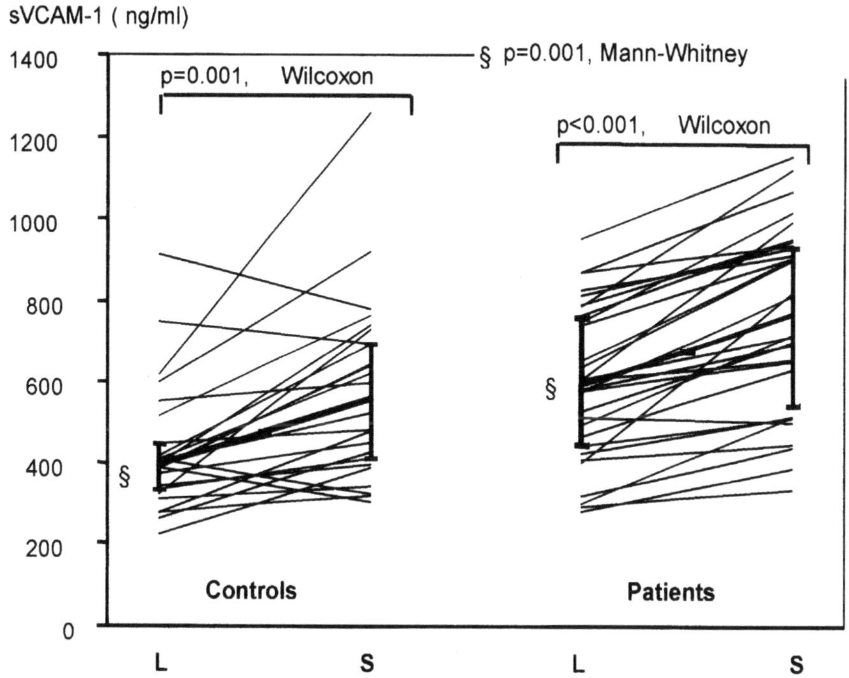

Fig. 6.10. Plasma VCAM-1 levels in normal controls and patients with chronic venous disease (with and without skin changes), before and after venous hypertension. Descriptors: medians and interquartile ranges; statistics: Wilcoxon and Mann–Whitney *U*-test for unpaired data. *L*, lying, *S*, standing.

Vascular Proliferation

The vascular proliferation seen in the skin of patients with venous disease has been known for many years [63] but has not been explained. Previously, this might have been ascribed to skin hypoxia, but in recent years many angiogenic factors have been recognised that stimulate the growth of blood vessels. Immunohistochemistry was used to evaluate the presence of a number of these factors in the skin of patients with chronic venous disease [64]. Skin biopsies were taken at the time of surgery for varicose veins from the legs of patients with and without skin changes as well as of breast skin in patients without clinical evidence of venous disease, for use as a control. Histology demonstrated no evidence of up-regulation of transforming growth factor β (TGFβ) in the skin of patients with venous disease. In contrast, there was some increase in platelet derived growth factor, sub-type BB (PDGF-BB) in patients with venous disease. This was found in the capillary wall in vessels of the dermal papillae. There was also considerable up-regulation of the production of vascular endothelial growth factor (VEGF) in the epidermis of patients with venous disease, most marked in those with skin changes. It seems likely that VEGF may account for at least some of the vascular proliferation seen in the skin of patients with venous disease. This growth factor is also responsible for increased vascular permeability to large molecules, a feature of the skin microangiopathy that has been reported from capillary microscopy studies [51]. The mechanism of stimulation of epidermal VEGF production is unclear at present.

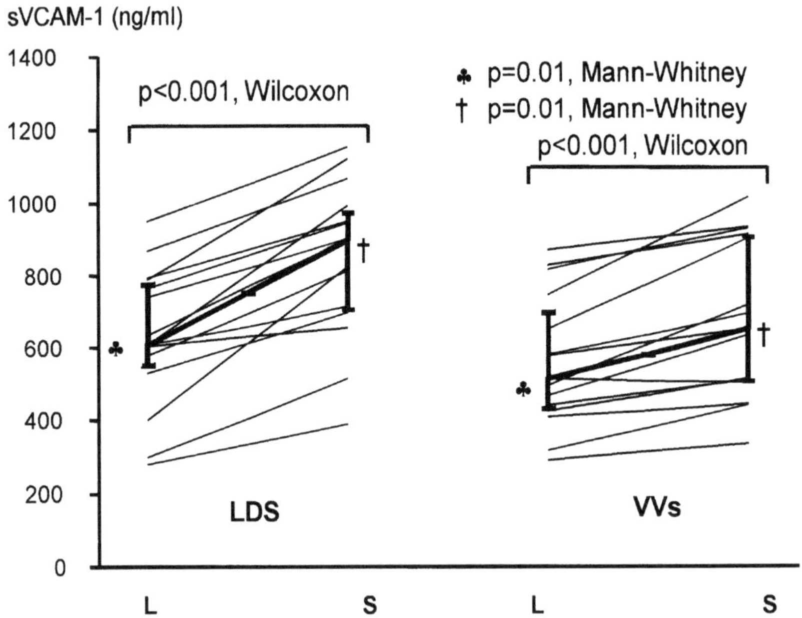

Fig. 6.11. Plasma VCAM-1 levels in patients with chronic venous disease, before and after venous hypertension. Descriptors: medians and interquartile ranges; statistics: Wilcoxon and Mann–Whitney *U*-test. *L*, lying; *S*, standing; *LDS*, lipodermatosclerosis; VVs, skin change absent.

Interpretation of Data from Published Studies

The studies referred to above suggest that a number of events are involved in the development of the microangiopathy of the skin which accompanies chronic venous disease of the lower limb.

Endothelial adhesion is a normal physiological activity of neutrophils and monocytes. During venous hypertension the fall in blood flow to the lower limb and increase in diameter of capillaries results in a fall in the shear rate in cutaneous capillaries. This favours leucocyte adhesion, which may be observed even in control subjects, but is of greater magnitude in patients with venous disease, presumably due to the perturbed state of the endothelium in chronic venous disease, in which increased amounts of endothelial adhesion molecules are expressed.

Measurements of leucocyte–endothelium interaction show that increased adhesion occurs during short-term venous hypertension (within 30 min). During this period neutrophil degranulation may be detected, releasing primary and secondary granule enzymes into the region of the endothelium. At the same time an increase in von Willebrand factor and soluble endothelial adhesion molecules can be found in the leg blood. These arguments apply to control subjects as well as to patients, although the magnitude of change is always greater in the patients than the control subjects. In fact, it is most unusual for a subject with normal veins to experience venous hypertension for a 30-min period. Small movements of the calf result in rapid reduction of lower limb venous pressure in a normal subject, so the circumstances of our experiment are not usually experienced by people with normal lower limb veins. However, the experiments do show that when the venous system becomes deranged, endothelial injury may result. I have also observed the egress of activated leucocytes in the blood from the lower limbs of control subjects following removal of venous hypertension. In patients with venous disease, these cells appear to remain in the lower limb, perhaps attached to the abnormal endothelium.

The chronic changes seen in liposclerotic skin may be the response to sustained, low-grade endothelial injury by neutrophils and monocytes over many months or years. The perivascular infiltration of vessels in the papillary dermis by macrophages and T lymphocytes may simply be a tissue response to the chronic inflammatory processes referred to above. The vascular proliferation seen in this condition is also observed in patients with skin conditions such as psoriasis. A consistent pathological feature in patients at risk of venous ulceration is the development of vascular proliferation in the skin, and liposclerotic skin change. Whether this is simply an associated phenomenon or is crucial to subsequent ulceration remains unclear at present. VEGF is probably one of the angiogenic factors involved in the development of this change.

The progression from chronic skin damage to actual ulceration also remains difficult to understand. Whilst many skin conditions are associated with inflammatory changes, few result in chronic non-healing skin ulceration. This is clearly the cumulation of long-term skin injury attributable to all the processes which I have described above. The progress from the chronic inflammatory state to ulceration is difficult to investigate and there is no animal model. A possible answer is that an initiating stimulus causes massive activation of the peri-vascular macrophages resulting in extensive tissue and blood vessel destruction. This may be a spontaneous event such as thrombosis of one of the capillary loops, which has been observed using capillary microscopy [65]. Alternatively minor trauma to the region may set in motion the series of events which leads to ulcer formation.

The data collected in the studies of neutrophil, monocyte and endothelial cell activity have so far failed to identify major differences between those patients who develop skin changes and are at risk of ulceration and those who do not. Clearly a fairly limited range of processes has been studied so far, and many areas have been left untouched. I have concentrated on the processes which may cause damage, and have so far neglected the defence or response mechanisms.

Other Systems Involved in the Disease Process

Although I have described the events in the microcirculation in CVI at length, it is clear that several other skin structures become damaged in patients with this condition. The regulation of the microcirculation is dependent on intact innervation. It has been known for some time that the vasodilatation response of the microcirculation is impaired in the leg skin of patients with venous disease. The presence of a peripheral neuropathy was sought in patients with venous disease, to determine whether venous disease is associated with nerve injury. Normal thresholds of sensation were found in the foot to vibration (A_{α} fibre) and cooling (A_{δ} fibre), but substantially increased thresholds for skin warming (C fibre) (Patients: median, 3.4 °C, interquartile range, 2.4–5.8; control: median, 1.2 °C, interquartile range, 2.1–1.1). This suggests that this nerve fibre type is particularly susceptible to injury in patients with venous disease. The consequence of this finding for the microcirculation is unclear, but implies a loss of external regulation. We have investigated this by making measurements of the vasomotion (cyclical fluctuations in flow assessed by laser Doppler fluxmetry) and performing frequency analysis by Fourier transform analysis. This revealed that the main vasomotion component was increased in magnitude and frequency in patients with liposclerotic skin compared with control subjects [66]. This finding may also suggest a loss in neuronal regulation of the microcirculation.

Bollinger et al. [67] have elegantly demonstrated that the lymphatic capillaries in the skin are abnormal and damaged in venous disease, with dilatation and incompetence of their valves. Eventually the lymphatic vessels become destroyed and cannot be found in the most severely affected skin. This may result in impairment of lymphatic drainage, which may account for some features of the leg in patients with CVI. It seems probable that the changes reported by Bollinger et al. are a consequence of the inflammatory and destructive mechanisms described in the sections above. However, the precise relationship of the lymphatic abnormality to the ulceration process is unclear and warrants further elucidation.

Why Do Ulcers Fail To Heal?

The discussion above presents the reasons why ulcers may form in the first place. However, it is less clear why ulcers may fail to heal subsequently. Certainly vigorous healing processes are detectable in histological sections of leg ulcers, with many tissue growth factors present in abundance. It is not clear whether there is any defect in the healing process or not. It has been suggested that the peri-vascular fibrin cuff traps tissue growth factors, preventing them from reaching the region where they are required to produce healing [68]. However, it has never been conclusively demonstrated that any growth factor is absent or so severely reduced in quantity that healing might be impaired. There is some evidence to suggest decreased levels of some tissue growth factors in slowly healing venous ulcers [69]. Biological systems are usually very robust, so it would probably take the absence or reduction of several growth factors before wound healing was impaired. Nevertheless this possibility has led to a number of attempts to treat venous ulcers using topically applied tissue growth factors [70,71]. A number of small studies have been reported in the wound-healing literature, but convincing evidence that this method of treatment is of any use is hard to find. Certainly there are technical problems in delivering a sustained dose of growth factor in a satisfactory way to the region of a venous leg ulcer. However, even if these problems could be overcome it is unclear whether ulcer healing would be more speedy or the resulting healed region less susceptible to further episodes of ulceration.

The presence of an ulcer does not remove the factors that led to its formation in the first place. It is therefore perfectly possible that the continuing presence of these prevents ulcer healing. Certainly when superficial venous surgery is performed in the treatment of patients with venous incompetence confined to the superficial veins, rapid ulcer healing is seen and there is a low recurrence rate [72,73]. This strongly suggests that the skin changes seen in chronic venous disease are partially or totally reversible if venous hypertension can be corrected. This type of treatment addresses only the causative factors and does not influence faulty wound healing, suggesting that it is the factors which caused the ulcer in the first place which are responsible for its failure to heal.

Implications for Pharmacological Treatment in Venous Disease

Although bandaging and stockings have been used effectively in the treatment of CVI for many years, modern pharmacological science may provide assistance in healing venous ulcers. Enhancing fibrinolysis has been attempted to promote removal of the fibrin cuff [74]. This particular treatment did not improve ulcer healing. Drugs which reduce white cell activation may be useful in healing venous ulcers, assuming that this mechanism is important in the perpetuation of ulceration. Pentoxifylline (Trental, Hoechst, Germany), has already been evaluated. This drug reduces the likelihood of white cell activation by an effect which appears to be independent of other known activators of neutrophils such as TNFα, resulting in a much lower likelihood of endothelial adhesion [75]. In a multi-centre study in which 82 patients were entered, pentoxifylline has been shown to result in better healing rates of ulcers than placebo [76]. A further randomised, placebo-controlled study in 200 patients has now been completed where higher levels of compression were used [77]. Here, although a trend towards improved venous ulcer healing was seen in the active treatment group, statistical significance was not reached. Clearly, effective compression has a greater effect on wound healing than does pentoxifylline. However, this drug may still be useful in resistant ulcers [78]. Prostaglandin E_1 inhibits the respiratory burst of neutrophils, preventing the release of superoxide radicals. A preliminary study has suggested that this too is effective in healing venous ulcers [79].

In continental Europe, "venotonic" drugs are widely used in the management of all stages of venous disease. The origins of these are plant extracts, although some synthetic drugs are currently in use. Drugs based on plant extracts including aescin (horse chestnut extract), hydroxyrutoside, diosmin and hesperidine. Synthetic "oedema-protective" drugs include calcium dobesilate and tribenoside. All these appear to reduce oedema associated with venous disease as well as symptoms attributable to varicose veins. Comparatively little work has been done on the efficacy of these drugs on leg ulcers. In 138 patients with recently healed venous ulcers, Wright et al. [80] compared the efficacy of below-the-knee elastic stockings combined with hydroxyrutosides (Paroven 500 mg b.d.) or placebo. The recurrence rates at 12 months were 23% with hydroxyrutosides and 22% with placebo. At 18 months the figures were 34% and 32%. These results show no evidence that hydroxyrutosides prevent ulcer recurrence when combined with elastic compression. The effect of Daflon 500 mg (Servier, France) in a venous ulcer healing study has been recently reported [81]. Patients were randomised to receive Daflon 500 mg or placebo combined with standard compression bandaging during an 8-week follow-up period. In 91 patients with an ulcer diameter of 10 cm or less, 14 of 44 (32%) patients receiving Daflon 500 mg compared with 6 of 47 (13%) receiving placebo healed their ulcers ($p = 0.028$, chi-squared) after 8 weeks of treatment. This pilot study indicates that Daflon should be further investigated to establish the clinical usefulness of any ulcer healing effect.

The development of other drug treatments to encourage venous ulcer healing will depend upon a better understanding of how ulcers form and the pathological processes involved. In the future, drug treatment for venous ulcers may well be helpful in achieving healing and the prevention of recurrence.

Conclusions

Venous ulceration continues to be a problem which eludes simple cures. A considerable amount of work has been done to elucidate the pathological mechanisms at work in this disease, but the exact sequence of events which leads to leg ulceration has yet to be established. Further work in this area may lead to development of new treatments for leg ulcers. The most effective non-surgical treatment remains compression bandaging, a method which has been in use for thousands of years.

References

1. Cornu-Thenard C, Boivin P, Baud J-M, de Vincenzi I, Carpentier PH. Importance of the familial factor in varicose disease. J Dermatol Surg Oncol 1994;20:313–326.
2. Grossman D, Heald DW, Wang C, Rinder HM. Activated protein C resistance and anticardiolipin antibodies in patients with venous leg ulcers. J Am Acad Dermatol 1997;37:409–413.
3. Wille-Jorgensen P, Jorgensen T, Andersen M, Kirchhoff M. Postphlebitic syndrome and general surgery: an epidemiologic investigation. Angiology 1991;May:397–403.
4. Mudge M, Leinster SJ, Hughes LE. A prospective 10-year study of the post-thrombotic syndrome in a surgical population. Ann R Coll Surg Engl 1988;70:249–252.
5. Baker SR, Stacey MC, Jopp-McKay AG, Hoskin SE, Thompson PJ. Epidemiology of chronic venous ulcers. Br J Surg 1991;78:864–867.
6. Strandness DE, Langlois Y, Cramer M, Randlett A, Thiele BL. Long-term sequelae of acute venous thrombosis. JAMA 1983;250:1289–1292.
7. Franzeck UK, Schalch I, Jager KA, Schneider E, Grimm J, Bollinger A. Prospective 12-year follow-up study of clinical and hemodynamic sequelae after deep vein thrombosis in low-risk patients (Zurich study). Circulation 1996;93:74–79.
8. Cornwall JV, Doré CJ, Lewis JD. Leg ulcers: epidemiology and aetiology. Br J Surg 1986;73:693–696.
9. Baker SR, Stacey MC, Singh G, Hoskin SE, Thompson PJ. Aetiology of chronic leg ulcers. Eur J Vasc Surg 1992;6:245–251.
10. Fowkes FGR, Callam MJ. Is arterial disease a risk factor for chronic leg ulceration? Phlebology 1994;9:87–90.
11. Nicolaides AN, Zukowski A, Lewis R, Kyprianou P, Malouf GM. Venous pressure measurements in venous problems. In: Bergan JJ, Yao JST, editors. Surgery of the veins. Orlando: Grune and Stratton, 1985:111–118.
12. Dodd H, Cockett FB. The pathology and surgery of the veins of the lower limb. Edinburgh: Churchill Livingstone, 1976.
13. Hoare MC, Nicolaides AN, Miles CR, Shull K, Jury RP, Needham T, Dudley HAF. The role of primary varicose veins in venous ulceration. Surgery 1982;92:450–453.
14. Kistner RL. Primary venous valve incompetence of the leg. Am J Surg 1980;140:218–224.
15. Pollack AA, Taylor BE, Myers TT, Wood EH. The effect of exercise and body position on the venous pressure at the ankle in patients having venous valvular defects. J Clin Invest 1949;28:559–563.
16. Nicolaides AN, Hussein MK, Szendro G, Christopoulos D, et al. The relation of venous ulceration with ambulatory venous pressure measurement. J Vasc Surg 1993;17:414–419.
17. Homans J. The aetiology and treatment of varicose ulcers of the leg. Surg Gynaecol Obstet 1917;24:300–311.
18. Fontaine R. Remarks concerning venous thrombosis and sequelae. Surgery 1957;41:6–24.
19. Blumhoff RL, Johnson G. Saphenous vein PpO_2 in patients with varicose veins. J Surg Res 1977;23:35–6.
20. Scott HJ, Cheatle TR, McMullin GM, Coleridge Smith PD, Scurr JH. A reappraisal of the oxygenation of the venous blood of varicose veins. Br J Surg 1990;77:934–936.
21. Pratt GH. Arterial varices: a syndrome. Am J Surg 1949;77:456–460.
22. Brewer AC. Arteriovenous shunts. BMJ 1950;ii:270.
23. Lindmayr W, Lofferer O, Mostbeck A, Partsch H. Arteriovenous shunts in primary varicosis: a critical essay. Vasc Surg 1972;6:9–14.
24. Browse NL, Burnand KG. The cause of venous ulceration. Lancet 1982;ii:243–245.
25. Browse NL, Gray L, Jarrett PEM, Morland M. Blood and vein-wall fibrinolytic activity in health and vascular disease. BMJ 1977l;i:478–481.
26. Michel CC. Oxygen diffusion in oedematous tissue and through pericapillary cuffs. Phlebology 1990;5:223–230.
27. Stacey MC, Burnand KG, Layer GT, Pattison M. Transcutaneous oxygen tensions as a prognostic indicator and measure of treatment of recurrent ulceration. Br J Surg 1987;74:545.
28. Clyne CAC, Ramsden WH, Chant ADB, Wenster JHH. Oxygen tension in the skin of the gaiter area of limbs with venous ulceration. Br J Surg 1985;72:644–647.
29. Dodd HJ, Gaylarde PM, Sarkany I. Skin oxygen tension in venous insufficiency of the lower leg. J R Soc Med 1985;78:373–376.
30. Schmeller W, Roszinski S, Tronnier M, Gmelin E. Combined morphological and physiological examinations in lipodermatosclerosis. In: Raymond-Martimbeaux, Prescott R, Zummo M, editors. Phlebologie '92. Paris: John Libbey Eurotext, 1992:172–174.

31. Hopkins NFG, Spinks TJ, Rhodes CG, Ranicar ASOA, Jamieson CW. Positron emission tomography in venous ulceration and liposclerosis. BMJ 1982;286:333–336.
32. Sjerson P. Blood flow in cutaneous tissue in man studied by washout of radioactive xenon. Circ Res 1969;25:215–29.
33. Cheatle TR, McMullin GM, Farrah J, Coleridge Smith PD, Scurr JH. Three tests of microcirculatory function in the evaluation of treatment for chronic venous insufficiency. Phlebology 1990;5:165–172.
34. Stibe ECL, Cheatle TR, Coleridge Smith PD, Scurr JH. Liposclerotic skin: a diffusion block or a perfusion problem? Phlebology 1990;5:231–236.
35. Braide M, Amundson B, Chien S, Bagge U. Quantitative studies of leucocytes on the vascular resistance in a skeletal muscle preparation. Microvasc Res 1984;27:331–352.
36. Engler RL, Dahlgren MD, Peterson MA, Dobbs A, Schmid-Schoenbein GW. Accumulation of polymorphonuclear leucocytes during three hour myocardial ischemia. Am J Physiol 1986;251:H93–100.
37. Romson JL, Hook BG, Kunkel SL, Abrams GD, Schork MA, Lucchesi BR. Reduction of the extent of ischemic myocardial injury by neutrophil depletion in the dog. Circulation 1983;67:1016–1023.
38. Wilson JW. Leucocyte sequestration and morphologic augmentation in the pulmonary network following haemorrhagic shock and related forms of stress. Adv Microcirc 1972;??:197–232.
39. Linas SL, Shanley PF, Whittenburg D, Berger E, Repine JE. Neutrophils accentuate ischemia-reperfusion injury in isolated perfused rat kidneys. Am J Physiol 1988;255:F728–735.
40. Yamakawa T, Suguyama I, Niimi H. Behaviour of white blood cells in microcirculation of the cat brain cortex during hemorrhagic shock: intravital microscopic study. Int J Microcirc: Clin Exp 1984;3:554.
41. Braide M, Blixt A, Bagge U. Leukocyte effects on the vascular resistance and glomerular filtration of the isolated rat kidney at normal and low flow rates. Circ Shock 1986;20:71–80.
42. Weissman G, Smolen JE, Korchak HM. Release of inflammatory mediators from stimulated neutrophils. N Engl J Med 1980;303:27–34.
43. Babior BM. Oxidants from phagocytes: agents of defense and destruction. Blood 1984;64:959–966.
44. Moyses C, Cederholm-Williams SA, Michel CC. Haemoconcentration and the accumulation of white cells in the feet during venous stasis. Int J Microcirc: Clin Exp 1987;5:311–320.
45. Thomas PRS, Nash GB, Dormandy JA. White cell accumulation in the dependent legs of patients with venous hypertension: a possible mechanism for trophic changes in the skin. BMJ 1988;296:1693–1695.
46. Scott HJ, McMullin GM, Coleridge Smith PD, Scurr JH. Venous ulceration and the role of the white blood cell. J Med Sci Tech 1990;14:184–187.
47. Bollinger A, Haselbach P, Schnewlin G, Junger M. Microangiopathy due to chronic venous incompetence evaluated by fluorescence videomicroscopy. In: Negus D, Jantet G, editors. Phlebology '85. London: John Libbey, 1986.
48. Franzeck UK, Speiser D, Haselbach P, Bollinger A. Morphologic and dynamic microvascular abnormalities in chronic venous incompetence (CVI). In: Davy A, Stemmer R, editors. Phlebologie '89. John Libbey Eurotext, 1989:104–107.
49. Coleridge Smith PD, Thomas P, Scurr JH, Dormandy JA. Causes of venous ulceration: a new hypothesis. BMJ 1988;296:1726–1727.
50. Burnand KG, Whimster I, Naidoo A, Browse NL. Pericapillary fibrin in the ulcer-bearing skin of the leg: the cause of lipodermatosclerosis and venous ulceration. BMJ 1982;285:1071–1072.
51. Haselbach P, Vollenweider U, Moneta G, Bollinger A. Microangiopathy in severe chronic venous insufficiency evaluated by fluorescence video-microscopy. Phlebology 1986;1:159–169.
52. Wilkinson LS, Bunker C, Edwards JC, Scurr JH, Coleridge Smith PD. Leukocytes: their role in the etiopathogenesis of skin damage in venous disease. J Vasc Surg 1993;17:669–675.
53. Veraart JC, Verhaegh ME, Neumann HA, Hulsmans RF, Arends JW. Adhesion molecule expression in venous leg ulcers. Vasa 1993;22:213–218.
54. Herrick SE, Sloan P, McGurk M, Freak L, McCollum CN, Ferguson MW. Sequential changes in histologic pattern and extracellular matrix deposition during the healing of chronic venous ulcers. Am J Pathol 1992; 141:1085–1095.
55. Scott HJ, McMullin GM, Coleridge Smith PD, Scurr JH. A histological study into white blood cells and their association with lipodermatosclerosis and ulceration. Br J Surg 1990;78:210–211.
56. Falanga V, Kruskal J, Franks JJ. Fibrin- and fibrinogen-related antigens in patients with venous disease and venous ulceration. Arch Dermatol 1991;127:75–78.
57. Shields DA, Andaz S, Abeysinghe RD, Porter JB, Scurr JH, Coleridge Smith PD. Neutrophil activation in experimental ambulatory venous hypertension. Phlebology 1994;9:119–124.
58. Shields D, Andaz SK, Timothy-Antoine CA, Scurr JH, Porter JB. CD11b/CD18 as a marker of neutrophil adhesion in experimental ambulatory venous hypertension. In: Negus D, Jantet G, Coleridge Smith PD, editors. Phlebology '95. hlebology 1995;Suppl 1:108–109.
59. Saharay M, Shields DA, Porter JB, Scurr JH, Coleridge-Smith-PD. Leukocyte activity in the microcirculation of the leg in patients with chronic venous disease. J Vasc Surg 1997;26:265–23.

60. Shields DA, Andaz S, Abeysinghe RD, Porter JB, Scurr JH, Coleridge Smith PD. Plasma lactoferrin as a marker of white cell degranulation in venous disease. Phlebology 1994;9:55–58.
61. Shields DA, Andaz SK, Sarin S, Scurr JH, Coleridge Smith PD. Plasma elastase in venous disease. Br J Surg 1994;81:1496–1499.
62. Shields D, Saharay M, Timothy-Antoine CA, Porter JB, Scurr JH. Neutrophil CD11b expression in patients with venous disease. In: Negus D, Jantet G, Coleridge Smith PD, editors. Phlebology '95. Phlebology '95. Phlebology 1995;Suppl 1:108–109.
63. Burnand KG, Whimster I, Clemenson G, Thomas ML, Browse NL. The relationship between the number of capillaries in the skin of the venous ulcer-bearing area of the lower leg and the fall in foot vein pressure during exercise. Br J Surg 1981;68:297–300.
64. Pardoe HD. The expression of angiogenic growth factors in the skin of patients with chronic venous disease of the lower limb. MSc thesis, University College London, 1996:1–61.
65. Franzeck UK, Speiser D, Haselbach P, Bollinger A. Morphologic and dynamic microvascular abnormalities in chronic venous incompetence (CVI). In: Davy A, Stemmer R, editors. Phlebologie '89. Paris: John Libbey Eurotext, 1989:104–107.
66. Chittenden SJ, Shami SK, Scurr JH, Coleridge Smith PD. Vasomotion in the leg skin of patients with chronic venous insufficiency. VASA 1992; in press.
67. Bollinger A, Isenring G, Franzeck UK. Lymphatic microangiopathy: a complication of severe chronic venous incompetence. Lymphology 1982;15:60–65.
68. Falanga V, Eaglstein WH. The "trap" hypothesis of venous ulceration. Lancet 1993;341:1006–1008.
69. Lagattolla NR, Stacey MC, Burnand KG, Gaffney PG. Growth factors, tissue and urokinase-type plasminogen activators in venous ulcers. Ann Cardiol Angeiol (Paris) 1995;44:299–303.
70. Falanga V, Eaglstein WH, Bucalo B, Katz MH, Harris B, Carson P. Topical use of human recombinant epidermal growth factor (h-EGF) in venous ulcers. J Dermatol Surg Oncol 1992;18:604–606.
71. Burgos H, Herd A, Bennett JP. Placental angiogenic and growth factors in the treatment of chronic varicose ulcers: preliminary communication. J R Soc Med 1989;82:598–599.
72. Bass A, Chayen D, Weinmann EE, Ziss M. Lateral venous ulcer and short saphenous vein insufficiency. J Vasc Surg 1997;25:654–657.
73. DePalma RG, Kowallek DL. Venous ulceration: a cross-over study from non-operative to operative treatment. J Vasc Surg 1996;24:788–792.
74. Layer GT, Stacey MC, Burnand KG. Stanozolol and the treatment of venous ulceration: an interim report. Phlebology 1986;1:197–203.
75. Sullivan GW, Carper HT, Novick WJ, Mandell GL. Inhibition of the inflammatory action of interleukin-1 and tumour necrosis factor (alpha) on neutrophil function of pentoxifylline. Infect Immun 1988;56:1722–1729.
76. Colgan M-P, Dormandy JA, Jones PW, Schraibman IG, Shanik DG. Oxpentifylline treatment of venous ulcers of the leg. BMJ 1990;300:972–975.
77. Dale JJ, Ruckley CV, Harper DR, Gibson B, Nelson EA, Prescott RJ. A randomised double-blind placebo controlled trial of oxpentifylline in the treatment of venous leg ulcers. In Negus D, Jantet G, Coleridge Smith PD, editors. Phlebology '95. Phlebology 1995; Suppl 1:917–918.
78. Anon. Oxpentifylline for venous leg ulcers. Drug Ther Bull 1991;29:59–60.
79. Rudovsky G. Intravenous prostaglandin E_1 in the treatment of venous ulcers: a double-blind, placebo-controlled trial. Vasa 1989; Suppl 28:39–43.
80. Wright DD, Franks PJ, Blair SD, Backhouse CM, Moffatt C, McCollum CN. Oxerutins in the prevention of recurrence in chronic venous ulceration: randomised controlled trial. Br J Surg 1991;78:1269–1270.
81. Guilhou JJ, Dereure O, Marzin L, Ouvry P, Zuccarelli F, Debure C, et al. Efficacy of Daflon 500 mg in venous leg ulcer healing: a double-blind, randomised, controlled versus placebo trial in 107 patients. Angiology 1997;48:77–85.

Section II
Diagnosis and Measurement

7 How Should Venous Disease Be Classified?

John J. Bergan

Introduction

Progress in science depends upon classification of knowledge. It could be said that science begins with such classification. Therefore, further advancement in the science of treatment of venous disorders may depend upon an improved method of classification of those conditions that come under treatment. As Kistner emphasised, if progress is to be made in the management of chronic venous disease, it is necessary to define the cause, location, and pathophysiology of the disease process in each case, just as is done in the arterial system [1].

Attempts have been made to classify venous problems in general and venous insufficiency in particular. Widmer, in his much-quoted study [2], presented a clinical classification that related to appearance of the limb. A more comprehensive approached based on haemodynamic and phlebographic data was proposed in Russia and published in English in *International Angiology*, but did not gain universal acceptance [3]. Enrici in Argentina described a classification in 1992 based upon clinical presentation of the patient [4], much as the Ad Hoc Committee of the SVS/ISCVS did using anatomical regions, clinical severity, physical examination and functional assessments [5].

Hach in Germany classified greater saphenous reflux into four stages ranging from reflux in the proximal thigh (stage 1) to reflux in the ankle and foot (stage 4), and was able to correlate increased deep vein diameter, elongation and tortuosity with the progressive stages of reflux [6]. His classification has been used by many but has not achieved worldwide acceptance. Cornu-Thenard in France limited his contribution to venous classification exclusively to varicose veins and made no attempt to include more severe venous disorders [7]. In contrast, Widmer recognised that a modern view of chronic venous insufficiency must include both superficial and deep lesions regardless of their cause or their clinical presentation. He suggested a five-stage classification of chronic venous insufficiency that shows thoughtfulness and wisdom but has not had any clinical impact [8]. Others have also tried their hand at classification of venous dysfunction [9–11].

The most recent contribution to classification of venous insufficiency was drawn up by a large number of physicians and surgeons interested in venous problems. It has been referred to as the Hawaii classification in reference to its site of origination, the 1994 American Venous Forum meeting in Maui. It was approved by the Joint Councils of the American Vascular Societies, which published it with its blessing in the *Journal of Vascular Surgery* [12]. Subsequently, it has received wide attention elsewhere [13].

Attempts to use the initial SVS/NA-ISCVS clinical classification with its three stages proved disappointing. Investigators found in practice that stages 1 and 2 would be considered together haemodynamically. Only then were they separable from the more advanced stage 3 [14].

The Hawaii classification has been well published. It is probably unfortunate that it was circulated before being tried out and perhaps modified. The classification is based on clinical presentation of the patient (C), aetiology of the problem (E), anatomical abnormality(ies) found (A), and the pathophysiology encountered (P). A clinical severity score was proposed and a diagnostic process was suggested. This was not an integral part of the classification. By February 1997, the classification had been published in 20 journals worldwide as well as in the American Venous Forum *Handbook of Venous Disorders* [15].

Experience With the CEAP Classification

Labropoulos, in publishing his application of the CEAP classification to 250 limbs examined in London at St. Mary's Hospital and in Maywood, Illinois at the Loyola University Medical Center, characterised the classification as "practical and useful owing to its simplicity". His display of experience in applying the classification clinically (Fig. 7.1) appeared elegant and apparently informative [16]. On closer inspection, the analysis was seen to be a documentation of the obvious. There were more limbs with telangiectasias and varicose veins than healed or open ulcers. There was more reflux than obstruction. That there were more women than men was a fact not given by the CEAP classification and the finding that only 2% of the limbs had obstruction raised a serious question about the method used in making the diagnosis of obstruction. It is notable that this report made no mention of the anatomical segments which were afflicted nor was the severity score referred to. Ultimately, the vast amount of work that went into classification of each limb and the assembly of results yielded only information that these limbs depicted the population referred to those two laboratories.

We have used the Consensus Statement, the CEAP classification and its disability

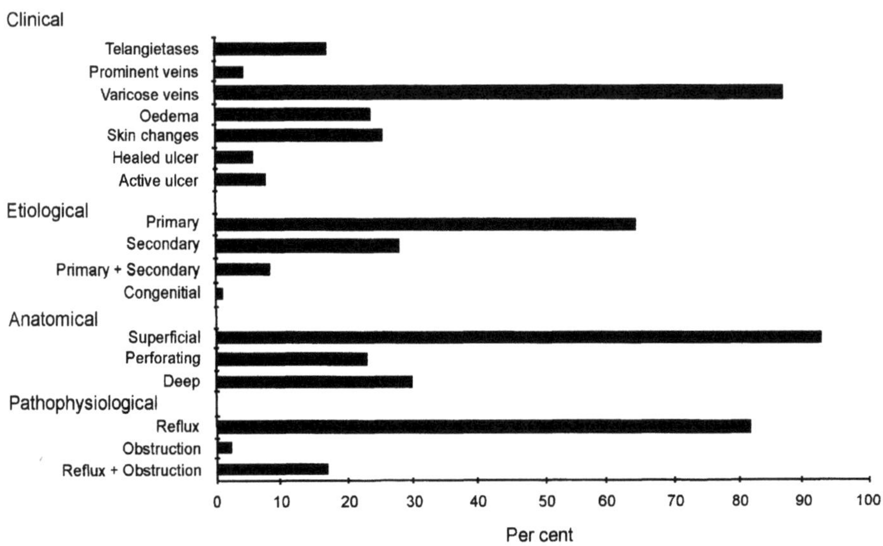

Fig. 7.1. Clinical, aetiological, anatomical and pathophysiological data from the 250 limbs in Labropoulos' study.

classification in three research efforts. These are typical of the studies which the originators of the classification had in mind. Therefore, a description of our experience may predict what others will encounter if they attempt to use the classification in its present form.

We found that the classification was most valuable when the number of limbs under study was the fewest. For example, 17 surgical specimens were removed for detailed study of leucocyte infiltration into venous walls and valves [17]. When the findings were positive and the distribution of the CD68 monocytic infiltration was more concentrated on proximal endothelial surfaces, it was informative to know how each limb supplying the specimen had been classified (Table 7.1). Each limb had been classified accurately using the CEAP classification, and exact sites of venous dysfunction were known – at least within the limitations of duplex testing.

It was found that a spectrum of venous dysfunction was present in the limbs which contributed the specimens. Only limbs with no venous disorder and those with only telangiectasias were absent. Therefore, it was disappointing to find that there was no relationship between the magnitude of the infiltrates nor the location of the monocytes on the endothelium or the macrophages in the venous wall, and the severity or duration of the venous insufficiency. Thus, the classification could be said to describe the clinical situation with some accuracy, but this did not correlate with histopathological findings.

Errors in CEAP

In addition, the apparent accuracy of the pathophysiological classification of each limb was seen to give a false feeling of veracity. This is also seen in the report by Labropoulos referred to above where venous obstruction must be under-represented. Unfortunately, in the present clinical/economic milieu, all patients cannot be subjected to the diagnostic testing which will provide truly accurate anatomical information regarding presence of obstruction versus reflux. In short, ascending phlebography to *include* the vena cava

Table 7.1 Clinical classification of specimens

Specimen no.	Sex	Age (years)	Disability score	CEAP classification
1 R	M	48	$C_1A_2D_2$	$C_{2s}E_pA_{4R,5R}P_R$
1 L[a]	M	48	$C_1A_2D_2$	$C_{2s}E_pA_{4R,5R}P_R$
2	F	39	$C_1A_3D_1$	$C_{2s}E_pA_{2R,17R,18R}P_R$
3	M	48	$C_5A_4D_6$	$C_{4s}E_sA_{13R0,14R0,16R,17R}P_{R0}$
4	M	67	$C_1A_2D_1$	$C_{2s}E_pA_{2R,3R}P_R$
5 R	M	48	$C_1A_3D_1$	$C_{3s}E_pA_{3R,17R,18R}P_R$
5 L	M	48	$C_1A_6D_1$	$C_{3s}E_pA_{1R,2R,3R,4R,17R,18R}P_R$
6	F	69	$C_1A_5D_2$	$C_{4s}E_pA_{1R,2R,3R,4R,5R}P_R$
7	F	53	$C_1A_2D_1$	$C_{2s}E_pA_{2R,3R,5R}P_R$
8	M	80	$C_1A_3D_1$	$C_{2s}E_pA_{2R,3R,5R}P_R$
9 r	F	60	$C_1A_2D_1$	$C_{2s}E_pA_{2R,3R}P_R$
9 l	F	60	$C_1A_2D_1$	$C_{2s}E_pA_{2R,3R}P_R$
10	F	71	$C_3A_5D_1$	$C_{4s}E_pA_{1R,2R,3R,17R,18R}P_R$
11 M	F	29	$C_1A_3D_1$	$C_{2s}E_pA_{2R,3R,17R}P_R$
11 ST	F	29	$C_1A_3D_1$	$C_{2s}E_pA_{2R,3R,17R}P_R$
12	F	33	$C_1A_2D_1$	$C_{2s}E_pA_{2R,3R}P_R$
13	F	63	$C_1A_2D_1$	$C_{2s}E_pA_{2R,3R}P_R$

M, Midsaphenous; St, subterminal.
[a] Lesser saphenous vein.

and iliac system simply cannot be done in every case. Similarly, descending phlebography cannot be applied to patients with relatively minor venous dysfunction. This is not a great defect however because duplex evaluation has proved to be accurate with regard to reflux.

Therefore, although the anatomical portion of the CEAP classification provides for designation of reflux or obstruction in the inferior vena cava and the common, internal and external iliac veins as well as pelvic, gonadal and broad ligament veins, in fact, today's practice, even in a research setting, gives information only from the femoral vein distally. Some will say that duplex study will detect proximal iliac venous obstruction, but experience in clinical practice has shown that this is not true. Even in our research experience using a very limited number of specimens, a false element of accuracy of classification of venous dysfunction was provided.

Simplifying CEAP

At the other end of the scale of experience with the CEAP classification was the report of the NA-SEPS Registry to the Society of Vascular Surgery [14]. This Registry seemed ideal for demonstrating the utility of the CEAP classification. By employing this classification and classifying each limb being subjected to the operation, experience derived from 17 institutions could theoretically be combined.

Ultimately, data from 151 patients having operations on 155 limbs at the 17 medical centres were submitted to the Registry office. The investigators used the Hawaii classification to the best of their ability. Quickly, it was learned that the entire CEAP designation for each limb could not be included in the analyses. Even assuming complete accuracy, the anatomical segment designation of reflux or obstruction or both was simply too cumbersome to work with.

Therefore, only the simplest form of the CEAP classification was used. This identified limbs as being in classes 4, 5 or 6, and this was more precise than the former classification previously approved by the Ad Hoc Committee of the Joint Councils of the Vascular Societies. However, in reporting to the Registry, investigators listed the anatomical segments which were studied as having reflux or obstruction but did not note the incomplete nature of their preoperative investigations. Logically, not all limbs were subjected to complete phlebography nor was it acknowledged that physiologically obstructing lesions are exceedingly hard to detect. Therefore, although the classification of limbs was clinically accurate, the anatomical classification could not have been.

The Disability Score

In this larger experience, perhaps the most valuable contribution of the new classification was the use of the disability score. Although the mean follow-up of limbs in this report was only 5.4 months, the average preoperative clinical score decreased from 9.4 (range 0–18) to 2.9 (range 0–12) ($p < 0.0001$) [18].

Finally, in a recent experience from our group reporting the effects of subfascial perforator vein interruption on ulcer healing, it has been possible to use the clinical and disability score assessed preoperatively and postoperatively [19]. As in the Registry report, the pathophysiological classification appeared to be entirely accurate. However, we know that this was flawed for the reasons indicated above. The lack of phlebologic evaluation of the abdominal and pelvic venous system must give an underestimation of the incidence of major venous obstruction in the limbs treated. Once again, however, the disability score as calculated preoperatively and postoperatively gave a clear indication of the results of the intervention. The average disability score preoperatively was 9.3 (range 0–18) and this decreased to a postoperative score of 3.5 with the follow-up extending to 24 months. This information gives subjective evaluation of the results of the intervention.

Discussion

The CEAP classification is a step forward in identifying precisely the clinical states of limbs afflicted by venous dysfunction. Its use clarifies the stages of venous stasis which are being treated. As indicated in the experience cited above, there are flaws in the system but this was predicted by the committee which proposed the classification.

Perhaps the greatest contribution of this classification will be a stimulus for a more sophisticated look at the causes of the venous valve and vein wall damage and an examination of the reasons for the cutaneous changes of severe chronic venous insufficiency, so that these can be incorporated as an integral part of a better system. An example of the need for this is our finding that while patient plasma, when reacted against a panel of naive leucocytes, causes neutrophil activation, the activation strength is not proportional to the severity of venous insufficiency. Only when classes 1, 2 and 3 are combined and compared with classes 4, 5 and 6 is there a statistically significant difference in neutrophil activation. Similarly, the CD68 monocyte infiltrate seen in the surgical specimens in the study described earlier is no greater in the advanced stages of venous stasis than in the less severe forms.

"The availability of accurate diagnoses and classification is basic to our understanding of the natural history of chronic venous disease and to its prognosis", said Kistner in describing the classification of venous disease which was later termed the CEAP classification. What he said is still true but the flaws of the system which he described lie in the accuracy of the evaluation and the discordance of the haemodynamic and histopathological findings with clinical staging of each limb.

Darke and Ruckley, in commenting on publication of the classification, expressed the views of many interested physicians. They cited demise of many medical classification schemes due to their intrinsic complexity. They saw no practical role for the anatomical classification.

In a constructive gesture, they suggested that only two basic classifications were necessary. The first would list a clinical presentation similar to the CEAP classification except that no distinction should be made between open and healed ulceration, the two being combined under the term "chronic ulceration". The second part of their suggested classification would divide morphology into two parts: primary and secondary (post-phlebitic/post-traumatic). Further, they suggested that primary insufficiency should be subdivided into isolated superficial incompetence and superficial incompetence combined with deep incompetence. They did not mention how venous obstruction would be incorporated into the classification. Perhaps this was in recognition of the difficulty in detecting and quantitating physiologic obstruction.

A New Proposal

A classification system of chronic venous insufficiency should have utility and simplicity if it is to achieve durability. It should not incorporate an element which will be incompletely evaluated such as the anatomical portion of the CEAP system. It should not rely on an evaluation method which is inaccurate. An example of this is duplex perforating vein identification, which has been shown to be in error in 20% of vessels [19].

Therefore, the following schema is suggested (Table 7.2). It should consist of three parts. The first should be a clinical classification ranging from 1 to 5. This adopts the best elements of CEAP and combines classes 5 and 6 into one, termed chronic ulceration. The second element should be the aetiology of the process. This should be simply primary or secondary, with all cases of thrombosis designated secondary even if a primary element had been present as a preliminary feature. The third element of the proposed method expresses pathophysiology. As shown in the table, superficial and deep reflux are indicated alone and in combination. They are also cited if combined with significant detectable obstruction.

Taking an example of the use of CEAP from Kistner's illustrative case would show how the systems of classification would differ [20]. In Kistner's case, advanced skin changes, oedema and open ulceration were due to prior deep vein thrombosis. His CEAP description was extremely informative, though cryptic. It was $C_{2,3,4,5\text{-}}sE_SA_{S,D,}P,PR_{2,3,11,12,13,14,15,0\text{-}9}$. In the proposed simplified classification this would be accurately described as $C_5E_2P_{D(A\&B)}$. This would state to an interested reader that the patient had chronic venous ulcer disease due to prior deep venous thrombosis and had venous obstruction with superficial and deep reflux.

Conclusions

Difficulty with devising a useful classification may be inherent in the nature of severe venous insufficiency. It may be that haemodynamic and haemostatic abnormalities act independently of leucocyte-induced skin damage and monocyte infiltration into venous valves and the venous wall. Perhaps only a better understanding of the effect of physiological obstruction as opposed to anatomical obstruction or a discovery of the fundamental cause of primary venous dysfunction will allow a simple practical classification to be constructed. However, a useful classification is proposed. This could be put to use today using existing knowledge and usual methods of evaluation.

Table 7.2. Proposed classification of venous dysfunction

Clinical class	Pathophysiology[a]
0 No abnormality	A Only superficial reflux
1 Telangiectasias[b]	B Only deep reflux
2 Varicose veins[c]	C Superficial and deep reflux
4 Lipodermatosclerosis[c]	D Obstruction[e]
5 Venous ulceration[d]	

[a] Aetiology should be indicated as primary (1°) or secondary (2°) (to thrombosis).
[b] No other abnormality; [c] includes lesser classes; [d] past or present.
[e] Combine with A, B or C.

Examples:		
Primary varicose veins	2 A	1°
Chronic venous ulcer	5 C	1°
Post-phlebitic state	4 D&C	2°

References

1. Kistner RL. Classification of chronic venous disease. Vasc Surg 1997;3:217–218.
2. Widmer LK. Classification of venous disorders. In: Peripheral venous disorders. Basle III. Bern: Hans Huber, 1978.
3. Sytchev GG. Classification of chronic venous disorders of the lower extremities and pelvis. Int Angiol 1985;4:203–206.
4. Enrici EA, Caldevilla HS. Classificacion de la insuficiencia venosa cronica. In: Enrici EA, Caldevilla HS, editors. Insuficiencia venosa cronicas de los miembros inferiores. Editorial Celcius 1992:pregnancies 109–114.
5. Porter JM, Rutherford RB, Clagett CP, et al. Reporting standards in venous disease. J Vasc Surg 1988;8:172–181.
6. Hach W, Schirmers U, Becker L. Veränderungen der tiefen Leitvenen bei either ner Starnmvarikose der Vein saphena magna. In: Müller, Wiefel H, editors. Mikrozirkulation und Blutrheologic. Baden Baden: Witzstrock, 1980.
7. Cornu-Thenard A, de Vincenzi, Maraval M. Evaluation of different systems for clinical quantification of varicose veins. J Dermatol Surg Oncol 1991;17:345–348.
8. Griton P, Widmer LK. Classification des varices et de l'insuffiance veineuse. J Mal Vasc 1992;17(Suppl B):102–108.
9. Partsch H. "Betterable" and "nonbetterable" chronic venous insufficiency: a proposal for a practice-oriented classification. Vasa 1980;9:165–167.
10. Pierchalia P, Tronnier H. Diagnosis and classification of venous insufficiency of the leg. Dtsch Med Wochenschr 1985;110:1700–1702.
11. Miranda C, Fabre M, Meyer P, Marescaux J. Evaluation of a reference anatomoclinical classification of varices of the lower limbs. Phlebologie 1993;46:235–239.
12. Porter JM, Moneta GL, and International Consensus Committee on Chronic Venous Disease. Reporting standards in venous disease: an update. J Vasc Surg 1995;21:635–645.
13. Beebe HG, Bergan JJ, Bergqvist D, et al. Classification of chronic venous disease in the lower limbs: a consensus statement. Eur J Vasc Surg 1996;12:487–492.
14. Iafrati MD, Welch H, Belkin M, O'Donnell T. Correlation of venous noninvasive tests with the SVS/ISCVS clinical classification of chronic venous insufficiency. Submitted for publication.
15. Gloviczki P, Yao JST. Handbook of venous disorders. London: Chapman & Hall, 1996.
16. Labropoulos N. CEAP in clinical practice. Vasc Surg 1997;31:224–225.
17. Ono T, Bergan JJ, Schmid-Schönbein GW, Takase S. Monocyte infiltration into venous valves. J Vasc Surg 1998;27:158–167.
18. Gloviczki P, Bergan JJ, Menawat SS, et al. Safety, feasibility, and early efficacy of subfascial endoscopic perforator surgery (SEPS): a preliminary report from the North American Registry. J Vasc Surg 1997;25:94–106.
19. Bergan JJ, Ballard JL, Sparks S, Murray JS. Subfascial surgery of perforating veins; SEPS. Phlebologie 1996;49:467–472.
20. Kistner RL. Clinical presentation and classification of chronic venous disease. In: Gloviczki P, Bergan JJ, editors. Atlas of endoscopic perforator vein surgery. Berlin Heidelberg New York: Springer, 1997.

8 How Do We Select the Appropriate Tests of Venous Function?

Andrew Nicolaides

Introduction

A careful clinical history and examination should reveal the patient's symptoms, their severity and whether these symptoms are due to venous disease rather than coexisting non-venous pathology (musculo-skeletal, arterial or neurological). The classic tourniquet tests provide some information about the sites of deep to superficial reflux but this is difficult to interpret when varicose veins are not prominent (poor refilling endpoint).

Because the history and clinical examination will not always indicate the nature and extent of the underlying pathology (anatomical extent, pathophysiology and aetiology), a number of diagnostic investigations have been developed. Provided they are performed and interpreted by doctors or technologists who have a good knowledge of venous disease, they can provide qualitative and quantitative information and offer answers to most questions posed in clinical practice. They elucidate whether there is calf muscle pump dysfunction, obstruction and/or reflux, and determine the anatomical extent and severity of the latter.

Chronic venous insufficiency is the result of venous hypertension which is produced by obstruction, reflux, calf muscle pump dysfunction or a combination of these abnormalities. For this reason a number of key pathophysiological questions should be asked. Is there any obstruction or reflux? If the answer is yes, then what is the anatomical extent of the abnormality or abnormalities present? What is the haemodynamic significance of each abnormality? Is there any calf muscle pump dysfunction and what is its haemodynamic significance? Finally, what is the overall haemodynamic effect of all the abnormalities present?

There is no single test that can provide answers to all the questions. For this reason a number of tests have been developed over the years that can answer several of the above questions. The selection of the appropriate tests will depend on the local facilities, the clinical presentation and the severity of the symptoms.

The information provided by the most popular tests used in clinical practice is summarised below.

Tests That Provide Information on Morphology

Ascending and Descending Phlebography

Until recently ascending phlebography has been the method of choice to visualise the venous system. It is still used as the "gold standard" to validate the accuracy of new investigations which determine the presence or absence of disease or its anatomical extent. However, the development of several accurate non-invasive tests, particularly duplex scanning, now makes phlebography unnecessary in the majority of cases. Phlebography does not provide quantitative information on venous function but allows the visualisation of old thrombus with residual obstruction and a collateral circulation. Recanalisation produces irregularity of the venous wall. Incompetent perforating veins can be identified by flow of contrast from deep to superficial veins.

Descending phlebography demonstrates reflux in either the superficial or deep veins and determines the points and extent of leakage from the pelvis to the lower limbs and from the deep to the superficial veins. It also provides information on the anatomical localisation and morphology of the venous valves, assesses the extent of reflux, delineates the venous anatomy in complex cases and differentiates primary from secondary disease.

The disadvantages of phlebography are that it is invasive and costly, and has potential complications. The development of duplex scanning which can detect the presence and anatomical extent of reflux has resulted in a decreased number of descending phlebograms. The latter are performed mainly when deep venous reconstruction is being considered or before repeat surgery for varicose veins when duplex scanning is not conclusive.

Continuous Wave Doppler Ultrasound

Continuous wave Doppler ultrasound is a useful method for detecting reflux at the saphenofemoral and saphenopopliteal junctions [1]. It has become routine in outpatient clinics for screening because it is quick, inexpensive and non-invasive.

Popliteal vein reflux can be detected by this method with a sensitivity of 100% and a specificity of 92%, i.e. a false positive rate of 8% [2]. False positive results are due to variations in the anatomy of the short saphenous vein and reflux in veins other than the popliteal vein.

A limitation of continuous wave Doppler ultrasound is that it cannot insonate an individual vessel because it detects flow in any artery or vein in the path of the ultrasound beam. At the level of the groin, reflux can be in the long saphenous vein, its tributaries or the common femoral vein. Doppler ultrasound cannot identify the exact site of reflux and the findings should be confirmed with duplex scanning if surgery is contemplated [3]. Continuous wave Doppler cannot detect the level of the saphenopopliteal junction [4]. Reflux in the gastrocnemius or the Giacomini vein can give false positive results indicating deep venous reflux despite the presence of competent popliteal valves. For this reason the finding of venous reflux in the popliteal fossa needs to be followed with duplex scanning if surgery is contemplated.

Duplex Scanning

Duplex scanning, has been used since the early 1980s for the diagnosis of deep vein thrombosis. It has now been extended to detect the presence and anatomical extent of obstruction or reflux [5]. (Semrow et al, 1986). Colour flow duplex imaging, which provides instant visualisation of blood flow and its direction, has speeded up the examination and improved its accuracy. It has become conventional to show cephalad flow as blue and distal flow as red. The extent of reflux in the superficial or deep veins can be detected as well as deep-to-superficial reflux at the saphenofemoral and saphenopopliteal junctions and the thigh or calf perforating veins. Also, it can provide information on collateral flow and can delineate the variable anatomy in the popliteal fossa. Gastrocnemial vein reflux can be diagnosed quickly and with great accuracy.

Recent Applications of Duplex Scanning

Recent studies have shown that duplex scanning is an ideal method for serial examinations to monitor the evolution of thrombi and to check for the appearance of reflux following acute deep vein thrombosis [6]. These studies indicate that reflux develops progressively and that even a complete occlusion may alternately partially recanalise and reocclude before a final complete recanalisation. However, the factors causing reflux to develop in some patients and not in others remain unclear.

In the absence of deep venous obstruction, limbs with reflux confined to the proximal veins (above the knee) rarely develop skin changes or ulceration [7]. In contrast, even in the presence of normal deep veins, symptoms and signs of chronic venous insufficiency are more often found when the entire length of the greater saphenous vein is involved or when reflux is present in both the long and short saphenous veins [7]. Multisegmental reflux is significantly more prevalent in legs with ulcers than in non-ulcerated limbs (75% vs 22%) [8] and the patterns of reflux involve at least two of the venous systems (superficial and deep, superficial and perforating, superficial and perforating and deep) in about two-thirds of the patients in CEAP classes C4–6 [8,9].

The available data suggest that there is a strong association between the severity of chronic venous insufficiency and the anatomical distribution and extent of venous reflux. However, the information is fragmented in multiple studies that use different classifications and methods of reporting. Therefore, further studies with uniform criteria combining the anatomical information provided by duplex scanning with quantitative pressure or plethysmographic measurements are needed to establish such associations

The importance of gastrocnemial reflux was recognised by Dodd in 1965 [10] and May and Nissl in 1959 [11], but only recently has obtained general recognition as a cause of primary venous insufficiency and more importantly as a common cause of recurrence [12]. When gastrocnemial vein incompetence is suspected, the demonstration of reflux by duplex is mandatory because reflux can be eliminated by surgical ligation [13].

Tests That Provide Haemodynamic Information

Ambulatory Venous Pressure

Ambulatory venous pressure (AVP) measurements can be used to supplement the anatomical information provided by phlebography and duplex scanning. AVP is the most direct method for assessing venous hypertension. The pressure at rest (P_0), the mean ambulatory venous pressure during the steady state towards the end of the 10 tiptoe movements (P_{10}), the calculated difference between the two (P_0-P_{10}) and the refilling time are the most useful measurements.

Because AVP testing is invasive, it cannot easily be repeated nor used for screening. For this reason, non-invasive screening tests such as photoplethysmography, Doppler ultrasound, air-plethysmography and foot volumetry are more frequently used for routine investigation. Nevertheless, AVP testing remains the gold standard for overall haemodynamic function and for validation of non-invasive tests. As a research tool it needs to be used in the assessment of the haemodynamic effect of surgical reconstructive procedures in the deep veins and to improve selection of patients.

Arm/Foot Pressure Differential

The arm/foot pressure differential (ΔP) provides haemodynamic information on the severity of obstruction and the adequacy of recanalisation or the collateral circulation [14]. The method consists of recording the venous pressure in a vein of the foot and the hand simultaneously with the patient in the supine position at rest. The measurements are repeated during reactive hyperaemia of the lower limb. On the basis of these measurements, limbs with venous obstruction can be classified into four grades. The more proximal the obstruction the poorer is the compensation and the higher the grade. The technique is a global measure of haemodynamic obstruction due to outflow blockage in one or more proximal veins. Venous obstructions involve more than one anatomical segment in 75% of limbs [15]. When multisegment obstruction is present, additional direct femoral pressure measurements may be necessary for more precise assessment of functional obstruction at different levels. Measurements can be carried out before and after papaverine injection [16].

This method has the disadvantage that it is invasive and requires two venepunctures. In clinical practice its main value is in the selection of patients for venous reconstruction. There is no indication for a bypass procedure unless a high arm/foot pressure differential exists and grade 3 or 4 obstruction is present [17].

Photoplethysmography, Light Reflection Rheography and Digital Photoplethysmography

Photoplethysmography (PPG) is a non-invasive technique that can detect local changes in the blood content of tissues and has found its principal application in the study of blood flow and blood volume changes in the skin. In the 1980s, PPG had a limited application for quantitative measurements because of inability to calibrate the signal and inability of the recorded signal to return to the same baseline [18]. Only time measurements such as the post-exercise refilling time could be used. Light reflection rheography [19] and digital-PPG [20] are more recent descendants of PPG. They incorporate modern computer technology with self-standardisation allowing measurements not only of the time-related parameters but also of the amplitude. The most frequently performed examinations of quantitative photoplethysmography in the investigation of chronic venous insufficiency are the muscle pump test to assess dysfunction and the vein occlusion test to diagnose venous outflow obstruction [20,21].

In practice, photoplethysmography is performed when valvular incompetence is suspected. Although the PPG refilling time without and with occlusion of superficial veins can help to distinguish between limbs without major venous pathology, those with superficial venous incompetence and limbs with deep venous incompetence, it is not considered to be a good indicator of the severity of deep venous insufficiency. This is because any abnormal AVP in the range of 45–100 mmHg can be associated with a short refilling time (2–10 s) [18]. Refilling time depends upon several physical factors including the size of the reservoir to be filled and the diameter of the vein in which the reflux occurs. A long refilling time may be observed when reflux occurs in small-diameter veins because the rate of reflux in millilitres per second would be low.

In contrast, when reflux occurs in large-diameter veins in which the volume flow is large, reflux can be very short because the venous "reservoir" will fill quickly. The finding of an abnormally short refilling time in the absence of any reflux in the main superficial trunks or deep veins on duplex examination is suggestive of reflux through the pelvic and vulvar veins. It is hardly surprising that the refilling times correlate poorly with other methods [22,23].

Recent studies using digital-PPG have demonstrated that the measurements of venous refilling time and muscle pump efficiency have a better quantitative relationship with symptoms than conventional PPG or light reflection rheography [20].

PPG can be used as a screening test to detect the presence of chronic venous insufficiency or when an assessment of the overall physiological function of the lower limb veins is required without resorting to more invasive or expensive tests. Suspected reflux because of a short refilling time should always be confirmed by continuous wave Doppler or preferably by duplex sonography. The test should not be relied upon to identify the anatomical distribution of the disease.

Air-Plethysmography

Venous hypertension is the result of impaired venous return. The latter is often due to the combined effects of venous reflux, obstruction or poor calf muscle pump function. Air-plethysmography has the ability to measure each of these three components and by doing so it has contributed to our improved understanding of venous pathophysiology. Because measurements involve the whole leg, they are more reproducible than those from segmental plethysmographs such as strain-gauge or foot volumetry. Air-plethysmography has now become the most popular method of quantitation of venous haemodynamics.

Evaluation of Venous reflux

Venous reflux is less than 2 ml/s in normal limbs in which the veins fill slowly from the arterial side. It may increase up to 30 ml/s in limbs with severe venous reflux [24]. Venous reflux greater than 7 ml/min has a 73% sensitivity, a 100% specificity and a 100% positive predictive value of identifying limbs with venous ulceration [25]. The incidence of oedema, skin changes and ulceration increases with higher values of reflux irrespective of whether reflux was in the superficial or deep veins. When measurements were repeated after reflux in the superficial veins was abolished by finger compression of the long saphenous vein at the level of the knee, reflux was reduced to less than 5 ml/s in limbs with primary varicose veins but not in limbs with reflux in the deep veins. Reflux through the short saphenous vein is difficult to eliminate by finger compression.

Evaluation of Venous Outflow

Venous outflow is evaluated using the venous occlusion technique with the patient supine [25]. A thigh tourniquet (10–12 cm wide) is placed as proximally as possible and inflated to 80 mmHg. Volume increases to a new plateau. The tourniquet is then deflated suddenly and the venous outflow curve is recorded. The outflow fraction at 1 s (OF_1) is the venous outflow expressed as a percentage of the total venous volume. The procedure is repeated after occluding the long saphenous vein at the knee. In clinical practice OF_1 greater than 38% is considered to indicate absence of any functional obstruction, OF_1 in the range of 30–38% indicates moderate obstruction and OF_1 of less than 30% indicates severe obstruction [26].

Evaluation of the Ejecting Capacity of the Calf Muscle Pump

The ejection fraction (EF) of the calf muscle pump after one tiptoe movement is over 60% in limbs without venous disease, 30–70% in limbs with primary varicose veins and may be as low as 10% in limbs with deep venous disease [27]. The ejection capacity is as important as reflux for development of venous ulceration. A good EF (> 40%) was associated with a low incidence of ulceration despite marked reflux and a poor EF (< 40%) was found with ulceration even in limbs with minimal reflux [28]. The combined EF and reflux measurements have a good correlation with the incidence of ulceration and offer the potential for selecting patients most likely to benefit from deep vein reconstruction. They also offer a means of haemodynamic follow up in natural history studies.

The Overall Performance of the Calf Muscle Pump

The combined effect of venous reflux, obstruction and ejection capacity is evaluated by measuring residual volume fraction after 10 tiptoe movements. The residual volume fraction is in the range of 5–35% in normal limbs, 20–70% in limbs with primary varicose veins and up to 100% in deep venous disease. It has a linear relationship with measurements of ambulatory venous pressure and the incidence of ulceration [27,28].

Recent Applications of Air Plethysmography

In contrast to duplex scanning, which detects abnormalities in individual veins, air-plethysmography provides information derived from the whole leg, and in contrast to segmental devices it avoids errors due to muscle movements during exercise. Although it can be used as a simple screening test, it has the potential to can offer a complete analysis of venous haemodynamics. Thus it is useful for routine clinical practice as well as research.

Venous hypertension usually results from the combined effect of reflux, obstruction and poor ejection. By using air-plethysmography the contribution of each parameter can be measured so that the appropriate intervention can be considered. Overall it would appear that the severity of reflux is strongly associated with the grade of disease. Surgical abolition of venous reflux in the deep or the superficial system has already been shown to normalise venous haemodynamics in properly selected patients with no obstruction and unimpaired calf muscle ejection [22,29,30].

Practical Applications

A clinician managing a patient with suspected chronic venous insufficiency should ask whether reflux or obstruction is present and what their anatomical extent and severity are. Different tests provide different information and there is not a single test that can provide all the information needed to make clinical decisions and to plan a management strategy.

By asking and answering relevant clinical questions more information becomes available and the diagnosis can be more precise. What is needed is a clear knowledge of the tests required to arrive at the correct clinical diagnosis with the minimum expense and inconvenience to the patient. Non-invasive venous investigations are performed by vascular technologists (or doctors) trained to apply the proper tests in order to provide answers to the key questions required by the clinician.

The initial evaluation of patients with chronic venous insufficiency consists of determining the presence or absence of reflux, obstruction or both in the venous system. As stated in the Introduction, the history and clinical examination will indicate the clinical presentation. The use of a pocket Doppler ultrasound by the physician in the outpatient clinic can provide information to confirm the presence of reflux at the saphenofemoral junction, popliteal fossa and superficial veins and obstruction at the femoropopliteal or iliofemoral segments in 80–90% of patients. A proportion (20–30%) will need further investigation because they are complicated cases. Many of these will have had a previous operation on their veins or the results of Doppler ultrasound are not clearcut. Those with reflux in the veins of the popliteal fossa and the group in which incompetent calf perforating veins are suspected need further clarification.

In the past, a phlebogram was required to localise venous obstruction, but duplex scanning has proved equally good, particularly for lesions distal to the common femoral vein. Phlebography also accurately localised the sites of deep-to-superficial reflux (saphenofemoral, saphenopopliteal, incompetent perforating veins) and the extent of reflux in the deep veins. Duplex scanning is proving to be a simpler and more accurate test – so much so that ascending and descending phlebography is now rarely performed. The main indication for phlebography is to detect floppy valves in the deep veins. Duplex scanning is the method of choice to localise the sites of incompetent perforating veins and the level of the saphenopopliteal junction.

Quantitative measurements of outflow obstruction and/or reflux may be needed for research, particularly to study the natural history of chronic venous insufficiency and to assess established and new methods for treatment. These quantitative measurements have now opened new avenues leading to a better scientific basis for patient management. Until recently, ambulatory venous pressure measurement was the only quantitative test available. Though invasive it indicated the severity of venous hypertension for it measured the end result of both reflux and outflow obstruction. However, new non-invasive tests can separate the relative contributions from venous obstruction, reflux in the superficial and/or deep veins as well as the calf muscle pump funcion, be it the result of intrinsic venous disease, a musculoskeletal problem, or both.

Five clinically relevant questions should be asked by the physician when a patient presents with symptoms and signs suggestive of chronic venous disease.

1. Is venous dysfunction responsible for the clinical picture?
2. Is venous dysfunction fully responsible? Are there any other contributory factors?
3. What is the prognosis for this patient?
4. What information is needed to make the correct therapeutic decision, and how to obtain can this information be obtained most efficiently?
5. How should the therapeutic results be evaluated?

A simple method is to categorise the diagnostic investications into three levels:

Level I *Clinical examination* (history, physical examination, hand-held Doppler, and including an evaluation of the arterial circulation).

Level II *Non-invasive investigations* (duplex scanning, plethysmography).

Level III *Invasive investigations* (ascending and descending phlebography, varicography, pressure measurements) *in addition to the above.*

A simple guide of the level of investigation in relation to the clinical CEAP classes is given below.

Class 0/1 (No visible or palpable signs of venous disease)
Level I is usually sufficient
Class 2 (Telangiectases or reticular veins)
Level I may be sufficient, but level II (duplex scanning) is utilised in many practices as indicated below.

In patients with reflux in the popliteal fossa, recurrent varicose veins, perforator incompetence and in surgery with planned preservation of the long saphenous vein, duplex scanning will provide the essential information for further management. Duplex scanning is also important for pre-operative marking of incompetent perforators and the level of the saphenopopliteal junction. If the duplex scan shows involvement of the deep venous system, level III may be considered.

Class 3 (Oedema)
Level I may be sufficient. In addition to the above considerations for class 2, level II (duplex scan) is utilised to determine whether reflux or obstruction in the deep veins is responsible for the oedema.

Isolated oedema. If level I is abnormal, levels II and III must be considered to investigate the deep venous and perforator systems. If obstruction is suspected, plethysmography is advisable. Lymphoscintigraphy should be considered.

Classes 4, 5, 6 (Skin changes with or without ulceration)
Level I and II investigations will be required in the majority of patients. Selected patients will proceed to level III, mainly the candidates for deep venous reconstruction.

Level I investigations may be sufficient in a group of patients with irreversible failure of muscle pump due to neurological disease, severe and non-correctable reduction of ankle movement or contraindication to surgical intervention. Some investigations may have to be postponed, particularly those using the tiptoe exercise (e.g. air-plethysmography) in patients with acute lipodermatosclerosis and painful active ulcers. The majority of patients will be subjected to level II investigations and in selected cases level III, mainly the candidates for deep venous reconstruction.

References

1. Barnes RW, Ross EA, Strandness DE. Differentiation of primary from secondary varicose veins by Doppler ultrasound and straingauge plethysmography. Surg Gynecol Obstet 1975;141:207–211.
2. Nicolaides AN, Fernandes e Fernandes J, Zimmerman H. Doppler ultrasound in the investigation of venous insufficiency. In: Nicolaides AN, Yao JST, editors. Investigation of vascular disorders. New York: Churchill Livingstone, 1981:478–487.
3. Vasdekis S, Clarke GH, Hobbs JT, Nicolaides AN. Evaluation of noninvasive methods in the assessment of short saphenous vein termination. Br J Surg 1989;76:929–932.
4. Hoare MC, Royle JP. Doppler ultrasound detection of saphenofemoral and sapheno-popliteal incompetence and operative venography to ensure precise sapheno-popliteal ligation. Aust NZ J Surg 1984;54:49–52.
5. Semrow C, Ryan TJ, Buchbinder D, Rollins DL, et al. Assessment of valve function using real-time B-mode ultrasound. In: Negus D, Jantet G, editors. Phlebology '85. London: John Libbey, 1986:352–355.

6. Markel A, Manzo RA, Bergelin RO, Strandness DE. Valvular reflux after deep vein thrombosis: incidence and time of occurrence. J Vasc Surg 1992;15:377–384.
7. Labropoulos N, Leon M, Nicolaides AN, Giannoukas A, Volteas N, Chan P. Superficial venous insufficiency: correlation of anatomic extent of reflux with clinical symptoms and signs. J Vasc Surg 1994;20:953–958.
8. Weingarten MS, Branas CC, Czeredarczuk M, Schmidt JD, Wolferth CC. Distribution and quantification of venous reflux in lower extremity chronic venous stasis disease with duplex scanning. J Vasc Surg 1993;18:753–759.
9. Labropoulos N, Delis K, Nicolaides AN, Leon M, Ramaswami G, Volteas N. The role of the distribution and anatomic extent of reflux in the development of signs and symptoms in chronic venous insufficiency. J Vasc Surg 1996;23:504–510.
10. Dodd H. The varicose tributaries of the popliteal vein. Br J Surg 1965;52:350–354.
11. May R, Nissl R. Die Phlebographie der unteren Extremität. Stuttgart: Thieme, 1959.
12. Vandendriessche M. Association between gastrocnemial vein insufficiency and varicose veins. Phlebology 1989;4:71–84.
13. Hobbs JT. The enigma of the gastrocnemius vein. Phlebology 1988;3:19–30.
14. Raju S. A pressure-based technique for the detection of acute and chronic venous obstruction. Phlebology 1988;3:207–216.
15. Raju S, Fredericks R. Venous obstruction an analysis of 137 cases with haemodynamic, venographic and clinical correlations. J Vasc Surg 1991;14:305–313.
16. Illig KA, Ouriel K, De Weese JA, Riggs P, Green RM. Increasing the sensitivity of diagnosis of chronic venous obstruction. J Vasc Surg 1996;24:176–178.
17. Raju S, Fredericks RK. Late haemodynamic sequelae of deep venous thrombosis. J Vasc Surg 1986;4:73–79.
18. Nicolaides AN, Miles C. Photoplethysmography in the assessment of venous insufficiency. J Vasc Surg 1987;5:405–412.
19. Hubner K. Is the light reflection rheography (LRR) suitable as a diagnostic method for the phlebology practice? Phlebol Proctol 1986;15:209–212.
20. Schultz-Ehrenburg U, Blazek V. New possibilities for photoplethysmography. Phlebol Digest 1993;5:5–11.
21. Schultz-Ehrenburg U, Blazek V. Quantitative digital photoplethysmography (D-PPG): first results with on line registration and significance of V0 (Venous Pump Power). In: Schultz-Ehrenburg U, Blazek V, editors. Advances in computer aided noninvasive vascular diagnostics. Dusseldorf: VDI Verlag, 1994.
22. Welch HJ, Faliakou EC, McLaughlin RL, Umphrey SE, Belkin M, O'Donnell TF. Comparison of descending phlebography with quantitative photoplethysmography, air plethysmography and duplex quantiative valve closure time in assessing deep venous reflux. J Vasc Surg 1992;16:913–919.
23. Bays RA, Healy DA, Atnip RG, Neumyer M, Thiele BL. Validation of air plethysmography, photoplethysmography and duplex ultrasonography in the evaluation of severe venous stasis. J Vasc Surg 1994;20:721–727.
24. Christopoulos D, Nicolaides AN, Szendro G. Venous reflux: quantification and correlation with the clinical severity of venous disease. Br J Surg 1988;75:352–356.
25. Christopoulos D, Nicolaides AN, Duffy P, Georgiou I. Noninvasive diagnosis and quantification of outflow obstruction in venous disease. J Cardiovasc Surg 1989;30:72–73.
26. Nicolaides AN, Sumner DS, editors. Investigation of patients with deep vein thrombosis and chronic venous insufficiency. Med-Orion 1991;39–43.
27. Christopoulos D, Nicolaides AN, Szendro G, et al. Air-plethysmography and the effect of elastic compression on the venous haemodynamics of the leg. J Vasc Surg 1987;5:148–159.
28. Christopoulos D, Nicolaides AN, Cook A, Irvine A, Galloway JM, Wilkinson A. Pathogenesis of venous ulceration in relation to the calf muscle pump function. Surgery 1989;106:829–835.
29. Gillespie DL, Cordts PR, Hartono C et al. The role of plethysmography in monitoring the results of venous surgery. J Vasc Surg 1992;16:674–678.
30. Bry JDL, Muto PA, O'Donnell TF, Isaacson LRN. The clinical and hemodynamic results after axillary-to-popliteal vein valve transplantation. J Vasc Surg 1995;21:110–119.
31. Harada R, Katz M, Comerota A. A non-invasive screening test to detect "critical" deep venous reflux. J Vasc Surg 1995;22:532–537.

9 Imaging of Chronic Venous Disease

P.L. Allan

Introduction

The imaging of venous disease has developed significantly over the last few years. In particular, the role of ultrasound has been discovered and developed, contributing significantly to both the anatomical and functional understanding of the pathophysiology of acute and chronic venous disorders. Magnetic resonance imaging and magnetic resonance angiography show promise for imaging the venous system of the limbs and hold potential for the future. Computed tomography has also developed significantly over recent years and has become increasingly valuable in the diagnosis of pulmonary embolus associated with deep venous thrombosis. However, these techniques have yet to establish a useful role in the investigation of chronic venous disease. The older techniques of venography and varicography have not been completely replaced by ultrasound and still have an important role to play in the diagnosis and assessment of a variety of disorders that affect the veins of the lower limb.

The spectrum of venous diseases covers deep vein thrombosis, primary and recurrent varicose veins, and chronic venous insufficiency, together with a variety of less common conditions that affect the veins of the upper and lower limbs. This book concentrates on venous insufficiency in the lower limb and therefore this will be the main subject for this review of imaging techniques.

Aims of Imaging in Patients with Chronic Lower Limb Venous Disease

The aims of imaging in patients with chronic lower limb venous disease are:

1. Identification of incompetent venous segments in the deep and superficial systems together with clarification of the overall pattern of incompetent channels.
2. Identification of points of leakage and incompetence which are amenable to surgery.
3. Confirmation that the deep veins are patent and competent in patients with a history of possible previous deep vein thrombosis.
4. Identification of evidence of post-thrombotic sequelae from previous deep vein thrombosis.
5. Clarification of patterns of recanalisation and recurrence following previous surgery.
6. Clarification of the anatomy in cases of atypical clinical findings on examination and hand-held Doppler.

Ultrasound

The development of duplex ultrasound over the last 15 years and subsequently colour Doppler ultrasound has allowed this non-invasive technique to be used to obtain both anatomical and functional information in relation to venous disease. Duplex ultrasound allows the operator to locate and identify specific structures using real-time imaging and then obtain information on the presence, direction and velocity of blood flow from a specific location or vessel within the image (Fig. 9.1). This is in distinction to the hand-held Doppler equipment used in the clinic and ward, which registers Doppler shifts from any vessel in the line of the ultrasound beam but is unable to separate and distinguish these; this can be a problem after previous surgery, or in areas of complex venous anatomy, such as the popliteal fossa.

Colour Doppler systems also combine imaging and blood flow information as part of the visual display. An area of interest is defined on the image using a box which can be varied in size and shape; any Doppler shifts registered within this area are converted into a colour map. The resultant colour map is laid over the image so that the blood flow information can be related to the structures seen on the image. The presence of moving blood is represented as a colour; the colour used represents the direction of flow in relation to the transducer face, with the tone of the colour representing the velocity of the flow, usually paler shades correspond to regions of faster flow (Fig. 9.1). Power Doppler is a development of colour Doppler which looks primarily at the overall energy in the Doppler signal. The data- processing algorithm used makes it more sensitive to low velocity and low strength signals but at the expense of losing the directional

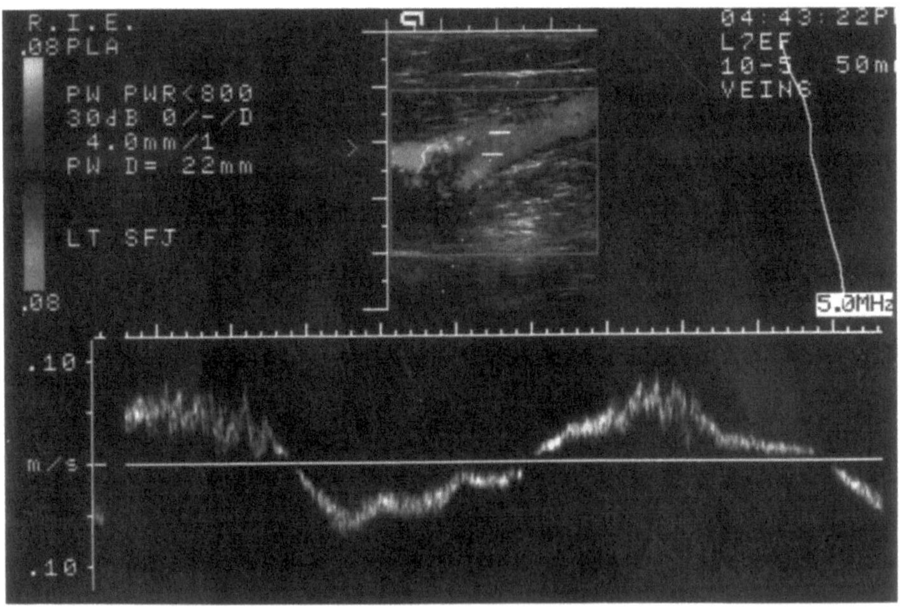

Fig. 9.1. Colour Doppler image of an incompetent sapheno-femoral junction and corresponding spectral display. The orange colour indicates flow towards the transducer and the spectral display shows bidirectional flow: flow towards the patient's head is shown below the baseline, whereas reflux with flow back towards the transducer is shown above the baseline. *(See also Plate I)*

information, although modern systems now combine colour and power information in order to obtain the advantage of high sensitivity and directional information.

Several pharmaceutical companies are developing ultrasound echo-enhancing agents which can be injected into the peripheral venous circulation and then traverse the pulmonary capillaries and recirculate around the cardiovascular system for several minutes. Following injection, these agents increase the echogenicity of the blood and therefore improve the signal-to-noise ratio. Using these agents in conjunction with power Doppler or sensitive colour Doppler should allow more accurate assessment of smaller vessels and slower rates of blood flow but their role in venous ultrasound, particularly in relation to chronic venous disease, has not been established.

Applications and Technique of Venous Ultrasound in Patients with Chronic Venous Disease

Ultrasound allows the non-invasive assessment of patients with a variety of chronic or recurrent venous diseases. In practice, these patients fall mainly into two groups: patients with recurrent varicose veins and patients with signs and symptoms of chronic venous insufficiency. In both cases the deep and superficial veins of the affected leg must be examined from the groin to the ankle in order to establish the patency and competence of the various venous segments and to identify clinically significant pathways of collateral or incompetent flow. The examination is best done with the patient standing but it may take up to half an hour or more for each leg in complex cases; many patients will find this excessively tiring and it may therefore be necessary to use a combination of sitting and standing depending on the segments of vein being imaged at any particular time. Some degree of patient verticality is necessary in order to use the effect of gravity in the demonstration of reflux. Three features of the examination are used in the assessment of lower limb veins: (1) the anatomical information provided by the high-resolution imaging, (2) the effect of light or moderate transducer on the calibre of the vein (a thrombosed vein will not collapse) and (3) information provided by spectral and colour Doppler on the direction of blood flow in the segment under review, allowing demonstration of reflux and some assessment of its severity.

Imaging, compression and colour Doppler can all show changes resulting from previous deep vein thrombosis if there is persistent occlusion of the vein, or partial recanalisation. In many cases, however, there may be no visible structural sequelae to the thrombotic episode, although there may be functional incompetence of the valves.

Techniques for the induction of reflux are varied. The simplest and most practical method is to give the calf a short, sharp squeeze with the hand whilst scanning the relevant vein above the level of calf compression; although this is fairly subjective, it can be adjusted quickly and easily with experience for the size of the leg, the amount of forward flow desired and the rate at which the compressions are applied. More objective and reproducible stimuli can be provided by using a cuff which inflates and deflates rapidly using compressed air [1]. Getting the patient to breathe in, cough, perform a Valsalva manoeuvre or blow into high-resistance spirometer circuit produce reflux by raising the intra-abdominal pressure to a varying degree. Unfortunately this only shows reflux down to the first competent set of valves; if there is a lower incompetent segment, it will be protected and masked by competent valves proximally.

Reflux is demonstrated when there is clear reversed flow occurring after the period of forward flow in the segment under examination. Reversed flow seen during a period of forward flow is usually due to turbulence and vortices, rather than reflux back through a damaged segment of vein. A short period of reversed flow as the valve cusps close may be seen but any reversed flow lasting for more than 0.5 s is generally held to be significant [1]. There is much discussion on the significance of reflux shown by ultrasound and it would seem that the presence of reflux in one or several segments of the lower limb veins is just one of several factors involved in the development and progression of signs and symptoms related to chronic venous insufficiency. Although 0.5 s. is an accepted measure of significant reflux, the relationship of this to the actual severity of the reflux and venous dysfunction is not clear. Rodriguez and colleagues [2] have shown that the volume of blood refluxing through an incompetent valve is not related to the duration of reflux measured by duplex ultrasound. However, the more severe and the more extensive the incompetence, the more likely it is to be associated with signs and symptoms of chronic venous insufficiency.

The ultrasound examination should include an assessment of the deep veins of the thigh and calf, the long and short saphenous veins, the presence of any incompetent perforators and the presence of any other significant communicating channels. The advent of colour Doppler has reduced the need to use tourniquets during the procedure in order to occlude a segment of vein, but occasionally they are useful in clarifying complex situations. Incompetent or enlarged perforating veins should be sought in both the thigh and calf segments; perforating veins may or may not show incompetent flow, but this is more likely with larger perforators of more than 4 mm diameter, when 60% will show incompetence [3]. It is useful if the location of significant perforators is related to anatomical landmarks such as the malleoli, patella or groin (Fig. 9.2). This is particularly important if sub-fascial endoscopic perforator surgery is being

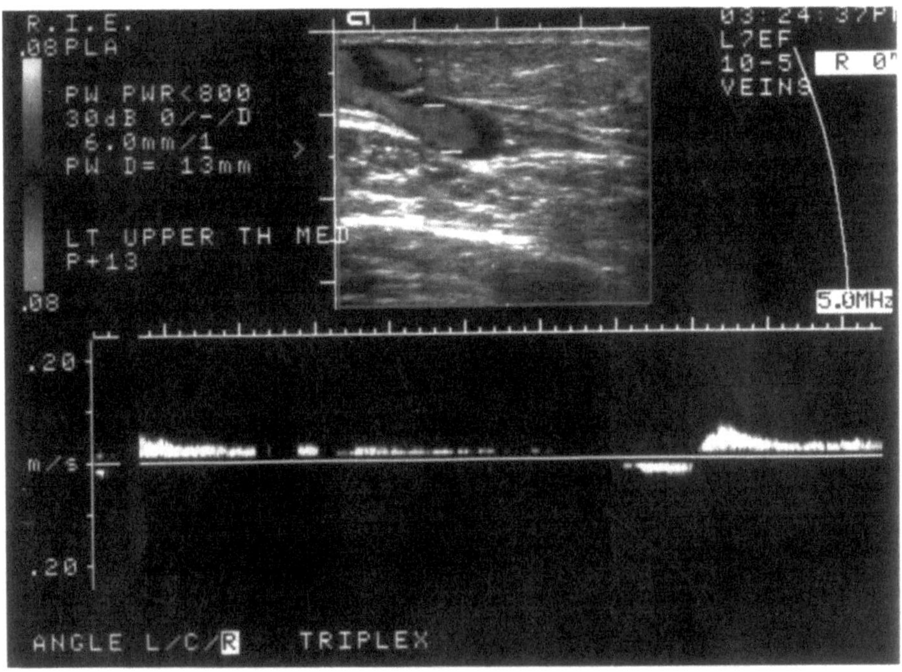

Fig. 9.2. Colour Doppler image of an incompetent perforating vein penetrating the fascia in the medial thigh, 13 cm above the patella, showing flow outwards towards the long saphenous vein. *(See also Plate II)*

contemplated, or if there is an atypical arrangement of the sapheno-popliteal junction, or some other aspect of the venous anatomy. Ideally, marking the sites of perforators with indelible ink prior to surgery should be considered. Some patients will have venous ulceration in the calf and abnormal perforators can lie under the ulcerated area, so that scanning of the ulcer bed using a sterile technique may be required.

Drawbacks in Relation to Doppler Ultrasound

The length of time needed to sort out complex cases can be excessive, with some examinations occasionally taking 30–40 min for each leg. This imposes a strain on both the patient and the sonographer. In patients with severe venous dysfunction it may be difficult to induce significant upward flow as the blood just moves from one compartment in the calf to another but does not pass up the leg. Connections to the pelvic and perineal veins or the profunda femoris vein can be difficult to image satisfactorily. Locating significantly incompetent perforating veins can be difficult unless time, care and attention are expended on the examination; even then significant perforators may be missed [3]. Complex patterns of multiple, incompetent venous channels can be difficult to sort out precisely on ultrasound and, if the sonographer has any doubts on the adequacy of the examination, a contrast study should be obtained if surgery is being considered.

Venography and Varicography

Prior to the advent of Doppler ultrasound techniques, contrast venography and varicography were the mainstay of imaging in patients with recurrent varicose veins and chronic venous insufficiency. The use of low-osmolar contrast agents has significantly reduced the discomfort for the patient and the small risk of contrast-induced thrombophlebitis developing as a result of the procedure [4].

The technique must be tailored to the diagnostic problem. For instance, the use of tourniquets will depend on whether the main problem is the exclusion of deep vein thrombosis, when they would be required; or the demonstration of deep to superficial incompetence, when they may or may not be needed, depending on the patterns of reflux demonstrated during the course of the examination. Similarly, the site of injection of contrast will depend on the clinical problem to be clarified; injection may be made into a foot vein (ascending phlebography), the femoral vein (descending phlebography) or a superficial varicose vein (varicography). The examination needs fluoroscopic control, with the position of the patient or the leg being altered to move the opacified blood through the venous channels being examined [5]. The contrast is usually injected with the patient in a semi-vertical position, this encourages the contrast to pool in the leg veins as it is denser than blood and venous flow is reduced with the patient in this position. The pattern of venous opacification during this period of passive filling is observed and any passive leakage of contrast through incompetent perforating veins can also be seen. The patient is then asked to contract the calf muscles to propel blood up the limb and help identify normal and abnormal patterns of flow (Fig. 9.3). Up to 80% of incompetent perforator veins will be shown using this technique [6] and a further 10% will be shown by performing a varicogram on the same legs [7]. Incompetent superficial and deep venous segments can be identified by the passage

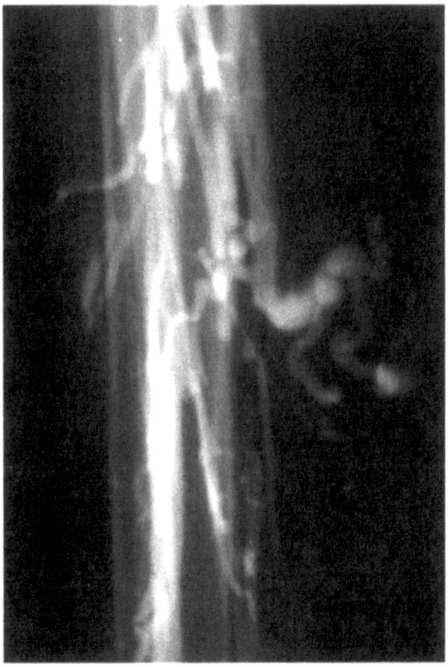

Fig. 9.3. Incompetent perforating veins shown on ascending venography. (Courtesy of Dr. K. McBride.)

of contrast from deep to superficial systems, or by reverse flow on bringing the patient upright from a supine position.

Varicography entails the injection of contrast agent directly into the superficial veins and screening the channels it takes on its way to the deep system of veins in the leg (Fig. 9.4), or to the groin and perineum. Altering patient position and the application of compression or tourniquets can help direct contrast to some extent, so that there is some choice in the channels which are opacified. This technique will not identify incompetent perforators accurately as the normal direction of flow through perforating veins is from the superficial system to the deep system. However, any opacified perforating vein that is larger than 3 mm is likely to be incompetent [8].

Drawbacks in Relation to Venography and Varicography

Contrast-induced thrombophlebitis is much less of a problem following the introduction of low-osmolar contrast agents. Although small (20G–21G) needles are used there is still some discomfort for the patient. The examination is still limited to some extent by the amount of contrast which can be injected (up to 200 ml of 240–300 mg I/ml strength for a leg) and the time during which it provides adequate contrast enhancement before dispersing and disappearing.

Relationship Between Ultrasound and Venography/Varicography

It is reasonable to assess patients with Doppler ultrasound first, as this will provide the information required in many cases and is non-invasive. However, a contrast

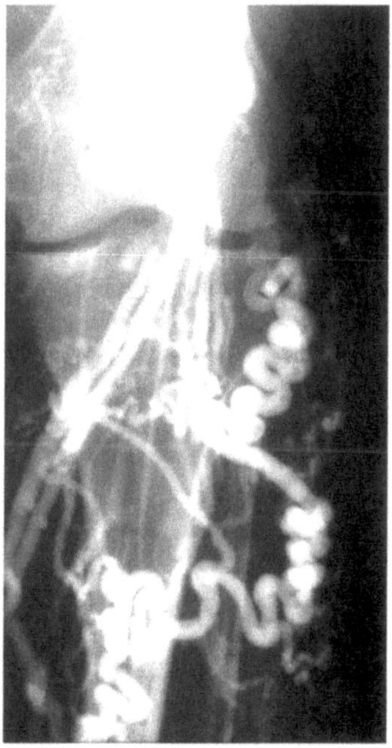

Fig. 9.4. Varicography with injection of radiographic contrast into a superficial varicose vein shows the complex nature of the multiple channels which connect with this segment. (Courtesy of Dr. K. McBride.)

examination should also be considered if the Doppler examination has not provided all the information required for a management decision to be reached. In practice the techniques of venography and varicography are complementary to Doppler ultrasound and are used together, as necessary, to answer any unanswered questions in relation to the clinical problem. Although some studies have suggested that ultrasound is up to 96% accurate at the identification of significantly incompetent perforator veins [9], other studies have questioned the reliability of ultrasound to identify all the relevant perforators, with sensitivities for incompetent calf perforators being in the region of 60–82% [8,10].

Magnetic Resonance Imaging and Computed Tomography

Magnetic resonance imaging (MRI) and computed tomography (CT) have not been widely applied to the assessment of peripheral venous disease in general, or to chronic venous disease in particular. Some attention has been given to their role in the diagnosis of deep vein thrombosis and this has shown that both have the ability to image the larger veins in the thigh and popliteal regions with sufficient resolution for the techniques to be comparable with venography or duplex ultrasound [11,12]. However, the temporal resolution required to obtain the dynamic real-time information needed for the assessment of venous function and incompetence cannot be achieved by CT or MRI at present. The spatial resolution of MRI for vessels the size of the normal superficial and deep veins in the calf is also currently less than satisfactory, but the technique is developing rapidly and improvements will continue to be made. Both CT and MRI are performed with the patient horizontal, rather than in the vertical position required for assessment of chronic venous insufficiency. In addition CT studies require the injection of contrast into distal veins in order to identify the patent venous channels. This makes the examination as uncomfortable as venography, without having the advantages of the latter as the patient cannot be moved into different positions, including head-up tilt, in order to influence the movement of contrast within the lower limb venous system. The use of appropriate MR contrast agents may improve the performance of this technique by improving the signal-to-noise ratio from slowly moving blood in relatively small vessels.

CT will show a variety of changes in the soft tissues of the lower limb in patients with chronic venous insufficiency. These include soft tissue oedema, fibrosis, atrophy and degeneration of muscle tissue and tendons, calcified phleboliths and, occasionally, ossification in the soft tissues; periosteal reactions and thickening are also seen on CT. MRI will show many of the connective tissue, muscle and tendon changes but it will not show calcification in the tissues as this does not give a signal on MRI.

Other Techniques

Radioisotopes are established as a potential technique for the diagnosis of developing deep vein thrombosis and following its growth or regression over a period of time. There have also been reports of radioisotopes being used to assess lower limb venous function by using labelled red blood cells in an isotope plethysmograph technique [13] that enables the rates of emptying and refilling of the vascular compartment to be measured. Isotopes can also be used to indicate the locations of incompetent perforating veins [14], but the technique is not practised widely and its potential value as a clinical diagnostic technique has yet to be assessed.

Conclusions

The underlying causes of chronic venous insufficiency signs and symptoms and the factors contributing to its development are multiple; in addition, they interact in a complex fashion. However, venous reflux, thrombosis, post-thrombotic changes and varicose veins have been shown to be significant factors in the development of these changes. Ultrasound and contrast phlebographic techniques can be used to clarify both the anatomy and the direction of blood flow in relation to the various segments of the lower limb veins, so that an accurate assessment of the relevant abnormalities can be developed and appropriate treatment decisions, both medical and surgical, can be reached.

References

1. Evans CJ, Leng GC, Stonebridge P, Lee AJ, Allan PL, Fowkes FGR. Reproducibility of duplex ultrasound in the measurement of venous reflux. Phlebology 1995;10:149–154.
2. Rodriguez AA, Whitehead CM, McLaughlin RL, Umphrey SE, Welch HJ, O'Donnell TF. Duplex-derived valve closure times fail to correlate with reflux flow volumes in patients with chronic venous insufficiency. J Vasc Surg 1996;23:606–610.

3. Phillips GW, Change LS. The value of ultrasound in the assessment of incompetent perforating veins. Aust Radiol 1996;40:15–18.
4. AbuRahma AF, Powell M, Robinson PA. Prospective study of safety of lower extremity phlebography with non-ionic contrast medium. Am J Surg 1996;171:255–260.
5. Lea Thomas M, Mcallister V, Rose DH, et al. A simplified technique of phlebography for the localisation of incompetent perforating veins of the legs. Clin Radiol 1972;23:486–491.
6. Fletcher EWL. Functional phlebography in venous disorders of the lower limb. In: Tibbs DJ, editor. Varicose veins and related disorders. Oxford: Butterworth-Heinemann, 1992:475–510.
7. Lea Thomas M, Bowles JN. Incompetent perforating veins: comparison of varicography and ascending phlebography. Radiology 1985;154:619–623.
8. Phillips GWL, Paige J, Molan MP. A comparison of colour duplex ultrasound with venography and varicography in the assessment of varicose veins. Clin Radiol 1995;50:20–25.
9. Stiegler H, Rotter G, Standl R, Mosavi S, von Kooten HJ, Weichenhain B, Baumann G. The value of colour duplex ultrasound in the diagnosis of insufficiency of perforating veins: prospective study of 94 patients (in German). Vasa 1994;23:109–113.
10. Pierik EG, Toonder IM, van Urk H, Wittens CH. Validation of duplex sonography in detecting competent and incompetent perforating veins in patients with venous ulceration of the lower leg. J Vasc Surg 1997;26:49–52.
11. Evans AJ, Sostman HD, Knelson MH, Spritzer CE, Newman GE, Paine SS, Beam CA. Detection of deep vein thrombosis: prospective comparison of MR imaging with contrast venography. AJR 1994;161:131–139.
12. Gartenschlager M, Klose KJ, Schmidt JA. Dignosis of floating venous thrombi by spiral CT phlebography (in German) Rofo 1996;164:376–381.
13. Whitehead S, Lemenson G, Browse NL. The assessment of calf pump function by isotope plethysmography. Br J Surg 1983;70:675–679.
14. Rulli F, Muzi M, Giordano A, Galli G, Zanella A. Radionuclide venography and the surgical treatment of chronic venous disease of the lower extremity. Ann It Chir 1997;68:61–64.

10 Venous Symptoms and Signs and the Results of Duplex Ultrasound: Do They Agree?

Andrew W. Bradbury

Introduction

Venous disease of the legs is common and comprises a wide spectrum of clinical severity from asymptomatic incompetence through hyphen-web, reticular and trunk varices to the skin changes of chronic venous insufficiency (CVI) and chronic venous ulceration (CVU) [1]. In the UK, more than 50 000 varicose vein (VV) operations are performed each year [2] and the direct annual health care costs of treating leg ulceration are estimated at £400–600 million [3]. In most developed countries venous disease accounts for 1–2% of total direct health care spending [4–6]. The indirect financial costs of venous disease are unknown but are almost certainly several-fold higher. It is perhaps surprising, therefore, how little information is available in the literature concerning the relationships between: (1) the presence of "venous" symptoms and objective evidence of venous disease on clinical examination (signs); (2) clinical status (symptoms and signs) and the results of venous investigations aimed at defining, functionally and anatomically, the pattern and severity of the venous disease; and (3) surgical intervention and improvements in clinical status and the results of such investigations.

Only when these questions are satisfactorily answered will it be possible to determine with certainty if, when, in whom and how health care resources should be directed towards the investigation and treatment of venous disease. For the present, the aim of this chapter to is examine how the results of venous investigations, specifically duplex ultrasonography, relate to the clinical status of the patient; and how duplex ultrasonography might provide added value in the assessment and treatment of patients with VVs, with or without the skin changes of CVI, and CVU.

Why Perform Investigations in Patients with Venous Disease?

Virtually every patient referred to a vascular surgeon with suspected venous disease, whether it be thrombo-embolic, VVs or CVI will undergo some form of investigation in addition to the normal clinical assessment. The most obvious conclusion to be drawn from this observation is that most surgeons regard history and examination alone to be inadequate, even potentially misleading, in the evaluation of venous pathology. By arranging for one or more investigations to be conducted, the surgeon hopes to be able to answer, more accurately than would be possible on the basis of clinical assessment alone, the following questions: (1) Are the symptoms of which the patient complains attributable to venous disease; and if not, what other pathological processes may be involved? (2) Is the patient's pattern of venous disease amenable to surgery and, if so, what operation should the patient have?

Although it is not common practice to perform investigations pre-operatively and then repeat them post-operatively for comparison, there may be merit in doing so for both clinical and academic reasons. Thus, apart from serving as a quality control [7,8], it may allow the surgeon to determine in the short term whether or not the patient will benefit from the operation in the medium and long term [9]. Such information may allow early decisions to be made regarding future prognosis as well as the requirement for, and nature of, any further follow-up or intervention. This will be discussed in more detail in later sections.

The Relationship Between Duplex Sonography and Other Forms of Non-invasive Venous Investigation

The relationships between the results of various forms of venous investigation and clinical status are the subject of a large literature in which the conclusions drawn are often conflicting [10,11]. Most observers have reported a reasonable degree of agreement between the extent and duration of venous reflux as defined by duplex ultrasonography and the results of air plethysmography (APG) [12–14], photoplethysmography (PPG) [15]; and foot volumetry (FV). Others have been less impressed by their concordance and advocate that most, if not all, patients should have both duplex ultrasonography and a plethysmographic test performed as part of their venous assessment [16,17]. Invasive studies such as various forms of phlebography and direct ambulatory venous pressure (AVP) measurements, long thought to represent the "gold standard", are now rarely employed, even for research purposes. Although understandable for reasons of convenience and patient comfort, in scientific terms this is perhaps a regrettable development as:

1. Not all investigators have found a good agreement between the results of non-invasive studies and AVP [18,19].
2. Non-invasive studies, including duplex ultrasonography, may not be able to distinguish patients with the symptoms and signs of different grades of CVI [20] with the same accuracy as, for example, AVP measurements [21].
3. Duplex ultrasonography may not be able to distinguish post-thrombotic from so-called primary deep venous incompetence as accurately as phlebography [22]. As these two disease processes may have different natural histories, prognoses and treatments this may be a serious deficiency of duplex ultrasound [23,24].

Nevertheless, duplex ultrasonography has virtually replaced all other forms of non-invasive venous assessment in day-to-day clinical practice, with plethysmographic tests being reserved for research purposes in most hospitals. For these reasons, as well as constraints on space, this chapter will focus on the relationship between the anatomical and functional information provided by duplex ultrasonography and the clinical status of the patient – both subjectively in terms of the leg symptoms they report, and objectively in terms of the physical signs of venous disease observed during clinical examination.

The Edinburgh Vein Study Methodology

Much of the data presented in this chapter originates from a preliminary analysis of the results of the Edinburgh Vein Study (EVS) performed by Dr. A.J. Lee, the study statistician. For that reason the EVS methodology is now briefly described. The study is described in greater detail in Chapter 1. The EVS is a cross-sectional population survey of an age-stratified random sample of men and women aged 18–64 years selected from the computerised age-sex registers of 12 general practices, whose catchment areas were geographically and socio-economically distributed throughout Edinburgh. Subjects were examined clinically, completed a self-administered questionnaire and underwent duplex ultrasound examination of both legs. Venous disease was classified and graded according to the Basle Study [25]. A total of 1566 subjects attended for examination (867 women and 699 men). The mean age of participants was 44.8 years for women and 45.8 years for men ($p > 0.05$). There was no significant difference between right and left legs with regard to any of the variables described in this chapter.

What Constitutes a Normal Venous Duplex Examination?

Before considering the relationships between the results of venous duplex ultrasonography and the present and future clinical status of patients with simple VVs and CVI, it is first necessary to define what constitutes a normal duplex examination. This is perhaps a more difficult question to answer than would at first appear to be the case as, to date, most duplex-based studies have involved the examination of patients presenting with venous disease and not normal subjects.

Professor Nicolaides' group from St. Mary's Hospital, London [26], used colour-flow duplex ultrasound to study of the lower limbs of 28 vascular surgeons (56 legs) and 25 normal volunteers (50 legs) who had no clinical signs or symptoms suggestive of venous disease, no history of deep or superficial venous thrombosis, and who had not undergone any venous operation or injection sclerotherapy. The authors defined pathological reflux as that which exceeded 1 s. Venous reflux was found in 29 limbs (52%) of vascular surgeons, and in 16 limbs (32%) in the control group ($p = 0.04$, χ^2 test). In the vascular surgeons, pathological reflux was present in both the superficial veins only in 22 of 56 limbs (39%), in deep and/or perforating veins only in 4 of 56 limbs (7%) and in the superficial and deep systems in 3 of 56 limbs (5%). In the control group superficial reflux was found in 9 of 50 limbs (18%), deep and/or perforator reflux in 3 of 50 limbs (6%) and superficial and deep venous reflux in 4 of 50 limbs (8%). Superficial reflux was thus present in 45% of limbs (25/56) of vascular surgeons compared with 26% of controls (13/50) ($p = 0.05$, χ^2 test). Long saphenous vein (LSV) reflux in the lower thigh accounted for 48% of superficial reflux in vascular surgeons and 39% in control subjects. The authors concluded that venous reflux is found more frequently in symptom-free vascular surgeons than in symptom-free age- and sex-matched controls. Perhaps more importantly, the study also demonstrates that, although deep venous reflux exceeding 1.0 s is unusual in symptom-free adult males, superficial reflux, predominantly in the lower LSV, is frequently present.

Professor Burnand's group at St. Thomas' Hospital, London, having observed that reverse flow > 0.5 s had become established in the literature as the cut-off for pathological reflux [27], but also that several published series had demonstrated a proportion of "normal" subjects to have flow exceeding this limit, performed a duplex assessment of the deep veins of 61 subjects who had normal venous function [28]. Their subjects had no history of venous thrombo-embolic disease, significant lower limb trauma, abdominal surgery, or symptoms or signs of venous disease. Furthermore, they had normal venous function on foot volumetry. Subjects were examined in three position: 10° and 45° of head-up tilt and standing. The duration of reverse flow was recorded following sudden release of cuff compression (Table 10.1) and during a Valsalva manoeuvre. Ninety-five per cent of all reverse flow was less than 0.65 s and 93% was within the 0.5 s cut-off. Importantly, reverse flow of more than 0.5 s was never observed in the posterior tibial veins of standing subjects, nor was it observed in the popliteal vein of any subject during a Valsalva manoeuvre. The authors concluded that reverse flow exceeding 0.5 s could not be used as a marker of deep venous disease in the superficial femoral vein, where a cut-off of 1.0 s might be more informative, but that in the popliteal and posterior tibial veins they could support the use of a 0.5 s cut-off provided that the patient was examined in the erect position and that a Valsalva manoeuvre was used to elicit reverse flow. Other workers have suggested 0.3 s [29] and confirmed 0.5 s [30,31] to be reliable cut-off points for defining abnormality. They have also stressed the influence of the subject's position, and how the reverse flow is elicited, on the duration of reflux observed.

The EVS is the first study to have used duplex ultrasonography to examine the venous systems of a randomly selected cross-section of the adult population and has confirmed that the prevalence of trunk varices [32], as well as the prevalence of significant reflux on duplex ultrasonography, is high. Thus, 284 of 699 (39.7%) male and 274 of 867 (32.2%) female subjects had trunk varices on clinical examination and duplex ultrasound revealed the presence superficial venous reflux ≥ 0.5 s in 18.6% of subjects. Superficial and deep reflux exceeding 1.0 s was found in 17.7% and 5% of subjects respectively (Table 10.2). However, when subjects with and without clinically apparent venous disease were separated, relatively few subjects with signs of venous disease were found to have superficial (or deep) reflux ≥ 0.5 s (Table 10.3). The only exception to this was in the LSV of the lower thigh, where prolonged reflux was frequently observed in the absence of obvious varices. The reasons for this remain unclear but, as similar data were reported in the St. Mary' s study described above, this may be a genuine finding.

It would seem, therefore, that in a non-patient population there is reasonably good agreement between a duplex scan which fails to demonstrate reflux ≥ 0.5 s in any superficial or deep venous segment, a normal clinical appearance of the leg and an absence of lower limb venous symptoms.

Table 10.1. Duration of deep venous reflux on duplex ultrasonography following removal of cuff compression in 61 limbs with normal venous function

Venous segment	Reflux (s)		
	10° head-up	45° head-up	Standing
SFV	0.21 (0–0.18)	0.14 (0.04–2.14)	0.10 (0–1.36)
PV above knee	0.15 (0–1.02)	0.13 (0–0.68)	0.10 (0–0.75)
PV below knee	0.15 (0.04–1.95)	0.13 (0.07--1.10)	0.10 (0–1.03)
PTV	0.08 (0–0.67)	0.07 (0–0.56)	0.09 (0–0.49)

After [28].
Values are the median (range).
SFV, superficial femoral vein; PV, popliteal vein; PTV, posterior tibial vein.

Table 10.2. Prevalence (%) of reflux ≥ 0.5 s and > 1.0 s in the legs of subjects in the Edinburgh Vein Study

Venous segment	Right leg		Left leg		Both legs	
	≥ 0.5 s (%)	> 1.0 s (%)	≥ 0.5 s (%)	> 1.0 s (%)	≥ 0.5 s (%)	> 1.0 s (%)
Superficial system						
LSV upper thigh	10.0	9.6	10.8	10.1	4.8	4.6
LSV lower thigh	18.6	17.7	17.5	16.7	8.0	7.5
SSV	4.6	3.7	5.6	4.2	1.6	1.1
Deep system						
CFV	7.8	2.1	8.0	2.1	2.5	0.6
SFV upper thigh	5.2	1.2	4.7	1.3	1.7	0.3
SFV lower thigh	6.6	2.5	6.4	2.7	2.2	0.8
PV above knee	12.3	5.0	11.0	5.3	3.9	1.3
PV below knee	11.3	4.7	9.5	4.6	3.3	1.0

CFV, common femoral vein; SFV, superficial femoral vein; PV, popliteal vein; LSV, long saphenous vein; SSV short saphenous vein.

Table 10.3. Duration of reflux (s) in Edinburgh Vein Study subjects with and without clinically apparent venous disease

Venous segment	No venous disease ($n = 861$)[a]			Venous disease ($n = 579$)[b]		
	Median	IQR	95th centile	Median	IQR	95th centile
Superficial system						
LSV upper thigh	0.00	0.00–0.10	0.29	0.15	0.00–4.3	8.00
LSV lower thigh	0.11	0.05–0.16	6.46	2.30	0.10–6.97	8.00
SSV	0.10	0.00–0.14	0.27	0.13	0.10–0.24	4.08
Deep system						
CFV	0.09	0.00–0.26	0.54	0.18	0.00–0.48	1.63
SFV upper thigh	0.11	0.00–0.25	0.52	0.15	0.00–0.33	1.14
SFV lower thigh	0.13	0.04–0.25	0.53	0.18	0.06–0.40	2.88
PV above knee	0.17	0.10–0.32	0.84	0.25	0.13–0.68	2.63
PV below knee	0.14	0.10–0.28	0.88	0.20	0.12–0.53	2.30

IQR, inter-quartile range; CFV, common femoral vein; SFV, superficial femoral vein; PV, popliteal vein; LSV, long saphenous vein; SSV, short saphenous vein.

[a]No clinically apparent trunk varices, perforators or skin changes of chronic venous insufficiency (CVI) and a maximum of grade I hyphen-web and/or reticular varices.

[b]Patients with clinically apparent trunk varices and/or skin changes of CVI.

Varicose Veins

The Basis for Treatment

Although many tens of thousands of operations are performed in the UK each year for simple (CEAP class 2) VVs, there is little evidence to support the contentions that:

1. Isolated and otherwise uncomplicated trunk VVs:
   (i) are the source of significant lower limb symptoms;
   (ii) predispose to the skin changes of CVI in a significant proportion of patients.
2. Operating on simple VVs leads to a significant amelioration of symptoms or clinically meaningful improvement in quality of life (QoL) [33].
3. Operating on simple VVs in the absence of skin changes will reduce the socioeconomic burden of venous ulceration in the long term when compared with a strategy of postponing surgery until the early skin changes of CVI become apparent.

4. Even in the presence of established CVI, including ulceration, surgery confers additional clinical and health economic benefits over and above best medical therapy.

This being the case, it is perhaps not surprising that health service funding bodies are becoming increasingly reluctant to pay for the surgical treatment of venous disease. Until the benefits (or lack of benefits) of VV surgery are satisfactorily demonstrated by long-term epidemiological and clinical studies, the surgeon must for the present attempt to target limited health care resources on those patients whom he or she believes have the most to gain from an operation. But, which patients with VVs merit surgical intervention and which do not? Should the decision to operate be based upon the patient's age; the nature, severity and chronicity of symptoms; or the extent and severity of trunk VVs on clinical examination? Can duplex ultrasonography aid clinical decision-making by defining those patterns of reflux most likely to give rise to symptoms in the present, and skin changes in the future?

A thorough understanding of the relationships between the patient's symptoms and signs and the results of duplex ultrasound is required to answer these clinically important questions.

"Venous" Symptoms and the Presence of VVs on Clinical Examination

Is there good agreement between the presence and severity of leg symptoms and the pattern and severity of trunk VVs on clinical examination in patients? Although many and various lower limb symptoms have been attributed, rightly or wrongly, to the presence of venous disease, few studies have addressed this clinically important issue.

The EVS has demonstrated the prevalence of lower limb symptoms in the general population to be extremely high, particularly in women (Fig. 10.1). On clinical examination the prevalence of trunk varices is equally high, especially in men. What is the concordance between those with symptoms and those with varices? How is the surgeon to know whether a particular patient's symptoms are truly venous in nature and, crucially, whether an operation will relieve them?

Most surgeons recognise that a significant proportion of patients with VVs seek an opinion because they are primarily concerned about the cosmetic appearance of their veins, but also that many such patients fear they may be denied treatment, or receive a lower priority, unless they complain of one of more lower limb symptoms. Many surgeons would also accept the fact that, even amongst those they consider to have "genuine" symptoms, frequently the only way of establishing whether the patient will benefit from surgery is to operate and await the outcome. This is an unsatisfactory situation for many reasons and a better understanding of the relationship between symptoms and signs in patients with VVs may allow scarce resources to be more appropriately focused.

Are some lower limb "venous" symptoms "hard" and others "soft"? Does the significance of a particular symptom depend upon the age and the gender of the patient? Can duplex ultrasound be used to aid clinical decision-making in this situation? The EVS has provided unique data which address some of these questions.

The prevalence of venous symptoms by presence and grade of trunk varices in the right legs of male and female subjects is shown in Table 10.4. Because of the higher prevalence of symptoms and trunk VVs in older subjects, the data have been age-adjusted to allow direct comparison of male and female subjects. In male subjects "itching" was the only symptom significantly related to the presence of trunk varices. However, despite the statistically significant result for linear trend, the observation may

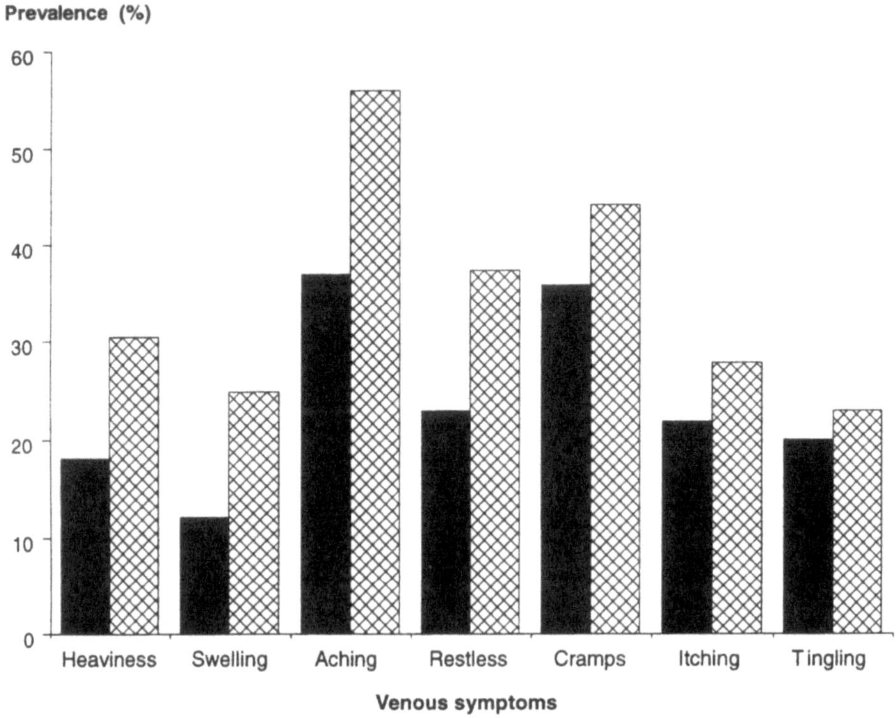

Fig. 10.1. Prevalence (%) of lower limb symptoms in male and female subjects of the Edinburgh Vein Study. *Black bars*, male subjects; *hatched bars*, female subjects. Gender differences were significant for all symptoms ($p \leq 0.01$) except for tingling ($p > 0.05$).

be of limited clinical value as only a third of patients with grade 2 and 3 trunk varices had "itching" compared with 15% of men who had no trunk VVs. In female subjects, heaviness and tension, aching and itching were all significantly related to the presence of varices. While the statistical strength of these relationships is greater than for the male subjects, the clinical value of the observations is again doubtful. In summary, therefore, while trunk VVs appear to be commoner in men, lower limb symptoms are much commoner in women. Furthermore, the presence of such symptoms is more closely associated with the presence of VVs in women than in men. Thus, not only do many asymptomatic subjects have trunk varices on clinical examination, but conversely others, especially men, experience a whole range of lower limb "venous" symptoms despite having little or no evidence of venous pathology on clinical examination. Such patients must, one presumes, have either deep venous, or non-venous, pathology to account for their symptoms.

"Venous" Symptoms and the Presence of Reflux on Duplex Ultrasonography in Patients with VVs

If there is a poor relationship between the presence of lower limb symptoms and the presence of trunk VVs on clinical examination, can duplex ultrasonography be used

Table 10.4. Age-adjusted prevalence (%) of venous symptoms by presence and grade of trunk varices in the right legs of male and female subjects in the Edinburgh Vein Study

"Venous" symptoms	None	Grade 1	Grades 2 + 3	p value[a]
Male subjects	($n = 476$)	($n = 191$)	($n = 32$)	
Heaviness/tension	14.1	15.7	18.7	NS
Feeling of swelling	6.1	7.9	14.1	NS
Aching	28.4	27.0	27.0	NS
Restless legs	19.6	18.7	18.5	NS
Cramps	30.9	31.7	37.1	NS
Itching	15.8	18.3	37.5	= 0.011
Tingling	12.4	13.2	15.8	NS
Female subjects	($n = 665$)	($n = 174$)	($n = 30$)	
Heaviness/tension	22.2	36.0	54.7	≤ 0.001
Feeling of swelling	17.6	21.6	24.6	NS
Aching	44.9	61.7	63.2	≤ 0.001
Restless legs	32.6	31.8	49.6	NS
Cramps	37.6	42.9	45.2	NS
Itching	20.6	27.5	38.0	= 0.005
Tingling	15.6	17.9	17.4	NS

[a]Test for linear trend; NS, not significant at the 5% level.

to aid clinical decision-making by identifying: (1) patterns of superficial reflux most likely to be associated with symptoms (and signs) and thus, perhaps, those patients most likely to benefit from its surgical correction; (2) patients whose symptoms may be due to deep venous disease; and (3) patients whose symptoms are likely to be of a non-venous aetiology?

Labropoulos and colleagues [34] used colour-flow duplex ultrasonography to define the pattern of venous reflux in 255 limbs (217 patients) with superficial venous reflux but normal deep and perforating veins. In 123 limbs (48.2%) reflux was confined to the LSV, in 83 limbs (32.6%) to the short saphenous vein (SSV), and in 49 limbs there was reflux exceeding 1 s in both systems. The authors conducted a careful study of the relationship between venous symptoms (ache and swelling) and signs (skin changes) and the pattern of superficial reflux (Table 10.5).

Ache and swelling were most clearly associated with full-length LSV reflux. By contrast, skin changes were related to below-knee LSV reflux, regardless of whether the LSV in the thigh was affected. Ache and swelling were also common in patients with SSV incompetence. Perhaps surprisingly, the prevalence of these symptoms was not increased by the presence of coexisting reflux in the gastrocnemial veins. The highest incidence of symptoms (and signs) was found in patients with full-length LSV and SSV reflux. However, even in the group with maximal superficial venous incompetence, the prevalence of ulceration was only 14%, 1 in 5 patients had normal skin and 1 in 10 was symptom-free.

Preliminary analysis of data from the EVS has also provided new insights into the relationships between symptoms and the presence of deep and superficial reflux on duplex ultrasonography, and suggests that a duplex examination may provide additional, clinically useful information regarding the aetiology of certain symptoms (Table 10.6). Thus, in men, whereas only itching was related to the presence of trunk varices on clinical examination, a feeling of swelling, of restless legs and of itching was related to the presence of superficial reflux ≥ 0.5 s on duplex ultrasonography. Furthermore, swelling and restless legs were significantly associated with the presence of deep venous reflux. In female subjects, heaviness, tension, swelling and itching were all significantly

Table 10.5. The prevalence (%) of symptoms and signs in relation to the pattern of superficial reflux

Pattern of reflux	Ache n (%)	Swelling n (%)	Skin changes n (%)	Ulceration n (%)
Reflux confined to LSV				
LSV AK only ($n = 24$)	11 (46)	8 (33)	1 (4)	0
LSV BK only ($n = 21$)	12 (57)	13 (62)	10 (48)	0
LSV full length ($n = 78$)	63 (81)	71 (91)	42 (58)	6 (8)
Total ($n = 123$)	86 (70)	92 (75)	53 (43)	6 (5)
Reflux confined to SSV				
Giacomini vein only ($n = 2$)	0	0	0	0
SSV only ($n = 46$)	29 (63)	36 (78)	24 (52)	0
MGV and/or LGV only ($n = 9$)	5 (56)	2 (22)	0	0
SSV + Giacomini ($n = 11$)	7 (64)	9 (82)	2 (18)	1 (9)
SSV + MGV or LGV ($n = 13$)	8 (62)	10 (72)	5 (38)	1 (8)
Total ($n = 83$)	49 (59)	57 (69)	31 (37)	2 (2)
Reflux in LSV and SSV				
SFJ + SSV ($n = 1$)	1	0	0	0
LSV-AK + SSV ($n = 5$)	3	4	1	0
LSV-BK + SSV ($n = 16$)	11 (69)	12 (75)	7 (44)	0
LSV-AK+BK + SSV ($n = 3$)	1	2	1	0
SFJ + LSV-AK + LSV ($n = 2$)	1	1	1	0
SFJ + LSV-AK+BK + SSV ($n = 22$)	19 (86%)	20 (91)	16 (73)	3 (14)
Total ($n = 49$)	36 (73%)	39 (80)	26 (53)	3 (6)

After [34].
LSV, long saphenous vein; SFJ, saphenofemoral junction; AK, above knee; BK, below knee; SSV, short saphenous vein; MGV, medial gastrocnemial vein; LGV, lateral gastrocnemial vein.

Table 10.6. The relationship between the presence of reflux ≥ 0.5 s on duplex ultrasonography and the presence of lower limb symptoms in the right legs of male and female subjects in the Edinburgh Vein Study

Symptom	Males		Females	
	Superficial venous reflux ≥ 0.5 s	Deep venous reflux ≥ 0.5 s	Superficial venous reflux ≥ 0.5 s	Deep venous reflux ≥ 0.5 s
Heaviness/tension	NS	NS	0.009	NS
Feeling of swelling	0.002	0.054	0.004	NS
Aching	NS	NS	0.045	0.059
Restless legs	0.052	0.03	NS	0.061
Cramps	NS	NS	0.057	0.044
Itching	0.033	NS	NS	NS
Tingling	NS	NS	NS	NS

NS, not significant at the 10% level.

associated with the presence of VVs on examination, and all but itching were associated with superficial reflux on duplex ultrasonography. Deep and superficial reflux in female subjects were also associated with the presence of cramps and aching. Further analysis examining the relationships between combinations of symptoms and the severity and pattern of reflux on duplex sonography is in progress.

Symptoms, Patterns of Reflux and the Development of Skin Changes

Using these and other data, the experienced clinician may be able relate age, gender, nature and severity of symptoms, signs and duplex findings in such as way as to make possible the identification of those patients who are most likely to benefit from VV surgery in terms of symptom relief.

But, which patients should be operated on to prevent the development of skin changes in the future? The fundamental question is whether operating on certain patients with VVs in the absence of skin changes will reduce the socio-economic burden of venous ulceration in the long term when compared with a strategy of postponing surgery until early skin changes become apparent. Clearly, if the answer were "yes" then it would be important to identify high-risk patients and offer them early prophylactic surgery.

There are no long-term epidemiological or clinical data presently available in the literature which can help answer this important question directly, although it is hoped that by conducting a long term of follow-up of the subjects within the EVS it will be possible to gain new insights into the natural history of VV disease, In the meantime, the issue must be addressed indirectly by defining the patterns of symptoms and reflux in patients who already have established CVI, on the basis that patients with simple VVs who have similar patterns of symptoms and reflux are more likely to be at increased risk of CVI in the future.

Symptoms

The relationship between the age-adjusted prevalence of various lower limb symptoms and the presence of skin changes on clinical examination in male and female subjects of the EVS is shown in Figs. 10.2 and 10.3. In male subjects only aching was significantly related to skin changes while there was a trend towards to a higher prevalence of skin changes in subjects complaining of heaviness. In females only heaviness was significantly related to the presence of skin changes but there was a trend with regard to all the other symptoms except tingling. At first sight, the almost complete absence of a statistical relationship between symptoms and skin changes is perhaps surprising. However, this was a population-based study and only 55 male and 38 female subjects had any evidence of CVI; and only 10 subjects had a history of ulceration. Nevertheless, these data do suggest that in patients with simple VVs no particular pattern of symptoms can be used to identify those patients at risk of developing skin changes in the future.

Patterns of Reflux

The St. Mary's group [35] have used duplex ultrasonography to examine the anatomical extent of pathological reflux in a large cohort of patients with increasing clinical severity of disease (Table 10.7). The development of skin changes and ulceration was associated with an increasing prevalence of mixed superficial and deep venous reflux. Amongst those with predominantly superficial disease there was an increase in multi-level disease affecting both the long and short saphenous systems. With respect to the deep system, skin changes and ulceration appear to associated with popliteal and crural, particularly posterior tibial vein, reflux. Other workers have reported similar results [36–38]. However, one must also note than, even in patients with apparently maximal superficial and deep venous reflux on duplex scanning, less than half had any evidence of skin changes. This may be because severity of reflux is only one of many factors which determine whether skin changes and ulceration develop; other, as yet ill-defined, microcirculatory or genetic influences may be equally important. Alternatively, it could be argued that reflux is important but that duplex ultrasonography is not the best way of quantifying it. Thus, the risk of future skin changes in patients with simple VVs may

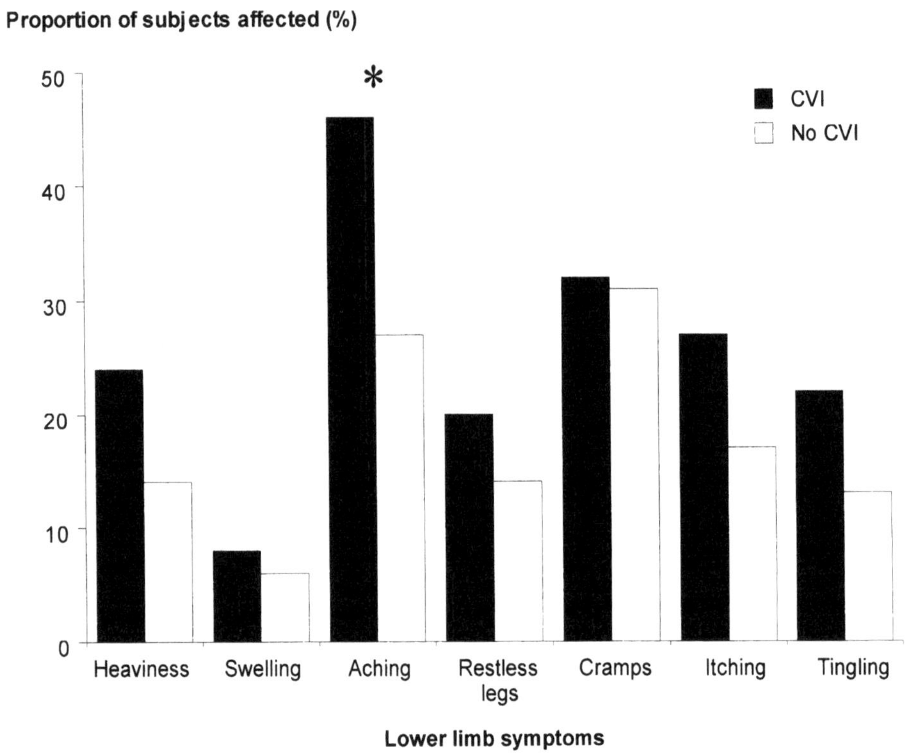

Fig. 10.2. The relationship between the age-adjusted prevalence (%) of lower limb symptoms and the presence of skin changes of chronic venous insufficiency (CVI) in male subjects in the Edinburgh Vein Study. * $p < 0.05$ by χ^2 test. No skin changes, 664 subjects; grade 1, 41 subjects; grades 2+3, 14 subjects.

be better defined by the venous filling as determined by plethysmography than by the anatomical pattern of reflux as shown by duplex ultrasonography [39,40].

The Leicester group have also used duplex ultrasonography to determine the pattern of venous reflux in 274 limbs and then employed multivariate logistic regression analysis to relate these finding to the clinical status of the leg in terms of the presence of ulceration [41]. Superficial femoral, profunda femoris and short saphenous reflux was not related to clinical status, while reflux in the common femoral, popliteal and long saphenous veins was. The adverse clinical impact of popliteal vein reflux was particularly apparent; the tibial veins were not specifically examined.

Conclusions

From the above data a number of tentative conclusions can be drawn regarding the relationship between symptoms, signs and duplex finding in patients with VVs:

1. A duplex scan which fails to demonstrate reflux exceeding 0.5 s can be considered normal, although this does not mean that subjects with superficial reflux exceeding 0.5 s will necessarily have symptoms or signs of venous disease.
2. The great majority of patients with clinically apparent trunk varices can be shown

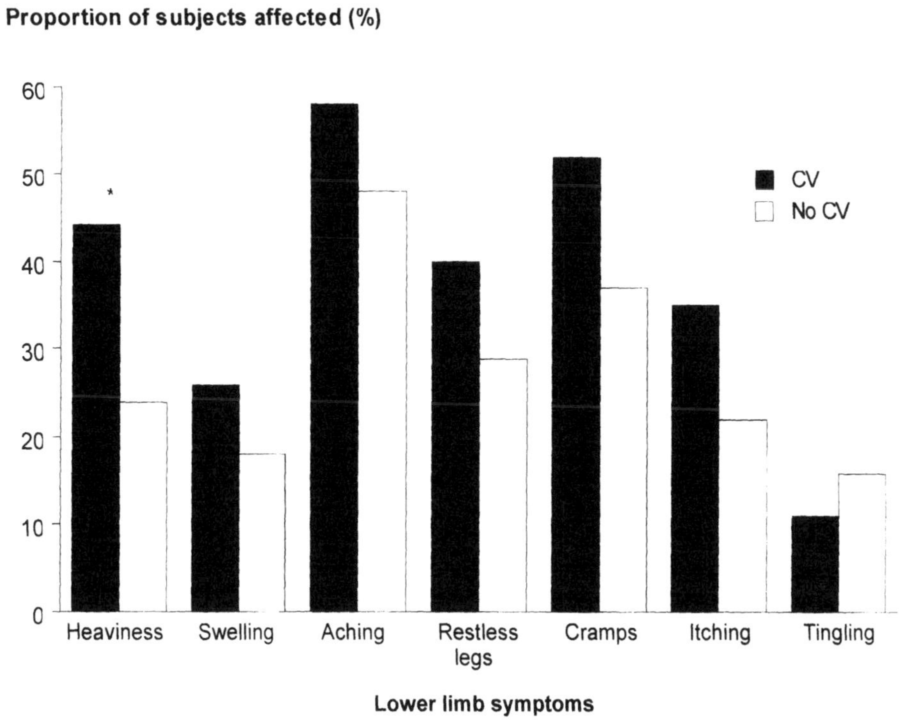

Fig. 10.3. The relationship between the age-adjusted prevalence (%) of lower limb symptoms and the presence of skin changes of CVI in female subjects in the Edinburgh Vein Study. *$p < 0.05$ by χ^2 test. No skin changes, 829 subjects; grade 1, 32 subjects; grades 2+3, 6 subjects.

on duplex ultrasonography to have reflux exceeding 0.5 s somewhere in their superficial venous system.

3. The prevalence of trunk varices is slightly higher in men but the prevalence of lower limb "venous" symptoms is very much higher in women.
4. In general there is a poor agreement between symptoms and signs in patients presenting with VVs, although:
   (i) there is a closer association between symptoms and presence of varices in women than in men;
   (ii) some symptoms appear more closely associated with venous disease than others.
5. There is a better agreement between symptoms and reflux as defined by duplex ultrasonography than there is between symptoms and examination findings.
6. There is a poor agreement between the presence of skin changes and symptoms in patients with VVs.
7. There is a good agreement between certain patterns of deep and superficial reflux on duplex and the presence of skin changes in patients who present with VVs [42]. However, in patients with VVs and no skin changes, a functional test may be a better predictor than duplex ultrasonography alone of whether skin changes will develop in the future.

Table 10.7. The site and extent of reflux in patients with increasing clinical severity of venous disease

Site of reflux	Normal (%)	VV (%)	Skin changes (%)	Ulcer (%)	Total (%)
	(*n* = 174)	(*n* =145)	(*n* = 155)	(*n* = 120)	(*n* = 594)
Superficial only	7	81	23	18	31
Perforator only	0	0	1	1	1
Deep only	2	3	5	4	3
Superficial and perforator	0	2	12	19	8
Superficial and deep	1	8	21	13	10
Perforator and deep	0	0	1	2	1
Superficial and perforator and deep	0	0	34	39	17
Normal	91	7	4	3	30
Extent of superficial reflux where present	(*n* = 13)	(*n* = 131)	(*n* = 138)	(*n* = 108)	(*n* = 390)
LSV-AK	23	20	14	10	15
LSV-BK	38	21	21	20	22
LSV full length	15	26	30	34	30
SSV	23	17	15	15	16
SSV + LSV-AK	0	2	2	3	2
SSV + LSV-BK	0	5	7	6	54
SSV + LSV full length	0	10	12	12	11
Extent of deep reflux where present	(*n* = 4)	(*n* = 17)	(*n* = 109)	(*n* = 89)	(*n* = 219)
Common femoral vein	25	18	16	12	15
Superficial femoral vein	0	6	9	8	8
Popliteal vein	0	29	31	36	32
Crural veins	75	47	44	44	45

After [35].
Abbreviations as in Table 5.

Chronic Venous Ulceration

The Basis for Treatment

The role of the surgeon in the management of CVU has yet to be defined because a randomised controlled trial of medical versus surgical therapy has not been conducted. At present, however, three patient groups can be distinguished on the basis of duplex ultrasound [43]:

Group I: isolated superficial reflux. Uncontrolled data suggest that saphenous surgery alone will augment healing and reduce recurrence [23]. Sub-fascial endoscopic perforator surgery (SEPS) probably confers no additional benefit as most incompetent medial calf perforating veins (IPV) regain competence following superficial surgery only (W.P. Stuart, personal communication).

Group II: Superficial and deep reflux. There may be a role for superficial venous surgery in this group. In the presence of deep venous disease, saphenous surgery does not restore competence to IPV and there may be a role for SEPS.

Group III: Isolated deep venous reflux. Attempts to restore deep venous competence surgically have not been widely taken up and remain experimental [44]. However, there may be a role for SEPS in preventing the transmission of deep venous pressure to the skin of the gaiter area.

As in the case of VVs by examining the relationship between symptoms, signs and the patterns of reflux in patients with venous ulceration, it may be possible to identify those patients who have the most to gain from surgical intervention.

The Relationship Between Symptoms and Duplex Findings in Patients with CVU

One might imagine that the relationship between symptoms and reflux in patients with CVU, particularly those in whom ulceration has occurred as part of the post-thrombotic syndrome, would be more straightforward than is the case in patients with simple VVs. However, in a study from this unit, the severity of symptoms and signs in 111 limbs (107 patients) with a history of phlebographically proven deep venous thrombosis showed no significant relationship with functional abnormalities detected by foot volumetry [45]. Furthermore. although patients with severe symptoms were more likely to have multi-segment deep vein reflux and/or combined long and short saphenous reflux on duplex ultrasonography, this trend did not attain statistical significance. There would appear to be a poor level of agreement between the severity of so-called post-thrombotic symptoms and objective evidence of deep and superficial venous disease following proven deep venous thrombosis, although in this study 8 patients with normal duplex scans were all symptom free. Again, these data can be interpreted in two ways. Firstly, it may be that reflux is only one of several factors that determine the presence and severity of symptoms in this patient group. Alternatively, it may be that duplex ultrasonography is not the best way of defining that reflux and that phlebography, AVP or a plethysmographic test would be more informative.

Reflux on Duplex Ultrasonography and Future Prognosis

As well as allowing the surgeon to tailor the operation to the patient's needs, there are data to suggest that defining the pattern of disease by means of duplex ultrasonography may provide important prognostic information with regard to the patient's response to both medical and surgical intervention.

In a recent study the relationship between deep and superficial reflux and the healing of venous ulceration in 155 patients treated non-operatively with compression bandaging was studied. At 24 weeks, 104 (67%) of ulcers had healed. There was no significant difference in the patterns of either deep or superficial reflux between healed and non-healed ulcers except with respect to the popliteal vein. In ulcers that healed, 39 (38%) of duplex scans indicated competence (reflux < 0.5 s) of the above-knee popliteal vein compared with 5 (10%) in the non-healing group ($p < 0.001$, χ^2 test). Similarly, 43 scans (42%) demonstrated below-knee popliteal vein competence in the ulcers that subsequently healed compared with only 5 (10%) in the legs that did not heal ($p < 0.001$, χ^2 test) [46]. These data suggest that the presence of popliteal vein reflux is an important adverse prognostic factor in patients with venous ulceration being treated non-operatively. Such information is of immediate relevance to the surgeon when making judgements about whether a particular patient may be managed entirely in the community or in a shared-care environment.

Popliteal vein reflux also appears to affect the outcome after surgical intervention for venous ulceration [47]. In a series of 43 patients undergoing superficial venous surgery and open perforating vein ligation (Linton's procedure) for chronic venous ulceration, 9 developed recurrent ulceration during a median follow-up of 66 (range 18–144) months. Of these, 6 had femoral vein incompetence and all had popliteal vein incompetence on duplex examination. By contrast, of the 34 patients who remained ulcer-free, 5 had femoral vein reflux and only one had popliteal vein reflux. This provides popliteal vein reflux with a positive predictive value for recurrent ulceration of 90%.

The importance of popliteal vein reflux in the development and chronicity of venous ulceration is demonstrated by a further study in which the duplex defined pattern of venous reflux was compared in the affected and non-affected legs of patients with unilateral ulceration [48]. In 54 patients with unilateral ulceration of "pure" venous aetiology, the only difference between the affected and non-affected legs was with respect to the popliteal segment.

Lastly, these data also underline how important it is that, when contemplating trials comparing non-operative and operative interventions for venous ulceration, the randomisation process must ensure that equal numbers of good-risk and bad-risk patients are entered in to each group. Stratifying on the basis of popliteal vein reflux appears to be one means of achieving this.

Conclusions

The following conclusions can be drawn regarding the relationships between the presence of CVU, symptoms and patterns of reflux as defined by duplex ultrasound:

1. There is poor agreement between symptoms and the distribution of venous reflux in patients with the post-thrombotic syndrome, skin changes only, or a history of previous ulceration. Even in those with open ulceration there is significant variation in the level of symptoms such as pain which is not easily explicable on the basis of the extent of venous disease alone. This is an area deserving of further research.
2. Duplex scanning provides invaluable information to the surgeon contemplating superficial venous surgery and SEPS.
3. The presence of popliteal reflux in patients with CVU is an important adverse prognostic factor whether that patient is treated medically with (multi-layer) compression bandaging or by means of surgery.

References

1. Beebe HG. Classification and grading of chronic venous disease in the lower limbs: a consensus statement. Eur J Vasc Endovasc Surg 1996;12:487–492.
2. Department of Health and Social Security. Hospital episode statistics 1987–88. London: DHSS, 1988.
3. Ruckley CV. Socio-economic impact of chronic venous insufficiency and leg ulcers. Angiology 1997;48:67–69.
4. Laing W. Chronic venous diseases of the leg. London: Office of Health Economics, 1992.
5. Bosanquet N, Franks P. Venous disease: the new international challenge. Phlebology 1996;11:6–9.
6. Kistner RL. Definitive diagnosis and definitive treatment in chronic venous disease: a concept whose time has come. J Vasc Surg 1996;24:703–710.
7. Pierik EGJM, Toonder IM, van Urk H, Wittens CHA. Validation of duplex ultrasonography in detecting competent and incompetent perforating veins in patients with venous ulceration of the lower leg. J Vasc Surg 1997;26:49–52.
8. Pierik EGJM, van Urk H, Wittens CHA. Efficacy of subfascial endoscopy in eradicating perforating veins of the lower leg and its relation with venous ulcer healing. J Vasc Surg 1997;26:255–259.
9. Akesson H, Bridin L, Cwikile W, Ohlin P, Plate G. Does the correction of insufficient superficial and perforating veins improve venous function in patients with deep venous insufficiency? Phlebology 1990;5:113–123.
10. Moulton S, Bergan JJ, Beeman S. Gravitational reflux does not correlate with clinical status of venous stasis. Phlebology 1993;8:2–6.
11. McMullen GM, Scott HJ, Coleridge-Smith PD. A comparison of photoplethysmography, Doppler ultrasound and duplex scanning in the assessment of venous insufficiency. Phlebology 1989;4:75–82.

12. Neglen P, Raju S. A rational approach to detection of significant reflux with duplex Doppler scanning and air plethysmography. J Vasc Surg 1993;17:590–595.
13. Bays RA, Healy DA, Atnip RG, Neumyer M, Thiele BL. Validation of air plethysmography, photoplethysmography, and duplex ultrasonography in the evaluation of severe venous stasis. J Vasc Surg 1994;20:721–727.
14. Weingarten MS, Czeredarczuk M, Scovell S, Branas CC, Mignogna GM, Wolferth. A correlation of air plethysmography and colour-flow assisted duplex scanning in the quantification of chronic venous insufficiency. J Vasc Surg 1996;24:750–754.
15. Sarin S, Shields DA, Scurr JH, Coleridge Smith PD. Photoplethysmography: valuable non-invasive tool in the assessment of venous dysfunction. J Vasc Surg 1992;16:154–162.
16. van Bemmelen PS, van Ramshorst B, Eikleboom BC. Photoplethysmography re-examined: lack of correlation with duplex scanning. Surgery 1992;112:544–548.
17. van Bemmelen PS, Mattos MA, Hodgson KJ, Barkmeier DE, Faught WE, Sumner DS. Does air plethysmography correlate with duplex scanning in patients with chronic venous insufficiency? J Vasc Surg 1993;18:796–807.
18. Rosfors S. A methodological study of venous valvular insufficiency and musculovenous pump function of the lower leg. Phlebology 1992;7:12–19.
19. Payne SPK, Thrush AJ, London NJM, Bell PRF, Barrie WW. Venous assessment using air plethysmography: a comparison with clinical examination, ambulatory venous pressure measurement and duplex scanning. Br J Surg 1993;80:967–970.
20. Iafrati MD, Welch H, O'Donnell TF, Belkin M, Umphrey S, McLaughlin R. Correlation of venous non-invasive tests with the Society for Vascular Surgery/International Society for Cardiovascular Surgery clinical classification of chronic venous insufficiency. J Vasc Surg 1994;19:1001–1007.
21. Nicolaides AN, Hussein MK, Szendro G, Christopoulos D, Vasdekis S, Clarke H. The relation of venous ulceration with ambulatory venous pressure measurements. J Vasc Surg 1993;17:414–419.
22. Baker SR, Burnand KG, Sommerville KM, Lea Thomas M, Wilson NM, Browse NL. Comparison of venous reflux assessed by duplex scanning and descending phlebography in chronic venous disease. Lancet 1993;341:400–403.
23. Darke SG, Penfold C. Venous ulceration and saphenous ligation. Eur J Vasc Surg 1992;6:4–9.
24. Janssen MCH, Wollersheim H, van Austen WNJC, de Rooij MJM, Novakova IRO, THien Th. The post-thrombotic syndrome: a review. Phlebology 1996;11:86–94.
25. Widmer LK, editor. Peripheral venous disorders: prevalence and socio-medical importance. Bern: Hans Gruber, 1978:1–90.
26. Labropoulos N, Delis KT, Nicolaides AN. Venous reflux in symptom-free vascular surgeons. J Vasc Surg 1995;22:150–154.
27. van Bemmelen PS, Bedford G, Beach K, Strandness DE. Quantitative segmental evaluation of venous valvular reflux with duplex ultrasound scanning. J Vasc Surg 1989;10:425–431.
28. Lagatolla NRF, Donald A, Lockhart S, Burnand KG. Retrograde flow in the deep veins of subjects with normal venous function. Br J Surg 1997;84:36–39.
29. Araki CT, Back TL, Padberg FT, Thompson PN, Duran WN, Hobson RW. Refinements in the ultrasonic detection of popliteal vein reflux. J Vasc Surg 1993;18:742–728.
30. Sarin S, Sommerville K, Farrah J, Scurr JH, Coleridge Smith PD. Duplex ultrasonography for the assessment of venous valvular function of the lower limb. Br J Surg 1994;81:1591–1595.
31. Masuda EM, Kistner RL, Eklof B. Prospective study of duplex scanning for venous reflux: comparison of Valsalva and pneumatic cuff techniques in the reverse Trendelenberg and standing positions. J Vasc Surg 1994;20:711–720.
32. Callam MJ. Epidemiology of varicose veins. Br J Surg 1994;81:167–173.
33. Baker DM, Turnbull NB, Pearson JCG, Makin GS. How successful is varicose vein surgery? A patient outcome study following varicose vein surgery using the SF-36 health assessment questionnaire. Eur J Vasc Endovasc Surg 1995;9:299–304.
34. Labropoulos N, Leon M, Nicolaides AN, Giannoukas AD, Volteas N, Chan P. Superficial venous insufficiency: correlation of anatomic extent of reflux with clinical symptoms amd signs. J Vasc Surg 1994;20:953–958.
35. Labropoulos N, Delis K, Nicolaides AN, Leon M, Ramasawami G, Volteas N. The role of the distribution and anatomic extent of reflux in the development of signs and symptoms in chronic venous insufficiency. J Vasc Surg 1996;23:504–510.
36. Hanrahan LM, Araki CT, Rodriguez AA, Kechejian GJ, LaMorte WW, Menzoian JO. Distribution of valvular incompetence in patients with venous stasis ulceration. J Vasc Surg 1991;13:805–812.
37. Lees TA, Lambert D. Patterns of venous reflux in limbs with skin changes associated with chronic venous insufficiency. Br J Surg 1993;80:725–728.

38. Myers KA, Ziegenbein RW, Zeng GH, Matthews PG. Duplex ultrasonography scanning for chronic venous disease: patterns of reflux. J Vasc Surg 1995;21:605–612.
39. Vasdekis SN, Clarke GH, Nicolaides AN. Quantification of venous reflux by means of duplex scanning. J Vasc Surg 1989;10:670–677.
40. Nicolaides AN, Sumner DS. Investigation of patients with deep venus thrombosis and chronic venous insufficiency. London: Med-Orion, 1991.
41. Payne SPK, London NJM, Jagger C, Newland CJ, Barrie WW, Bell PRF. Clinical significance of venous reflux detected by duplex scanning. Br J Surg 1994;81:39–41.
42. Sakurai T, Gupta PC, Matsushita M, Nishikimi N, Nimura Y. Correlation of the anatomic distribution of venous reflux with clinical symptoms and venous haemodynamics in primary varicose veins. Br J Surg 1998; in press.
43. Scriven JM, Hartshorne T, Bell PRF, Naylor AR, London NJM. Single-visit venous ulcer assessment clinic: the first year. Br J Surg 1997;84:334–336.
44. Raju S, Fredericks RK. Durability of venous valve reconstruction techniques for "primary" and post-thrombotic reflux. J Vasc Surg 1996;23:357–367.
45. Milne AA, Stonebridge PA, Bradbury AW, Ruckley CV. Venous function and clinical outcome following deep venous thrombosis. Br J Surg 1994;81:847–849.
46. Brittenden J, Bradbury AW, Allan PL, Prescott RJ, Harper DR, Ruckley CV. Popliteal vein reflux reduces the healing of chronic venous ulceration. Br J Surg 1998;85:60–62.
47. Bradbury AW, Stonebridge PA, Callam ML, Ruckley CV, Allan PL. Foot volumetry and duplex ultrasonography after saphenous and sub-fascial perforating vein ligation for recurrent venous ulceration. Br J Surg 1993;80:845–848.
48. Bradbury AW, Brittenden J, Allan PL, Ruckley CV. Comparison of venous reflux in the affected and non-affected leg in patients with unilateral venous ulceration. Br J Surg 1996; 83:5135.

Section III
Clinical Management

11 Compression Therapy: Is It Worthwhile?

H. Partsch

Introduction

Empirical experience shows that compression is a very effective therapy which has been in use for several centuries. Some important mechanisms of its action have only recently been studied and controlled clinical trials to prove its efficacy are sparse. However, compression therapy is not old-fashioned and will certainly remain the basic management for patients with chronic venous disorders of the lower extremities for the foreseeable future.

Types of Compression Therapy

Various modalities of compression are summarised in Table 11.1, and the four main categories of compression material are listed in Table 11.2. *Inelastic bandages* such as

Table 11.1. Types of compression devices

Graduated compression stockings
Custom made
Standard size
Knee length
Thigh length
Compression tights
Bandages
Inelastic
Short-stretch
Medium-stretch
Long-stretch
Single layer
Multi-layer
Intermittent pneumatic compression
Single chamber
Sequential chambers
Foot pump
Lower leg
Full leg
Intermittent static pressure
"Mercury bath"

Table 11.2. Categories of compression material

	Inelastic	Short-stretch	Medium-stretch	Long-stretch
Stretch	0	< 70%	70–140%	>140%
Application	Trained staff	Trained staff	Trained patient	Patient
Stays on the leg	Day and night	Day and night	Daytime	Daytime

zinc plaster (Unna boot), and rigid gaiters such as Circ-Aid, are examples of completely non-elastic material which may remain on the leg for several days. *Elastic bandages* or compression stockings are applied in the morning, preferably before getting up, and are removed before going to bed at night. Several layers of elastic material (*four-layer bandage*) have properties resembling short-stretch material and may also be worn day and night (Fig. 11.1).

What Is the Evidence for Optimal Pressure and Gradients?

Effective Pressure Range

The range of pressure applied during compression therapy covers a very broad spectrum from the 15 mmHg exerted by stockings designed for prophylaxis of deep vein thrombosis (class I according to the CEN, Commission Européen de Normalisation) to the suprasystolic pressure peaks produced by intermittent compression machines such as the "mercury bath" for treating patients with lymphoedema. The pressure measured by different devices changes with the measuring site (radius of the leg segment), body position (lying, sitting, standing) and with the elastic properties of the compression material.

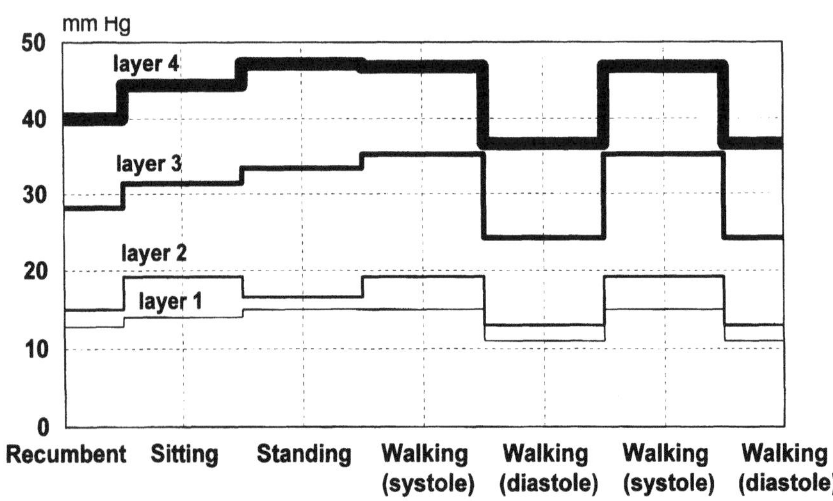

Fig. 11.1. Midcalf pressure measurement using the CCS 1000 instrument [2] after application of each layer of a four-layer bandage. The third and the fourth layers contribute most to the high pressure of the bandage. The large difference between the pressure at muscle systole and muscle diastole during walking is similar to the effect of a short-stretch bandage.

A pressure level of 60 mmHg measured in the standing position will immediately fall to less than 40 mmHg in the horizontal position if inelastic material is used but only to 50 mmHg if elastic bandages are applied [1]. This latter pressure level may be too high to be tolerated by the patient, which explains why elastic material should be removed at night. After 24 h there is a pressure drop of 10 mmHg on average with completely inelastic zinc plaster bandages but of only 5 mmHg with four-layer bandages [2].

The idea of using higher compression in patients with severe forms of chronic venous insufficiency than with the mild stages is based more on experience than on evidence from clinical studies [3,4]. Ulcer recurrence rate would be significantly lower if compression with higher pressure were performed [5].

Importance of Graduated Compression

According to Laplace's law the pressure on the leg is indirectly proportional to the radius of the extremity. This means that due to the cone shape of the lower extremity the pressure of a bandage applied with the same strength will be higher on the distal lower leg than on the thigh. While a graduated pressure decrease from the distal to the proximal parts of the leg is reasonable for the recumbent patient wearing class I stockings to prevent thrombosis, its importance has not been proven for higher compression in the walking situation. Laplace's law also comes into play when venous ulcers are situated in the retromalleolar fossa or at the flat medial portion of the distal lower leg. By decreasing the radius of the circumference differently shaped rubber foam pads and pelottes increase *local pressure*, which is a critical practical prerequisite for ulcer healing.

What Is the Evidence for the Physiological Effects of Compression Therapy?

Various effects of compression have been demonstrated, as listed in Table 11.3 and discussed in more detail below.

Decrease in Oedema

Short-stretch bandages and Unna's boots are able to reduce the circumference of a swollen leg by several centimetres per week. This reduction of oedema is the reason

Table 11.3. Compression effects proved by different methods

Compression effect	Investigative method
1. Decrease in oedema	Volumetry, measuring tape, isotopes
2. Softening of lipodermatosclerosis	Ultrasound, CT, durometer
3. Decrease in venous volume (narrowing of veins)	Phlebography, blood pool scintigraphy, APG
4. Increase in venous velocity	Circulation time (isotopes), duplex ultrasonography
5. Blood shift into central compartments	Blood pool scintigraphy, cardiac output
6. Reduction in venous refluxes	Duplex ultrasonography, APG
7. Improvement of venous pumping	Foot volumetry, APG, venous pressure
8. Influence on arterial flow	Duplex ultrasonography, xenon clearance, laser Doppler
9. Improvement of microcirculation	Capillaroscopy, $tcPO_2$, laser Doppler
10. Improvement in lymph drainage	Isotopic and indirect lymphography

APG, air plethysmography.

for the drop in bandage pressure after 24 h that means the bandage has to be renewed. Walking exercises induce a kind of massage [1]. Similar effects may be obtained by four-layer bandages and by intermittent pneumatic compression. To prevent refilling of the leg with oedema fluid continuous and permanent compression is essential. To maintain the oedema-free condition elastic stockings may be sufficient, although they are not usually able to decrease oedema in a massively swollen limb.

Softening of Lipodermatosclerosis

Structural skin changes after intermittent pneumatic compression have been reported using computed tomography (CT) and ultrasound [6]. The durometer [7] is a simple device for demonstrating changes in the consistency of dermal tissue.

Decrease in Venous Volume (Narrowing of Veins)

It may be demonstrated by phlebography that firm compression is able to reduce the diameter of superficial and deep veins to the dimension of a thin cord [1]. Measuring radioactivity over the legs after labelling of red blood cells shows that blood volume decreases with increasing external pressure up to 40 mmHg in the horizontal position [1]. This may also be demonstrated by air plethysmography (APG) in the upright position. Non-elastic material applied with the same pressure leads to a more intense volume reduction [8]. With elastic material a pressure of 40 mmHg is needed to obtain a similar volume reduction to that obtained by 20 mmHg with a non-elastic material (Fig. 11.2). Short-stretch bandages empty the veins almost completely with a pressure of 40 mmHg and a higher pressure of 60 mmHg adds little to volume reduction (Fig. 11.2b).

Acceleration of Venous Flow

Due to the narrowing of the venous diameter blood flow velocity will increase when the arterial inflow remains unchanged. This may be demonstrated by measuring circulation times after injection of a radioactive tracer into a dorsal foot vein with and without leg compression. Using anti-thrombosis stockings it can be demonstrated that venous flow velocity increases by a factor of 1.5 on average, both in the leg and in the iliac veins [9]. Duplex investigations reveal conflicting results, probably due to technical problems [10].

Blood Shift into Central Compartments

Compression of both legs leads to a shift of blood into central vascular compartments, to an increase in the preload of the heart and to an increase in cardiac output. Therefore compression therapy must be performed with caution in patients with severe cardiac failure [1]. Diuresis may be improved by mobilising fluid from the extravascular compartment.

Reduction of Venous Refluxes

Popliteal venous refluxes due to valvular incompetence play a central role in the pathophysiology of chronic venous insufficiency [11]. They may be measured by duplex

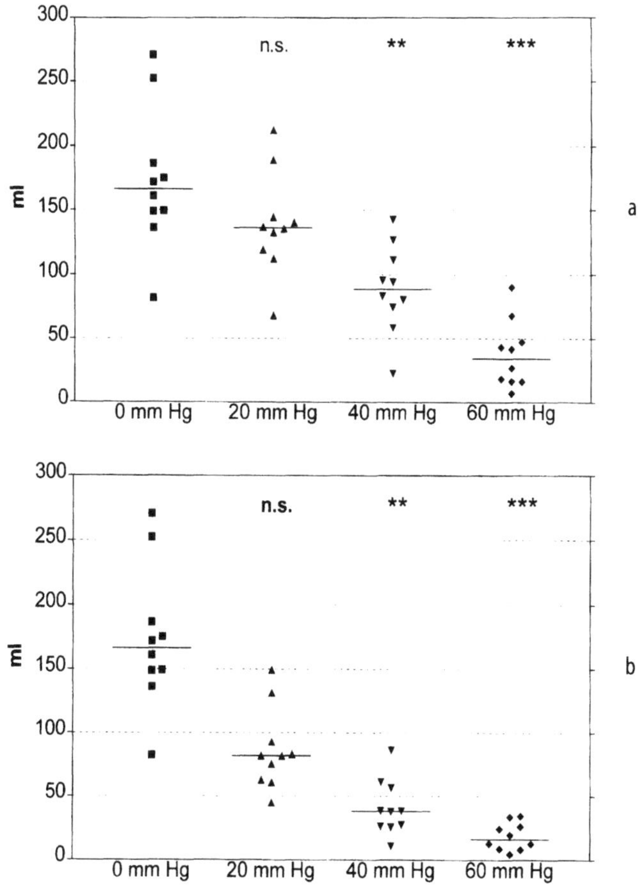

Fig. 11.2a,b. Venous volume (VV) measured by air plethysmography (APG) in 10 patients with venous ulcers and popliteal reflux proved by duplex ultrasonography. Elastic bandages (**a**) applied with increasing pressure (*x*-axis) are less effective in reducing VV than inelastic bandages (**b**). n.s., no significant difference; $^{**}p < 0.01$; $^{***}p < 0.001$.

ultrasound and by plethysmography, preferably APG [8]. Compression decreases reflux in the upright position. Again, with the same pressure inelastic material is more effective than elastic [8,12]. (Fig.11.3). Reduction of venous refluxes by external compression is also observed in completely avalvular segments and may therefore be explained not only by a coaptation of valve leaflets [13].

Improvement of Venous Pumping

Using foot volumetry, expelled volume reflects the amount of venous blood pumped up from the foot during standardised knee-bending exercises. This parameter, which is reduced according on the degree of venous incompetence, shows a steady improvement with increasing external compression pressure [14]. Individuals with varicose veins show significant improvement of expelled volume with class I or II compression stockings while patients with severe post-thrombotic syndrome benefit most from class III stockings [15].

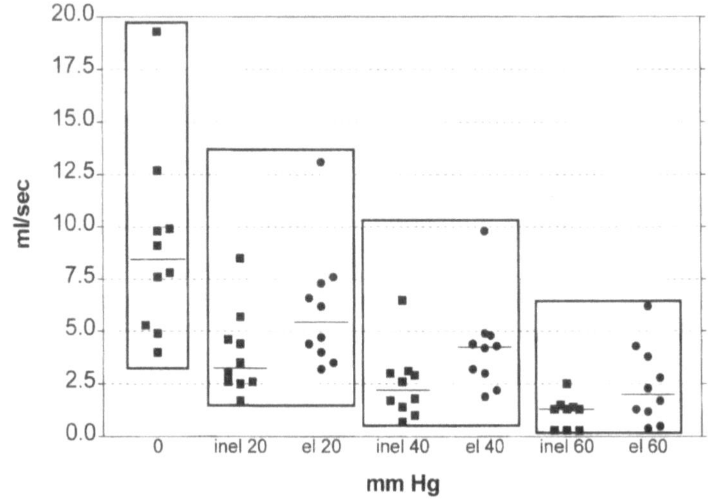

Fig. 11.3. Venous filling index (VFI) measured by APG in 10 patients with venous ulcers and popliteal reflux. Applied with the same pressure, inelastic bandages (*inel*) are more effective than elastic bandages (*el*) at reducing venous reflux. Inelastic bandages with a pressure of 20 mmHg on average diminish VFI more than elastic bandages exerting a pressure of 40 mmHg.

Peripheral venous pressure measurement has shown that a significant decrease in ambulatory venous hypertension can only be obtained with strong inelastic bandages, not with elastic compression (Fig. 11.4) [14]. This effect may be explained by the more intense narrowing of deep veins by inelastic material as demonstrated by APG (Figs. 11.2, 11.3)

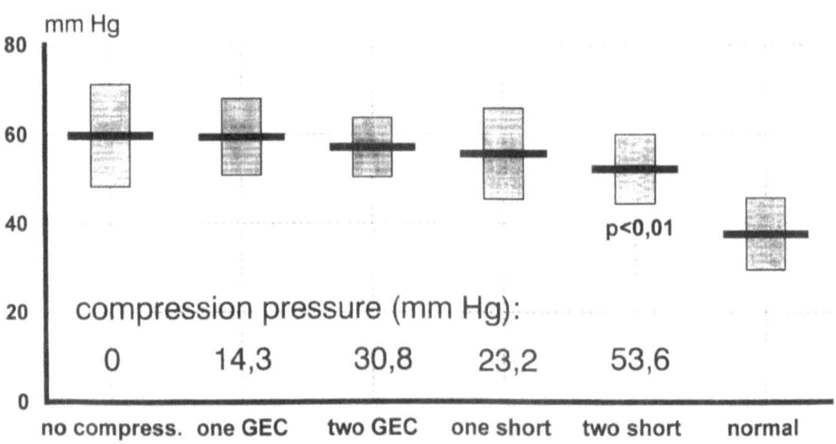

Fig. 11.4. Mean ambulatory venous hypertension [(systolic + 2 × diastolic pressure/3] measured in 13 patients with chronic venous insufficiency in a dorsal foot vein during 20 standardised knee-bends in 40 s (mmHg, $x \pm$ SD). Normal values are lower than 50 mmHg (*right column*). Significant improvement ($p < 0.01$) can be only obtained by firm two-layer short-stretch bandages with an average pressure of 53.6 mmHg on the distal lower leg. One-layer short-stretch bandages with a mean pressure of 23.2 mmHg are on average more effective than two graduated elastic compression stockings (*GEC*) applied over each other, despite their higher pressure of 30.8 mmHg [14].

and could not be found when elastic compression stockings were used [10]. This important finding disproves the widely accepted theory that venous incompetence cannot be reversed in large veins by the external application of compression to the lower leg. It also shows that conclusions drawn from experiments made by compression stockings should not be extrapolated to other compression devices which are more effective.

Influence on Arterial Flow

Firm static compression reduces arterial inflow, as can be demonstrated by different methods. In patients with arterial occlusive disease severe skin damage may be caused by external compression. However, intermittent pressure waves with pressure peaks at the systolic ankle pressure have been shown to increase blood flow in the large arteries and in the skin [16]. Rigid bandages applied with low pressure may exert similar effects when the ankle pump is moved, actively or passively [17] (Fig. 11.5). Especially when arterial obstruction as well as oedema impedes the nutrition of the skin, a reduction in leg swelling by a careful intermittent compression regime may improve the condition.

Improvement of Microcirculation

Some important mechanisms of compression at the microcirculatory level have been described in the last few years. Blood flow in the enlarged capillary loops is accelerated, capillary filtration is reduced and reabsorption increased due to enhanced tissue pressure. Effects on mediators involved in the local inflammatory response may explain both the immediate pain relief that occurs with good compression, and ulcer healing [18].

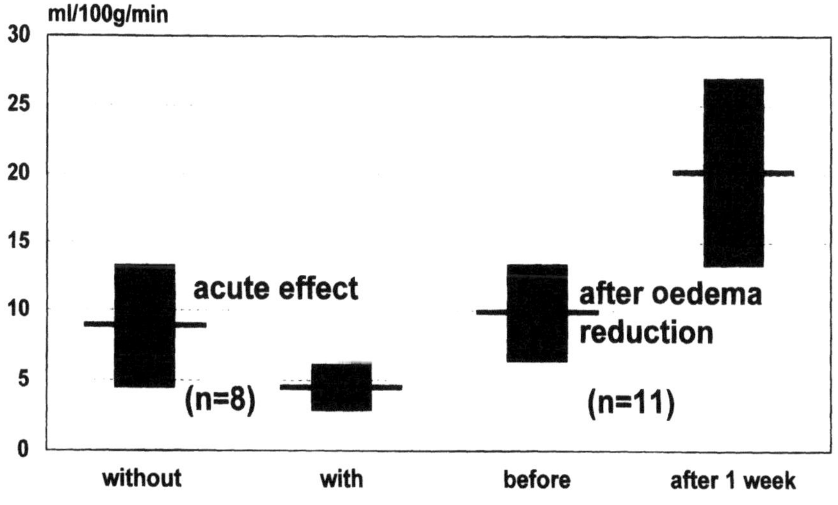

Fig. 11.5. Measurement of maximal flow in the tibial anterior muscle by histamine–xenon-133 clearance in 8 patients before and immediately after application of a firm inelastic bandage and in 11 patients before and 1 week after the bandage. All patients had post-thrombotic syndrome and leg swelling. Compression causes an immediate decrease in muscular blood flow. After reduction of oedema by walking with inelastic bandages, the arterial blood flow shows a significant increase 1 week later.

Improvement in Lymph Drainage

Intermittent pneumatic compression enhances prefascial lymph drainage [1]. Unna boots are able to increase subfascial lymph transport, which is reduced in post-thrombotic syndrome. Consequent compression leads to a morphological improvement in lymphatics in patients with lipodermatosclerosis. This can be demonstrated by indirect X-ray lymphography [1].

What Is the Clinical Evidence that Compression is Worthwhile?

Primary Prophylaxis of Deep Vein Thrombosis

Several controlled clinical trials have proved that compression stockings are effective in preventing deep vein thrombosis (DVT). In comparison with control groups graduated compression stockings are able to reduce the frequency of DVT in different risk categories of patients. It has also been demonstrated that this kind of physical prophylaxis is cost-effective [19]. Intermittent pneumatic compression has also been proved to be an effective measure for mechanical prophylaxis [19].

Secondary Prophylaxis after DVT

In a randomised control trial Brandjes and co-workers [20] showed that about 60% of patients with a first episode of proximal DVT develop post-thrombotic syndrome within 2 years. A sized-to-fit compression stocking reduced this rate by about 50% [20].

Acute DVT

For the acute stage of DVT early ambulation with firm compression bandages seems to impede thrombus extension more effectively than bed-rest [21]. More work has to be done to demonstrate that prevention of stasis is an important therapeutic target, not only for primary prevention but also for treatment in the acute stage of thromboembolic disease.

Venous Leg Ulcers

Ulcer healing is a clear and important clinical parameter for effective treatment. In comparison with local therapy alone, compression resulted in significantly faster healing rates of venous ulcers [4]. Various high-compresssion regimens are more effective than low compression. After the ulcers are healed, non-compliance of the patient in wearing compression stockings is followed by a higher recurrence rate [22]. Additional sequential pneumatic compression promotes ulcer healing [23].

References

1. Partsch H. Compression therapy of the legs. Dermatol Surg Oncol 1991;17:799–805.
2. Partsch H, Menzinger G, Blazek V. Static and dynamic measurement of compression pressure. In: Blazek V, Schultz-Ehrenburg U, editors. Frontiers in computer-aided visualization of vascular functions,. Aachen: VDI Verlag, 1997:145–152.

3. Struckmann J. Compression stockings and their effect on the venous pump: a comparative study. Phlebology 1986;1:37–45.
4. Fletcher A, Cullum N, Sheldon TA. A systematic review of compression treatment for venous leg ulcers. BMJ 1997;315:576–580.
5. Harper DR, Ruckley CV, Dale JJ, Callam MC, Allan P, Brown D, et al. Prevention of recurrence of chronic leg ulcer: a randomised trial of different degrees of compression. In: Raymond-Martinbeau P, Prescott R, Zummo M, editors. Phlebology '92 London Paris: John Libbey, 1992:902–903.
6. Gniadecka M. Dermal oedema in lipodermatosclerosis: distribution, effects of posture and compressive therapy evaluated by high frequency ultrasonography. Acta Derm Venereol 1995;75:120–124.
7. Falanga V, Bucalo B. Use of a durometer to assess skin hardness. J Am Acad Dermatol 1993;29:47–51.
8. Menzinger G, Horakowa M, Mayer W, Partsch H. Reduction of venous reflux by compression: a comparison between short and long stretch material. Phlebology 1995;[Suppl 1]:888–891.
9. Partsch H, Kahn P.Venöse Strömungsbeschleunigung in Bein und Becken durch "Anti-Thrombosestrümpfe". Klinikarzt 1982;11:609–615.
10. Mayberry JC, Moneta GL, DeFrang RD, Porter JM. The influence of elastic compression stockings on deep venous hemodynamics. J Vasc Surg 1991;13:91–99.
11. Brittenden J, Bradbury AW, Allan PL, Prescott RJ, Harper DR, Ruckley CV. Popliteal vein reflux reduces the healing of chronic venous ulcer. Br J Surg 1998;85:60–62.
12. Spence RK, Cahall E. Inelastic versus elastic leg compression in chronic venous insufficiency: a comparison of limb size and venous hemodynamics. J Vasc Surg 1996;24:783–787.
13. Partsch B, Mayer W, Partsch H. Improvement of ambulatory venous hypertension by narrowing of the femoral vein in congenital absence of venous valves. Phlebology 1992;7:101–104.
14. Partsch H. Improvement of venous pumping function in chronic venous insufficiency by compression depending on pressure and material. Vasa 1984;13:58–64.
15. Stöberl C, Gabler S, Partsch H. Indikationsgerechte Bestrumpfung-Messung der venösen Pumpfunktion. 1989;18:35–39.
16. Eze AR, Comerota AJ, Cisek PL, Holland BS, Kerr RP, Veeramasuneni R, Comerota AJ Jr. Intermittent calf and foot compression increases lower extremity blood flow. Am J Surg 1996;172:130–134.
17. Mayrowitz HN, Larsen PB. Effects of compression bandaging on the leg pulsatile blood flow. Clin Physiol 1997;17:105–117.
18. Abu-Own A, Shami SK, Chittenden SJ, Farrah J, Scurr JH, Smith PD. Microangiopathy of the skin and the effect of leg compression in patients with chronic venous insufficiency. J Vasc Surg 1994;19:1074–1083.
19. Nicolaides AN, Bergqvist D, Hull R. Prevention of venous thromboembolism. Inernational Consensus Statement (guideline according to scientific evidence). Int Angiol 1997;16:3–38.
20. Brandjes DPM, Büller H, Hejboer H, Huismann MV, de Rijk M, Jagt H, ten Cate JW. Incidence of the postthrombotic syndrome and the effects of compression stockings in patients with proximal venous thrombosis. Lancet 1997;349:759–762.
21. Partsch H, Kechavarz B, Köhn H, Mostbeck A. The effect of mobilisation of patients during treatment of thromboembolic disorders with low-molecular-weight heparin. Int Angiol 1997;16:189–192.
22. Wright DDI, Franks PJ, Blair SD, Backhouse CM, et al. Oxerutins in the prevention of recurrence in chronic venous ulceration: randomized controlled trial. Br J Surg 1991;78: 1269–1270.
23. Coleridge Smith P, Sarin S, Hasty J, Scurr JH. Sequential gradient pneumatic compression enhances venous ulcer healing: a randomized trial. Surgery 1990;108:971–975.

12 What is the Place of Sclerotherapy?

John H. Scurr

Introduction

The role of sclerotherapy in the management of patients with varicose veins is currently determined by the country in which you live and the doctor you consult. There have been relatively few controlled trials, and our understanding of sclerotherapy techniques is based on craft rather than science. Three names are associated with three techniques, and although the underlying principles may be similar, the application is very different. The three techniques – the Fegan (the Irish school) [1,2], the Sigg (the Swiss school) [3] and the Tournay (the French school) [4] – form the basis of treatment. Every doctor employing sclerotherapy will have devised his own methods and will claim exceptional results, but will have no scientific data or clinical trials to support his claim.

Sclerotherapy may be used as a primary management of varicose veins, in a secondary supporting role and in the management of recurrent varicosities. It can be applied to all veins ranging from dermal flares to reticular veins [5] and varicosities. Whilst the principles may be similar, the techniques involve different injection procedures, differing needles and differing sclerosants. In attempting to identify the place of sclerotherapy it is necessary to have some understanding of the basic pathophysiology of venous disorders, the different disease processes and the results of sclerotherapy.

Which Patients Are Suitable for Sclerotherapy?

Patients with varicose veins can now be fully assessed non-invasively. A full patient history should be taken and a physical examination performed. The non-invasive investigations available include Doppler ultrasound, duplex ultrasound imaging and plethysmography. Duplex ultrasound imaging provides the most information, and although not performed routinely, is being used more frequently. Early indications suggest that this leads to better patient selection, a lower incidence of recurrence and the ability to classify patients for the purposes of scientific studies.

Patients can be divided into those with junctional incompetence, perforator incompetence, truncal varicosities with reflux, truncal varicosities without reflux and isolated varicosities. Patients with junctional incompetence are probably better treated surgically. Similarly those with truncal incompetence are better treated with the removal of varicosities, usually in association with junctional ligation. Only those patients with truncal varicosities and no reflux or isolated varicose veins, capillary or reticular flares, are suitable for sclerotherapy. Using an objective non-invasive vascular assessment patients can be accurately allocated to two groups: those who require surgery followed by sclerotherapy, and those who require sclerotherapy alone.

Any doctor treating patients with varicose veins should be prepared to offer the full range of treatment. A combination of surgery and sclerotherapy will probably achieve the best results. Sclerotherapy should not be employed because a patient cannot afford to come into hospital to undergo surgical treatment, or because the doctor offering to treat the patient has no facilities or ability to carry out surgery. Similarly surgeons should not assume that surgical treatment is appropriate in all cases.

Principles of Sclerotherapy

The principal objective of sclerotherapy is to destroy the superficial veins. The injection of a sclerosant solution into a vein will produce a thrombophlebitis, unless the vein is empty, in which case it will produce an endothelial reaction, resulting in fibrosis and complete venous destruction. The importance of injecting into a vein with accurate positioning of the needle, and then injecting into an empty segment, was stressed by Fegan. Fegan's original hypothesis that the injection needs to be in proximity to perforating veins is probably not valid, provided the superficial veins are obliterated over a significant length. The volumes of sclerosant involved are small, provided the vein is empty and endothelial contact is maintained. The reaction is rapid, and endothelial damage occurs in a very short period of time.

Fegan advocated compression. We would not disagree with that although differences of opinion have occurred over the years [6–8]. The duration of compression has never been subjected to a proper clinical trial. We know that luminal obliteration occurs in days, and therefore compression is probably not needed for more than a few days [9]. In those patients with junctional incompetence and truncal reflux, maintaining endothelial contact to produce obliteration can be extremely difficult. Much of Fegan's work was carried out before we had the ability to examine patients non-invasively and a number of his patients would therefore have had junctional incompetence and significant truncal reflux. Although three separate schools have been described, the principles remain the same: the sclerosant needs to be injected into a vein and the concentration of sclerosant needs to be sufficient to produce an endothelial obliteration.

Excessive concentrations of sclerosant will produce a severe reaction. If the sclerosant is injected in sufficient concentration outside a vein and close to the skin, the skin will break down forming an ulcer. Extravasation of sclerosant from the vein will not cause an ulcer.

Having injected the sclerosant into an empty vein by elevating the leg, compression to the vein then needs to be applied until the reaction is complete (Fig. 12.1). The duration of compression is probably related to the size of the vein, although there are no studies to confirm this. If the injection of sclerosant is given into a full vein or blood leaks back into the vein soon after the injection has been given, a thrombophlebitis will occur. This can be painful and can be associated with considerable local skin staining. The larger the vein the more difficult it is to produce an endothelial reaction and the greater the risk of producing a thrombophlebitis

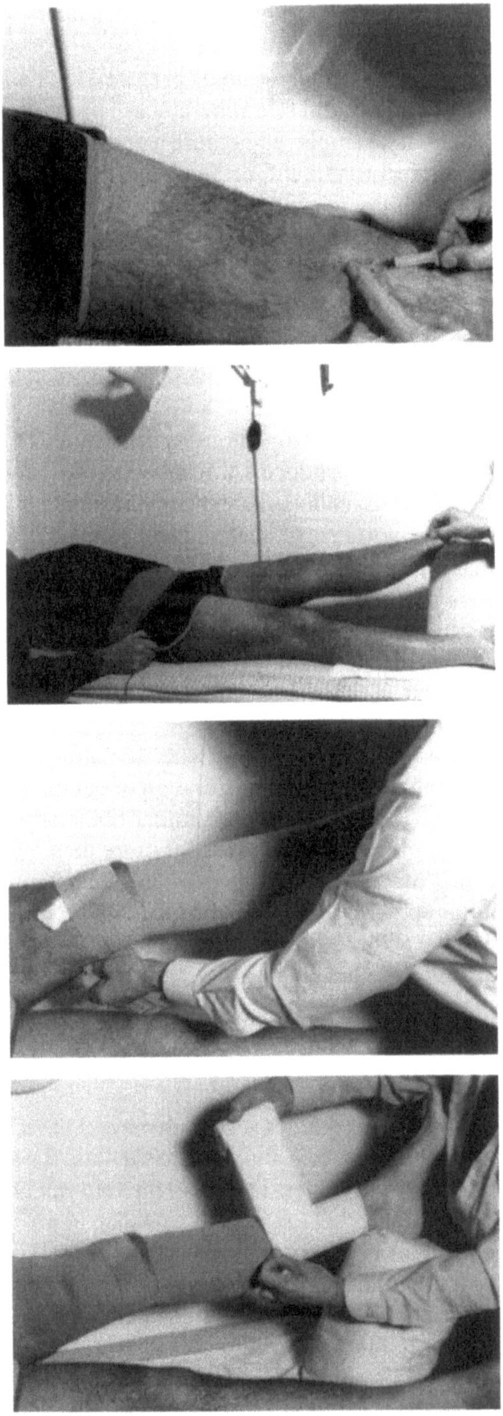

Needle inserted into vein – leg semi dependent.

Limb elevated to empty vein before injecting sclerosant.

Crepe bandage is applied over cotton pads at each injection site.

The crepe bandage is now locked together by elastic adhesive bandage. A gap is left to permit knee flexion.

Fig. 12.1. Compression sclerotherapy.

with skin staining. Under these circumstances consideration should be given to surgical removal of the vein.

Echosclerotherapy is a technique which allows the vein to be punctured under ultrasound control. This allows accurate localisation of junctions. There is no consensus as to whether this offers any true benefit in the treatment of patients with varicose veins by sclerotherapy.

Complications of Sclerotherapy

Sclerotherapy is simple and, provided simple guidelines are followed, is safe. The technique can be carried out in a general practitioner's surgery, or in a hospital following surgical treatment. The commonest complication involves technical failure and the persistence of veins. This is closely followed by superficial thrombophlebitis, pain and local discoloration. Ulceration can also occur following sclerotherapy. To produce an ulcer 1 cm in diameter or greater a significant quantity of sclerosant has to be injected into the wrong place. Extravasation of sclerosant following the correct administration does not produce a large ulcer. Compression bandaging is important, but overzealous compression can result in neurological complications including footdrop. Patients should be advised to report pain in the leg and foot following sclerotherapy. When a patient does complain the bandages should be removed and the leg inspected. Inadvertent intra-arterial injections have occurred, particularly in the region of the medial malleolus. When this occurs extensive skin loss follows. This is an extremely rare complication and can be avoided by taking care not to inject in the region immediately above the medial malleolus, by noting the colour of blood that comes into the syringe, and by stopping the injection immediately when the patient complains of any pain or discomfort.

Microsclerotherapy

Many patients who have undergone quite successful varicose vein surgery complain about dermal flares. In 30% of cases dermal flares are associated with significant underlying superficial venous insufficiency. This should be addressed before starting microsclerotherapy. In patients with no underlying superficial venous insufficiency microsclerotherapy proves extremely successful for the treatment of dermal flares. Techniques using 32 gauge needles, often specially modified and employing an intravascular technique, have proved effective. Because the veins are very small, dilute concentrations of sclerosant should be used. Higher concentrations are associated with skin staining and may result in blistering and ulceration. The technique involves inserting a fine needle into the veins, withdrawing it until blood is seen at the base of the needle, and then carefully injecting until the patch of veins disappears (Fig. 12.2). The veins initially disappear followed by a small area of erythema. A careful, slow injection is required to achieve the best results. A sudden injection will result in extravasation locally. Provided a dilute concentration of sclerosant is employed there is seldom a problem.

There are two principal complications which occur with microsclerotherapy. First, following treatment blood may persist in the small veins or may leak back into the small veins, setting and producing a dark line. If this happens, puncturing the vein

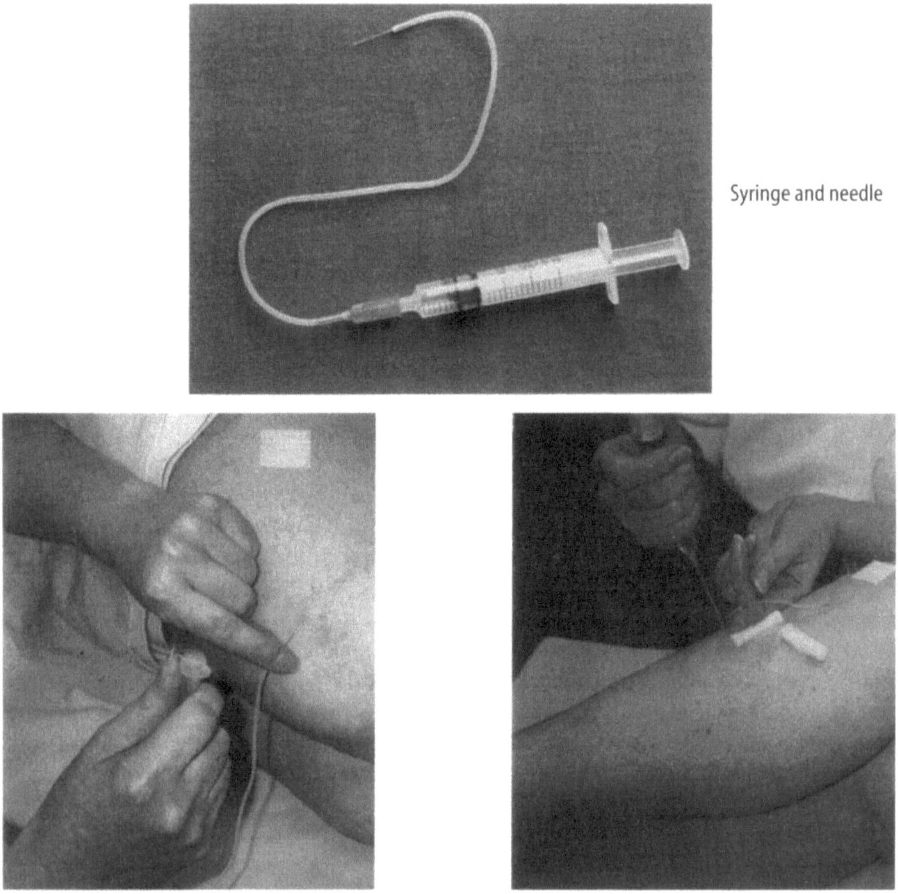

Syringe and needle

Needle inserted into vein by transfixing and then pulling back

Slow injection until large area of vein disappears

Fig. 12.2. Microsclerotherapy.

with a small needle and massaging the blood from the vein will minimise the effect and reduce the chance of brown discoloration developing. If the blood remains within the vein, it will cause a pale brown stain when it breaks down. Although these stains usually disappear, they may take 1 or 2 years to go. The other complication which may occur is the development of a small ulcer. These occur at the injection site and are probably associated with local infection. Before the ulcer appears there is an area of redness. If the patient is treated with antibiotics at this stage, the redness settles and no ulcer will occur. If the redness is ignored then an ulcer measuring 2–4 mm across can occur. Although these ulcers always heal they are associated with a degree of depigmentation and scarring. Given that microsclerotherapy is used in patients with dermal flares to achieve a good cosmetic result, these complications can be upsetting.

If the dermal flares are not associated with an underlying superficial venous insufficiency then these flares will return. Patients should be warned of this and expect to receive treatment on a regular basis.

References

1. Fegan W. Continuous compression technique for injecting varicose veins. Lancet 1963;II:109.
2. Fegan W. Varicose veins: compression sclerotherapy. London: Heinemann, 1967.
3. Sigg K. Treatment of varicose veins by injection sclerotherapy as practised in Basle. In: Hobbs JT, editor. Treatment of venous disorders in the lower limb. Lancaster: MTP Press, 1976.
4. Tournay R. La sclérose des varices. Expansion scientific française, 4th ed. Paris: 1985.
5. Goldman M. Sclerotherapy for superficial venules and telangiectasias of the lower extremities. Dermatol Clin 1987;5:369–379.
6. Conrad P. Continuous compression techniques of injecting varicose veins. Med J Aust 1967;1:1011–1014.
7. Dormandy J. A randomized trial of bandaging after sclerotherapy for varicose veins. Phlebologie 1982;35:125–131.
8. Fraser I, Perry E, Hatton M, Watkin D. Prolonged bandaging is not required following sclerotherapy of varicose veins. Br J Surg 1985;75:488-490.
9. Scurr J, Coleridge-Smith P, Cutting P. Varicose veins: optimum compression following sclerotherapy. Ann R Coll Surg Engl 1985;67:109-111.
10. Consensus paper on sclerotherapy of lower limb varicose veins. Task Force on Venous Disorders, 1994.

13
Perforator Surgery: What Is Its Role?

Wesley P. Stuart

Introduction

Minimally invasive surgical interruption of calf perforating vessels is now widely utilised in the management of the complications of chronic venous insufficiency (CVI) [1–4]. However, the precise role of incompetent calf perforating veins (IPV) in the pathogenesis of the skin changes of CVI has never been defined and, as a result, the indications for subfascial endoscopic perforator surgery (SEPS) remain controversial [5].

What Is Known About the Role of the Perforator in the Pathogenesis of Venous Disease?

Essentially the evidence regarding the role of the perforator in the pathogenesis of venous disease can be divided into two categories: the relationship between the number of incompetent calf perforators and clinical status, and haemodynamic studies of the contribution of incompetent perforating veins to CVI.

Association Between Incompetent Calf Perforators and Clinical Status

Using duplex ultrasonography, Hanrahan et al. [6] sought to identify the nature of venous reflux in the limb affected by venous ulceration. They found that in 46% of cases there was no duplex evidence of any venous abnormality in the ulcer bed itself or within 2 cm of the ulcer margin. More specifically, although they identified a mean of 2.43 IPV per limb in the ulcer group, only 27% of the limbs had IPV in the ulcer base itself.

A similar study was performed by Nicolaides' group at St. Mary's Hospital, London [7]. Thirty-four limbs with a history of venous ulceration were examined using duplex ultrasonography. This study reported that only 17% of limbs failed to demonstrate local venous reflux. In only 12 of 43 ulcers (28%) could an IPV be seen in the base or within 2 cm of the edge. IPV could be demonstrated in 15 of the 34 limbs (44%). Taking these two studies together it would be possible to argue that there is a poor association between the presence of either local, or any, IPV in a limb and venous ulceration. Certainly, there seems little to support the concept of an IPV feeding every ulcer crater as argued by Robert Linton [8].

However, later work by Labropoulos et al. [9] suggests a stronger link between the presence of IPV and venous ulceration. Dividing 594 limbs into four clinical groups based upon severity of venous disease, he demonstrated an increasing burden of venous reflux in the limbs with deteriorating clinical status. In particular he demonstrated an increase in the number of limbs demonstrating IPV and an increase in the mean number of IPV per limb. In 174 disease-free limbs there were no IPV. In 145 limbs with varicose veins only 2% demonstrated IPV. Seventy-five of 155 limbs with lipodermatosclerosis demonstrated IPV (a mean of 1.8 per limb) and 73 of 120 limbs with ulceration demonstrated IPV (2.1 per limb).

Work from Edinburgh also suggests a closer association between the number of IPV and clinical status (personal data). Three hundred and eleven limbs were divided into four clinical grades: grade 0, no venous disease; grade I, varicose veins only with no skin changes of CVI; grade II, lipodermatosclerosis but no ulcer history; and grade III, limbs with open or healed ulcers. The results are summarised in Table 13.1.

It is possible that improvements in ultrasound technology have allowed a larger number of perforators to be seen in these later studies.

Haemodynamic Evidence

Zukowski et al. [10] attempted to unravel the complexities of the possible contribution of IPV to abnormal venous haemodynamics. They examined 221 limbs from 149 patients with different degrees of skin changes ranging from simple varicose veins to ulceration. Patients were assessed for the anatomical extent of the disease (venography and ultrasound) and for the functional contribution at various sites of reflux (ambulatory venous pressure, AVP). Patients were divided into three groups based upon the anatomical distribution of reflux: group A, varicose veins only with no evidence of incompetent perforating veins; group B, varicose veins with incompetent perforating veins; and group C, presence of deep venous disease, regardless of the state of the superficial system. The sites of deep to superficial incompetence were sequentially occluded using tourniquets at the below-knee level and at the ankle level. Subgrouping of the group B limbs was performed based on the 90% venous refill times (VR90) and AVPs after the placement of tourniquets at the below-knee and ankle levels.

The following conclusions were drawn from the group B limbs. In subgroup I, the placement of a below-knee tourniquet normalised the haemodynamics of the leg, i.e. the IPV were not haemodynamically compromising the limb. In subgroup II the ankle tourniquet, but not the below-knee tourniquet, normalised the haemodynamics of the leg and the IPV were judged responsible for some of the haemodynamic compromise of the limb. Subgroup III was considered to represent undiagnosed deep system pathology as tourniquets failed to normalise the haemodynamics.

Akesson et al. [11] examined the effect on limb haemodynamics of staged surgical procedures. This comprised superficial system reflux eradication followed, after at least

Table 13.1. The association between clinical grade and number, competence and diameter of calf perforating veins

Clinical grade	Grade 0 ($n = 50$)	Grade I ($n = 95$)	Grade II ($n = 58$)	Grade III ($n = 108$)
No. of limbs with perforators (%)	44 (88)	90 (95)	57 (98)	106 (98)*
No. of limbs with IPV (%)	3 (6)	49 (52)	48 (83)	97 (90)**
Median (IQR) no. of perforators per limb	1 (1–2)	2 (1–3)	2 (1–3)	2 (2–3)†
Median (IQR) no. of IPV per limbs	0 (0–0)	1 (0–2)	1 (1–2)	2 (1–2)†
Median perforator diameter (range) (mm)	2 (1–4)	3 (1–8)	4 (1–11)	4 (1–8)†

IQR, inter-quartile range; IPV, incompetent perforating veins.
* $p < 0.05$, ** $p < 0.001$, χ^2 test; † $p < 0.001$ Kruskal–Wallis test.

6 months, by perforator surgery [11]. The limb haemodynamics were assessed using occlusion plethysmography, foot volumetry and AVP after the superficial surgery and then again after perforator interruption. The addition of the second perforator procedure conferred no measurable haemodynamic benefit over superficial surgery alone.

Bradbury and Ruckley [12] examined the long-term haemodynamic trends in a group of patients who had undergone superficial venous extirpation, as required, combined with subfascial perforator ligation. Foot volumetry was used to measure the VR50 (venous half refilling time) and ejection fraction, before and at intervals following operation. In the group that remained ulcer-free, the significant improvements in the VR50 and ejection fraction seen with surgery were sustained. Conversely, in the group in which ulcers recurred (26%), both the VR50 values and ejection fraction were seen to deteriorate to pre-operative values. Furthermore, earlier work had demonstrated that the recurrence group consisted almost exclusively of those patients in whom there was popliteal segment reflux and that only one patient with popliteal reflux remained ulcer free [13] . These findings concerning the importance of the popliteal segment support the earlier findings of Burnand et al. [14].

Clinical Studies

Zukowski et al. [10] successfully demonstrated a haemodynamic effect attributable to IPV. However, subsequent studies have demonstrated difficulty in measuring the haemodynamic benefits of perforator surgery in both the short and long term.

The search turns to clinical data to explain or support these findings. Darke and colleagues [15,16] examined the effects of surgery on the superficial system alone in patients with venous ulcers in whom there was demonstrable superficial and perforator system reflux but intact deep vessels. In papers examining the short- and long-term outcomes they demonstrated that if the deep system is intact lasting healing can be achieved by saphenous extirpation alone.

Two studies now offer an explanation of why, in patients with intact deep systems, perforator surgery may be superfluous. Campbell and West [17] presented data in 1995 demonstrating that saphenous surgery alone may correct perforator abnormalities in most patients. They reported that in a population of 185 legs 80.5% of the 226 perforators that were incompetent pre-operatively regained competence on extirpation of the saphenous system.

A similar study was performed in Edinburgh, with particular attention to the condition of the deep vessels (personal data). Sixty-two limbs underwent duplex scanning before and after saphenous surgery in which no attempt was made to interrupt perforators. Fourteen of these limbs demonstrated deep venous reflux and this, together with limbs in which saphenous reflux abolition was incomplete, meant that post-operatively 21 limbs still demonstrated mainstem reflux. The effects of surgery on the number perforators and their competence is summarised in Table 13.2. In a substantial minority,

Table 13.2. Pre-operative and post-operative perforator characteristics after saphenous surgery alone

	Pre-operative	Post-operative
Limbs demonstrating IPV	40	23*
Total no. of perforators	130	120^{NS}
Total no. of IPV	68	34*
Median diameter of perforators (range)	4 (1–11) mm	3 (1–8) mm†

IPV, incompetent perforating veins.
* $p < 0.01$ χ^2 test; ^{NS} not significant, χ^2 test; † $p < 0.01$, Mann–Whitney *U*-test.

IPV remained post-operatively. The relationship of this to remaining mainstem reflux is demonstrated in Fig. 13.1. It is clear that saphenous surgery alone will correct abnormal IPV physiology in the majority of cases if the deep system is intact.

The questions therefore remains whether IPV associated with deep venous incompetence have a role in the development and intractable nature of venous ulcers, and whether surgical interruption of IPV improve the prognosis for short- and long-term ulcer healing.

Review of the Results of Perforator Surgery

Some of the results from the published series of surgical interruption of perforators are presented in Table 13.3. There is a wide range of quoted rates of ulcer recurrence. Two series in particular deserve mention. From St. Thomas' Hospital, London, Burnand et al. [14] reported a 100% ulcer recurrence rate in those patients with popliteal vein reflux. This compares with a recurrence in only 1 of the 17 patients with an intact popliteal segment. As mentioned before, the prognostic importance of deep venous disease in the popliteal segment is echoed in the data reported from Edinburgh. The 26% of cases with ulcer recurrence were all in the group with popliteal segment reflux [13].

The results from these series show a wide variation in both recurrence rates (range 2–34%) and wound complication rates (1–44%). There are several crucial flaws in these series, leaving the question regarding the impact of subfascial ligation largely unanswered for the following reasons:

1. None of these studies is a randomised trial or controlled.
2. There is poor control of confounding factors, principally other ulcer aetiology.
3. Many of the trials pre-dated duplex ultrasonography, and therefore there was poor

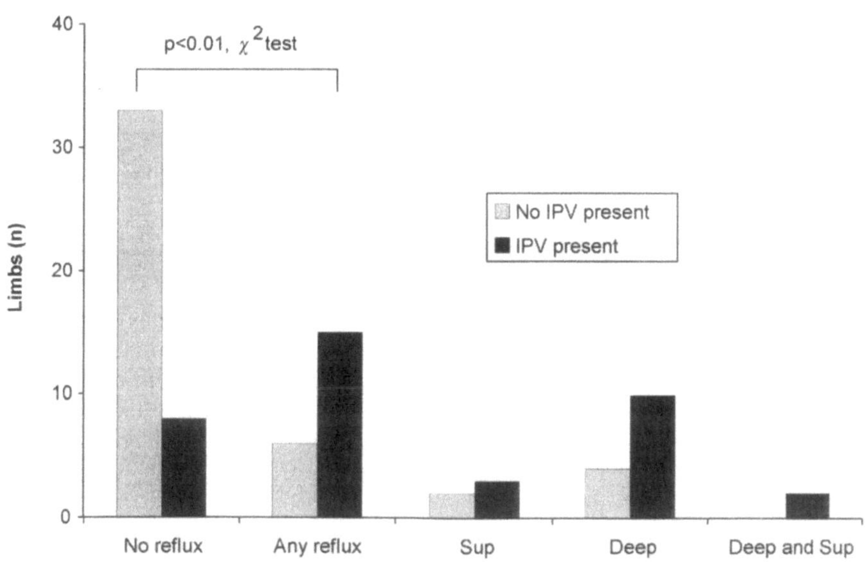

Fig. 13.1. The effect of residual post-operative reflux on the proportion of limbs demonstrating incompetent perforating veins (IPV) following saphenous surgery. *Sup*, superficial system reflux; *Deep*, deep system reflux.

Table 13.3. Published series of perforator surgery outcome

Author (year)	Ref. no.	Patients (*n*)	Limbs (*n*)	Wound comps (%)	Recurrence (%)	Follow-up period
Silver (1971)	[18]	28	31	13	10	64% > 5y
Field (1971)	[19]	51	57	–	2	1–8y (mean 6y)
Thurston (1973)	[20]	89	102	12	13	3–84m (mean 3y)
Bowen (1975)	[21]	55	71	44	34	6m–15y (48% > 3y)
Burnand (1976)	[14]	41	41		DVI 100% no DVI 1/17	up to 5 years
Blumenburg (1978)	[22]	16	25	4	4	6m–6y
DePalma (1979)	[23]	53	68	1	6	6m–12y
Almgren (1982)	[24]	57	41 ulcer 16 LDS	19	(48 ulcer free) 22%	?
Hyde (1981)	[25]	83	–	13	33	Mean 10y
Negus (1983)	[26]	77	108	19	13	6m–6y (76% > 3y)
Cheung (1985)	[27]	32	31 ulcer	22	34	5m–4y
Johnson (1985)	[28]	37	47	11	22% at 1y 41% at 3y 51% at 5y	
Wilkinson (1986)	[29]	108	134	24	2	6m–9y (80% < 5y)
Szostek (1988)	[30]	148	148	17.5	14.5	6m–10y (105 cases)
Cikrit (1988)	[31]	32	–	–	22	6m–10y (mean 4y)
Nash (1991)	[32]	90	–	–	18	3y
Robison (1992)	[33]	17	18	56	37	42m (life table)
Bradbury (1993)	[12]	53	53	–	26	median 60m (3–144m)

m, months; y, years; LDS, lipodermatosclerosis; DVI, deep venous insufficiency.

assessment of concomitant venous disease (i.e. deep and superficial venous insufficiency) and perforator competence.

4. Consequently, the concomitant venous surgery was not standardised with respect to timing or superficial system reflux eradication.
5. The ulcer status at the time of surgery is unclear in many cases.
6. The follow-up periods are variable and often inadequate.
7. Series are incomplete with cases missing from follow-up.
8. There is no life-table analysis.
9. The post-operative care is not standardised, particularly with respect to compression hosiery.
10. In the absence of a reliable non-invasive method of assessment there is no way of assessing the completeness of the surgery.

For the above reasons it is really not possible to form firm conclusions regarding the efficacy of perforator surgery from reported series. Furthermore, the data referred to earlier from Darke and colleagues [15,16] would suggest that in a significant proportion of patients saphenous surgery alone would yield good long-term results. Burnand's [14] and Bradbury's [13] series would indicate that those with post-phlebitic changes and popliteal vein reflux have a particularly poor prognosis.

What Are the Potential Indications for Perforator Surgery?

Taking into account the above evidence we have attempted to classify incompetent perforators to aid decisions regarding surgical interruption.

Type I IPV: These occur in the presence of superficial system disease only. Studies have demonstrated that in up to 80% of such cases the IPV will revert to normal physiology with complete eradication of saphenous system reflux. SEPS is probably not indicated for these patients.

Type II IPV: These occur in association with deep venous reflux alone. Saphenous system surgery will not correct the reflux in these vessels and SEPS is probably indicated.

Type III IPV: These occur in association with mixed deep and superficial system reflux. Saphenous surgery alone will not correct IPV reflux and SEPS is probably indicated.

Type IV IPV: The incompetence demonstrated by calf perforators occurs in association with deep venous obstruction. The abnormal blood flow through such vessels represents flow through collateral pathways bypassing the deep obstruction. Interruption of these vessels is potentially deleterious to the haemodynamics of the limb and SEPS may be contraindicated.

Type V IPV: In this rare group of patients incompetence occurs in the perforators alone in the absence of demonstrable deep or superficial main stem venous pathology. SEPS may be indicated for these patients.

What Studies Still Need To Be Done?

In the light of conflicting data regarding clinical outcome and the haemodynamic effects of perforator surgery, a randomised controlled trial (RCT) is required to assess the benefits of perforator surgery. However, before this can be undertaken the benefits of any kind of venous surgery must be demonstrated by RCT.

The questions to be addressed are the following:

1. Does surgery of any kind offer reduced ulcer healing times and sustained ulcer remission compared with conservative measures alone?
2. Does perforator interruption confer additional benefit over saphenous surgery alone in terms of either time to healing and/or sustained remission?
3. If so, does this apply to all groups or just patients with deep venous reflux?

References

1. Hauer G. Die endoscopische subfasciale Diszision der Perforansvenen: vorlaufige Hitteilung. Vasa 1985;14:59–61.
2. Jugenheimer M, Junginger T. Endoscopic subfascial sectioning of incompetent veins in the treatment of primary varicosis. World J Surg 1992;16:971–975.
3. Pierik EGJM, Wittens CHA, van Urk H. Subfascial endoscopic ligation in the treatment of perforating veins. Eur J Vasc Surg 1995;9:38–41.
4. Gloviczki P, Bergan JJ, Menawat SS, et al. Safety, feasibility, early efficacy of subfascial endoscopic perforator surgery: a preliminary report from the North American registry. J Vasc Surg 1997;25:94–105.
5. Ruckley CV, Makhdoomi KR. The venous perforator. Br J Surg 1996;83:1492–1493.
6. Hanrahan LM, Araki CT, Rodriguez AA, Kechejian GJ, LaMorte WW, Menzoian JO. Distribution of valvular incompetence in patients with venous stasis ulceration. J Vasc Surg 1991;13:805–812.
7. Labropoulos N, Giannoukas AD, Nicolaides AN, Ramaswami G, Leon M, Burke P. New insights into the pathophysiologic condition of venous ulceration with colour-flow duplex imaging: implications for treatment? J Vasc Surg 1995;22:45–50.
8. Linton RR. The communicating veins of the lower leg and the technique for their ligation. Ann Surg 1938;107:582–593.
9. Labropoulos N, Delis K, Nicolades AN, Leon M, Ramaswami G, Volteas N. The role of the distribution

and anatomic extent of reflux in the development of signs and symptoms in chronic venous insufficiency. J Vasc Surg 1996;23:504–510.
10. Zukowski AJ, Nicolaides AN, Szendro G, Irvine A, Lewis R, Malouf GM, Hobbs JT, Dudley HAF. Haemodynamic significance of incompetent calf perforating veins. Br J Surg 1991;78:625–629.
11. Akesson H, Brudin L, Cwikiel W, Ohlin P, Plater G. Does the correction of insufficient superficial and perforating veins improve venous function in patients with deep venous insufficiency? Phlebology 1991;5:113–123.
12. Bradbury AW, Ruckley CV. Foot volumetry can predict recurrent ulceration after subfascial ligation of perforators and saphenous ligation. J Vasc Surg 1993;18:789–795.
13. Bradbury AW, Stonebridge PA, Callam MJ, Allan P, Ruckley CV. Foot volumetry and duplex ultrasonography in patients with recurrent venous ulceration after superficial and perforating vein ligation. Br J Surg 1993;80:845–848.
14. Burnand K, Thomas ML, O'Donnell T, Browse NL. Relation between postphlebitic changes in the deep veins and the results of surgical treatment of venous ulcers. Lancet 1976;i:936–938.
15. Sethia KK, Darke SG. Long saphenous incompetence as a cause of venous ulceration. Br J Surg 1984;71:754–755.
16. Darke SG, Penfold C. Venous ulceration and saphenous ligation. Eur J Vasc Surg 1992;6:4–9.
17. Campbell WA, West A. Duplex ultrasound audit of operative treatment of primary varicose veins. In: Negus D, et al., editors. Phlebology '95. Phlebology 1995; Suppl 1:407–409.
18. Silver D, Gleysteen JJ, Rhodes GR, et al. Surgical treatment of the refractory post-phlebitic ulcer. Arch Surg 1971;103:554–560.
19. Field P, van Boxel P. The role of the Linton flap procedure in the management of stasis dermatitis and ulceration in the lower limb. Surgery 1971;70:920–926.
20. Thurston OG, Williams HTG. Chronic venous insufficiency in the lower extremity: pathogenesis and surgical treatment. Arch Surg 1973;106:537–539.
21. Bowen FH. Subfascial ligation (Linton operation) of the perforating leg veins to treat post-thrombophlebitic syndrome. Am Surg 1975;41:148–151.
22. Blumenburg RM, Gelfland ML. The posterior stocking seam approach to radical subfascial clipping of perforating veins. Am J Surg 1978;136: 202–205.
23. DePalma RG. Surgical treatment for venous stasis: results of a modified Linton operation. Am J Surg 1979;137:810–813.
24. Almgren B, Bowald S, Eriksson I, Forsberg O. The posterior approach for the subfascial ligation of perforating veins. Acta Chir Scand 1982;148:243–245.
25. Hyde GL, Litton TC, Hull DA. Long-term results of subfascial vein ligation for venous stasis disease. Surg Gynecol Obstet 1981;153:683–686.
26. Negus D, Friedgood A. The effective management of venous ulceration. Br J Surg 1983;70:623.
27. Cheung PS, Lim ST, Ng A. Evaluation of the posterior approach for subfascial ligation of perforator veins. Aust NZ J Surg 1985;55:369–372.
28. Johnson WC, O'Hara ET, Corey C, et al. Venous stasis ulceration: effectiveness of subfascial ligation. Arch Surg 1985;120:797–800.
29. Wilkinson JE, Maclaren IF. Long term review of procedures for venous perforator insuffiency. Surg Gynecol Obstet 1986;163:117–120.
30. Szoskek M, Skorski M, Zajac S, Kosicki S, Kosicki A, Zlotorowcz W, Fraczek M. Recurrences after surgical treatment of patients with post-thrombotic syndrome of the lower extremities. Eur J Vasc Surg 1988;2:191–192.
31. Cickrit DF, Nichols WK, Silver D. Surgical management of refractory venous stasis ulceration. J Vasc Surg 1988;7:473–478.
32. Nash TP. Venous ulceration: factors influencing recurrence after standard surgical procedures. Med J Aust 1991;154:48–50.
33. Robison JG, Elliot BM, Kaplan AJ. Limitations of subfascial ligation for refractory chronic venous stasis ulceration. Ann Vasc Surg 1992;6:9–14.

14 Can We Tailor Surgery to the Venous Abnormality?

Simon G. Darke

Introduction

The question posed in the chapter title is open to a variety of interpretations. At its most simple it addresses the feasibility of correcting a venous abnormality by means of an operation. However, when addressing the broader and practical consideration of patient management two important supplementary issues must be addressed: (a) the means by which the abnormality has been identified, and (b) whether this abnormality, and its surgical correction, is relevant to the clinical condition of which the patient complains. More properly, therefore, the question might be "Can we tailor surgery *to the patient's need*?" Clearly these are problems that continue to confront us today in many branches of surgery, but perhaps are particularly germane in the management of venous disease. Indeed some of the chapters in this book are targeted towards various such dilemmas.

These broad concepts can be illustrated with two contrasting examples of clinical settings and operative procedures. For instance, it is now possible with confidence to establish the presence of sapheno-femoral incompetence and its significance in relation to the patient's complaint of, say, painful and unsightly varicose veins. An operation has the prospect, at least in the medium term, of correcting the problem both morphologically and clinically. Surgery has been appropriately and effectively tailored to the venous abnormality and to the patient's clinical need.

By contrast, consider incompetence in the popliteal vein of a patient with a venous ulcer. There may be uncertainty as to how this "incompetence" might be recognised. And assuming that it is thought to be "present", its significance in this particular clinical setting may be unclear, particularly where there are coexistent abnormalities. Can an operation restore normal and durable valvular function? And even if the operation is technically successful in this respect, is the clinical state improved or benefited? Admittedly this second example is extreme, but nonetheless it remains real in practical terms and illustrates a number of relevant doubts and uncertainties. Thus it is apparent that in answering the question posed in the chapter title the whole gamut of venous appraisal and management is potentially under scrutiny.

Problems in Studying Chronic Venous Disease

The Classification of Venous Disease is Complex

In order to study any clinical problem it is essential to be able to identify groups of patients with certain features in common. This may be necessary to evaluate a procedure, compare outcomes or design prospective clinical trials. For venous disease it is complex and difficult [1], particularly because of the diversity of the subject. A full classification is addressed in detail elsewhere in this book, but let us consider the implications in the context of the question posed here. The essential components can be summarised as follows:

1. *Complaint*: Cosmesis, skin change, pain and swelling.
2. *Aetiology*: Congenital/inherent or acquired/post-phlebitic.
3. *Morphology*: Outflow obstruction; valvular incompetence; both the above; recurrence following previous intervention.
4. *Anatomical*: The morphology of (ii) and (iii) can be further divided into anatomical components: superficial – long and short saphenous, deep – iliac, femoral, popliteal, tibio-peroneal, calf perforator.
5. *Severity/quantification*: Quantification of (i) and (iii).

Even if this complex classification can be rationalised, other difficulties arise in answering the question posed.

Symptoms Are Subjective and Cannot Always Be Quantified

The evaluation of symptoms is subjective. If a patient insists that ostensibly trivial varicose veins are painful, yet our personal convictions are that they be mainly of cosmetic concern, there is no arbiter by which this uncertainty can be resolved. These difficulties may be particularly evident in the medico-legal setting where, for instance, a client may describe ill-defined symptoms and disabilities following a deep vein thrombosis or similar event.

Signs May Be of Uncertain Significance

Ankle ulceration is a distressing and common complaint which, in one UK study, was found to have a prevalence in the population of 0.15% [2]. Whilst the presence of an ulcer may not be in doubt, the cause and in particular the pathogenic relevance of venous disease may be difficult to determine even with detailed investigations because of the multiple factors that frequently contribute [3,4].

There May Be Inconsistent Correlation of Symptoms and Signs with Identifiable Morphology

There are sometimes inadequacies and paradoxes in relating clinical settings to demonstrable morphology. In studies that have explored the clinical long-term consequences of deep vein thrombosis, for instance, a poor correlation between the development of subsequent symptoms and the demonstration of morphological abnormalities has been found [5,6]. This is frustrating and difficult to understand and interpret. A more common and obvious example is why some patients with saphenous incompetence get ankle ulcers and others do not.

It Takes a Long Time to Recruit Patients to Trials, Treat Them and Follow Them Up for a Meaningful Period

Recruitment of clinical material takes time, as admittedly it does in many clinical studies. But, as already stated above, there is often the specific need to investigate and define groups of patients with features in common to form the basis for study. These often take a long time to find and require exhaustive investigation and sampling of large numbers of patients.

In some instances, the follow-up needs to be of particularly long duration to allow for realistic analysis and conclusions. For the results of varicose veins or venous ulcer surgery 5 or even 10 years are necessary. It takes a long time to complete a trial.

Follow-up Outcomes May Be Difficult to Define or Identify

Follow-up may be difficult to evaluate and quantify, with ill-defined end-points. There may, for instance, be clinically evident modest recurrent superficial varicosities that are no concern to the patient. How is that to be evaluated and quantified when assessing the outcome of surgery? An ulcer may break out again following minor trauma years after apparently successful surgery, and heal spontaneously after 3 months. How is this to be classified in terms of success? In contrast, in arterial disease the end-points are usually clear and easy to identify: stroke, amputation, death and graft occlusion.

Investigations Have Limitations and Uncertainties

The investigation of venous morphology has for years been rudimentary, relying on clinical signs, venography and, in the last 30 years, continuous wave Doppler. There is no doubt that the advent of duplex ultrasound has been of inestimable value and a number of chapters here bear testimony to that fact. But this modality of investigation is relatively new and incompletely evaluated. Debate still exists as to the criteria by which, for instance, we should regard a valve as "incompetent" and thus at what point it becomes clinically relevant. This is in part because we remain uncertain about what significance can be placed on these various findings in relation to the overall clinical picture. This is a problem compounded by, and a function of, the points made above.

The identification of previous deep vein thrombosis remains a real problem. When post-phlebitic change can be identified, by either ascending venography or duplex scanning, it is specific and beyond reasonable dispute. But when these investigations are normal it remains difficult to exclude a post-phlebitic state with certainty. It is a situation of high specificity and unknown sensitivity. Furthermore, we know from prospective studies that many limbs return to apparent normality after extensive proven deep vein thrombosis [7]. This area of investigation therefore is unsatisfactory, which is probably one reason why it remains largely ignored.

There May Be Complex Morphology Confusing the Outcome of Management Strategies

These complexities are further compounded by the multiplicity of factors that come into play when, as is often the case, more than one venous abnormality can be identified. What will be the benefit of ligating an incompetent saphenous system in a patient with a venous ulcer, where there is evidence of previous deep vein thrombosis and, as a consequence, coexistent reflux in the deep veins? Can we ascribe ulcer healing to calf perforator ligation or a valve repair when the incompetent saphenous system has been ligated synchronously? The venous literature abounds with studies attempting, but largely failing, to answer these questions.

Can Surgical Procedures Deliver their Technical Objectives?

An alternative approach to the question is to look at the surgical options open to us and whether technical operative objectives can be achieved.

Long Saphenous Surgery

Most surgeons would feel that the long saphenous system can be accurately and completely ligated with little difficulty. But how durable is ligation? In terms of recurrence of varicose veins there now seems little doubt that excision of the long saphenous trunk reduces the risks of recurrence [8]. However, recurrent reflux from the groin may occur principally by the phenomenon of neovascularisation [9]. Overall, though, this operation is simple to perform with satisfactory medium-term results.

Short Saphenous Ligation

The short saphenous system is anatomically more varied and technically demanding to identify and ligate. In general the custom is not to strip the short saphenous trunk because of the risk of damaging the sural nerve. The sapheno-popliteal junction can develop recurrent reflux in a manner identical to the long saphenous system, including neovascularisation. Little is known about the durability of surgery to this area. This is probably because it is less common, and more difficult to investigate. It is certainly a more difficult operation and what data there are suggest that the recurrence rate due to both incomplete ligation and neovascularisation is higher than for the long saphenous system [10,11].

Ankle and Calf Perforator Ligation

In the past ankle and calf perforator ligation has been done by a direct open procedure. The operation has received a degree of recent and renewed interest through the introduction of less invasive "endoscopic procedures" [12].

In purely technical terms a satisfactory result can be obtained by either method.

Split Skin Grafting

Obviously split skin grafting applies only to skin ulceration. By and large, with sufficient bed rest and nursing care, sometimes aided by debridement, ulcers can be successfully grafted. Surprisingly little has been written about the durability of this approach. It would seem a legitimate procedure to advance healing of a large ulcer if accompanied by adjunctive procedures to correct coexistent venous morphology. Its role in the management of venous ulcer where no potential exists to improve the underlying abnormalities (e.g. post-phlebitic limb: see below) is uncertain and to my knowledge uninvestigated. On an anecdotal basis it is common to see in such a limb an excellent result on departure from hospital but then to be disappointed by the rapid breakdown when the patient becomes ambulant once more.

Deep Valve Repair and Replacement

Deep valve repair and replacement was the focus of a lot of interest 10 or so years ago but has received little attention of late. A number of ingenious methods have been described to repair directly a valve which is thought to be primarily incompetent (as opposed to post-phlebitic). In purely technical terms this procedure seems to work in an acceptable proportion of cases. By and large, a valve rendered incompetent from the consequences of previous deep vein thrombosis cannot be directly repaired, and thus replacement is necessary. Although the brachial valve has been used as a free transplant, in due course most of these become incompetent. Valve transposition, usually by re-routing the incompetent superficial femoral vein below a competent valve in the deep femoral vein, has had poor results [13].

Reconstruction for Post-phlebitic Occlusive Disease

The Palma procedure has, in very selected cases, an acceptable technical success rate. In this operation the long saphenous trunk is detached in the lower thigh and anastomosed to the common femoral vein in the opposite groin leaving its anatomical connections to the ipsilateral femoral vein intact. This is to alleviate obstruction caused by a previous and persistent iliac vein occlusion. It can be difficult to perform and in technical terms may fail immediately or subsequently. It may not relieve symptoms. Other similar procedures are largely ad hoc and of anecdotal interest only [14].

These, then, are some of the limitations in answering the question "Can we tailor surgery to the venous abnormality?" They are some of the reasons why we have been slow and perhaps ineffective in the study of venous disorders.

The Surgical Management of Venous Ulcer

To try to apply the question of tailoring surgery to the venous abnormality over the full range of chronic venous disease is outside the remit of this chapter and a number topics have been considered by other authors in this book. It is proposed, therefore, to discuss how this question might be applied to the management of venous ulcer. In so doing two assumptions are made: (i) that venous hypertension is established as the cause of the ulcer and (ii) that the possible venous abnormalities (mentioned above) have been demonstrated as completely as possible.

Within this book is information as to the optimal way this might be achieved by clinical examination, continuous wave Doppler, duplex ultrasound and venography. By these means a number of venous abnormalities can be identified: long saphenous incompetence, short saphenous incompetence, ankle and calf perforating vein incompetence, deep vein incompetence and post-phlebitic change causing valve reflux or outflow obstruction. In any one limb there may be any combination of these. To consider further the question "Can we tailor the operation to the venous abnormality" in venous ulcer it is proposed that the underlying morphology be grouped into one of the following types:

Type 1: Perforator incompetence alone.

Type 2: Saphenous incompetence (with or without perforator incompetence).

Type 3: Primary deep vein incompetence (with or without saphenous and perforator incompetence).

Type 4: Post-phlebitic disease. This may include saphenous, perforator or deep incompetence with or without outflow obstruction.

Table 14.1 shows an analysis and interpretation of the published series that have investigated the underlying morphological patterns of venous ulceration to date and allocation into types 1–4 [15–23]. Clearly the data were not published according to these categories. In particular, most of these authors did not identify type 4 (post-phlebitic) patients as a separate group, which confuses the issue. However, what follows is the best possible interpretation of the data within these limitations.

Type 1: Perforator Incompetence Alone

It is apparent from Table 14.1 that to find nothing but ankle and/or calf perforator incompetence in a limb perceived to have a truly venous ulcer is unusual. Indeed it may be that on the rare occasions this is found to be the case, the true morphology may be a post-phlebitic state (type 4), because of the difficulty in identifying this situation (see above). Those that have described a few such cases did not specify post-phlebitic patients separately. The one exception is my own series where a limited number of such patients were found. However, this series was conducted without duplex scanning, which must be considered suboptimal evaluation [17]. In the subsequent series employing duplex ultrasonography no such patients have been seen [22].

But if such a patient, in theory at least, is found, what is the evidence that perforator ligation might be expected to bring about healing? It is of course true to say that interruption of incompetent ankle perforating veins has long had its protagonists. But the evidence from clinical outcome on which the convictions are based has often been where perforator ligation was combined with saphenous ligation [24–34]. It is therefore difficult to know what, if any, was the effect of the former procedure given that saphenous ligation alone may have achieved healing (see below). Furthermore the haemodynamic significance of "reflux" demonstrated at this site is now being questioned [35,36], as is the evidence for the benefits of perforator ligation [37]. There is no published analysis of the outcome of surgery for a group of patients such as these defined here. We therefore do not know for certain whether they exist as a group nor, if they do, how to treat them.

Table 14.1. Venous ulceration: morphology

Author (year)	Ref.	No. of limbs	Assessment	Type (%)			
				1	2	3 (Sup.)	4
McEnroe (1988)	[15]	118	Light rheology		12	80 (14)	?
Hanrahan (1991)	[16]	95	Duplex	8	36	49 (43)	?
Darke (1992)	[17]	235	Venography/CWD	4	39	35 (28)	22
Shami (1993)	[18]	59	Duplex		53	47 (32)	?
Lees (1993)	[19]	25	Duplex		52	48 (12)	?
Weingarten (1993)	[20]	148	Duplex		9	80 (55)	?
van Rij (1994)	[21]	120	Duplex/APG	2	67	31 (28)	?
Darke (1996)	[22]	81	Venography/CWD/duplex	0	59	28 (20)	12
Scriven (1997)	[23]	82	Duplex ("one-stop")	2	57	41 (37)	50

CWD, continuous wave Doppler; APG, air plethysmography; Sup., superficial.

Type 2: Saphenous Incompetence (Usually with Perforator Incompetence)

Hoare and colleagues [38] were the first to report a group of patients with venous ulceration in whom the only identifiable abnormality was saphenous and ankle perforator incompetence. Subsequently Sethia and Darke [39] showed that ligating the incompetent saphenous system normalised the dorsal vein foot pressures, thus anticipating that healing might be expected. There is now evidence to suggest that venous ulceration associated with isolated superficial (long or short saphenous) incompetence is durably healed by ligation of the appropriate saphenous system alone and, specifically, without ankle perforator ligation. In a study over an 8 year period 213 consecutive patients were recruited with venous ulceration of a minimum of 6 weeks' duration. These patients were evaluated by means of clinical examination, continuous wave Doppler and comprehensive ascending and descending venography. At that time, however, no duplex scanning was available so the accuracy in identifying deep incompetence is open to question. Nonetheless, within these limitations 39% were found to have type 2 morphology. These patients were treated by saphenous ligation and stripping to knee level, and in a mean follow-up of 3.5 years 49 of 54 limbs remained healed. In those 5 that failed to heal other factors were subsequently identified to possibly account for the persistent ulceration, including diabetes, leukaemia, and missed short saphenous and popliteal incompetence [17]. More recently, Bass [40] and colleagues have reported healing in 20 patients with lateral venous ankle ulceration and isolated sapheno-popliteal incompetence. Healing was achieved by short saphenous ligation within 12 weeks. On the basis of this information it seems reasonable to conclude that ligation of the perforating veins in these patients is unnecessary.

Type 3: Primary Deep Incompetence Usually Associated with Superficial and Perforator Incompetence

In many ways type 3 is the most interesting and challenging of the types because it introduces the possibility of a variety of operative procedures. But the first and most obvious question that needs to be addressed concerns the benefit that will occur from simple saphenous ligation where this coexists. It will be apparent from Table 14.1 that the majority of these patients are potentially in this category. If ligation were to be unsuccessful then a logical progression would be to consider perforator ligation. If in turn this failed to bring about healing then a group of patients would emerge in whom valve repair could be considered as a legitimate possibility. This of course would be on the assumption that suitable valves for repair could be demonstrated. In my original series [17] this possibility was explored by proceeding logically and stepwise along the lines indicated above. From the cohort of 231 patients, 52 such limbs with combined superficial and deep incompetence were treated by saphenous ligation. After a mean follow-up of 4 years 21 (40%) of these had healed. Nineteen of these unhealed patients then subsequently underwent sub-fascial ligation of perforating veins. Of these, 10 healed and 9 remained unhealed. On the face of it this did rather suggest a place for ankle perforator ligation in this highly refined group of patients and, furthermore, possibly even a further subgroup in whom valve repair might be considered. But these patients were, of necessity, recruited years earlier and thus before the days of duplex scanning. Deep incompetence had been diagnosed on the basis of descending venography and continuous wave Doppler of the popliteal vein. In truth these would not represent adequate evaluation by contemporary standards and any conclusions are open to doubt. This illustrates many of the frustrations of venous research referred to in the Introduction.

In a more recent study duplex ultrasound was used to identify deep incompetence, but the same philosophies of progressive management employed [22]. These patients are currently under observation. However, preliminary results are somewhat in contrast to the initial studies. The majority are at the moment healed with saphenous ligation alone and, in those who have not healed, other contributory circumstances may account for the failure. If in due course these findings hold to be correct then this questions the whole concept of primary deep incompetence being of clinical significance and casts doubt on the future for deep valve repair. It may be that the tests currently and somewhat arbitrarily employed to diagnose "incompetence" in the deep valves are too sensitive and therefore type 3 is no different in practice from type 2. As yet we do not know.

Type 4: Post-phlebitic Limb (Outflow Obstruction and Reflux in Saphenous, Perforators and Deep Systems)

This group poses the most dilemmas. As already stated there is the difficulty in diagnosis. Where there is incontrovertible evidence on imaging it is clear. Where there is a normal venogram/duplex, reliance might alternatively have to be placed on a history of a previous deep vein thrombosis. In the past these episodes have often been poorly documented at the time without appropriate definitive imaging. Increasingly in the future, however, this is likely to be less of a problem because of the changes in clinical attitudes and practice in the last 10–15 years with the routine use first of venography and more recently of duplex scanning in patients with suspected deep vein thrombosis. It is hoped, therefore, that this aspect will become clearer in the future.

Where the diagnosis of a post-phlebitic ulcer is established there is evidence on the outcome of surgical treatment. Burnand et al. [41], as long ago as 1976, showed no healing following calf perforating vein ligation in 23 of 24 limbs known to be post-phlebitic. Several of these patients underwent saphenous ligation as well. In contrast, and in support of the views expressed above, 17 of 18 limbs without post-phlebitic evidence healed with saphenous and perforator ligation [41]. One would question now, of course, whether saphenous ligation alone would have been adequate in this group, which according to the principles suggested here would be defined as types 2 and 3.

These findings have since been confirmed by Bradbury et al. [42], although they approached the problem in a different way. They analysed the finding of popliteal incompetence on duplex scan (i.e. type 3 or 4) as a discriminant factor in patients undergoing saphenous and perforator ligation for ulceration. In 9 of 10 with popliteal reflux the ulcer recurred early. All 33 with normal popliteal vein function (i.e. type 2) remained healed [42]. Again one might challenge the need to have added the ankle perforator ligation.

As will be apparent from both the above and other data, many of these (type 4) patients have saphenous incompetence in addition to other manifestations of post-phlebitic disease. This might be accounted for by one of three different situations: (i) incidental and coexistent saphenous reflux, (ii) a saphenous system rendered incompetent as a consequence of superficial as well as deep thrombosis, or (iii) a dilated and enlarged saphenous system acting as a collateral channel in response to persistent deep obstruction. These patients might be considered for saphenous ligation and the outcome will depend on which of these three situations exists. This can be tested by a variety of devices to quantify reflux and outflow with and without a superficial tourniquet to simulate the effects of saphenous ligation. Certainly, my anecdotal experience is that these tests reveal patients who would on this basis fall into all three categories. However, I remain to be convinced that patients in the post-phlebitic type, irrespective of the apparent status of the incompetent saphenous, are ever improved by saphenous ligation. Furthermore the two studies by Burnand and Bradbury alluded to above showed little if any improvement by a combination of perforator and saphenous surgery.

Summary

So where are we now and what does the future hold? Those with an interest in chronic venous disease will be much encouraged by the increasing interest as witnessed by the growth in numbers and status of national societies all over the world. There has been excellent research conducted in recent years and there is no doubt that the advent of the duplex scanner has done much to further the venous cause. But it is evident that there remain special difficulties in the study of venous disease and work still needs to be done, and easily could be done, to address the many persisting and important areas of ignorance. There are still many missing pieces in the venous jigsaw puzzle.

But what about our question and the surgical management of venous ulcer? There are some statements that can be made with reasonable confidence:

1. Fifty per cent or more of venous ulcers have superficial reflux as the main component and can be healed by appropriate ligation. They do not require perforator ligation. Indeed surgery can be tailored not only to the venous abnormality but also to the patient's need.
2. The significance of primary deep incompetence remains far from clear. Indeed it is possible that it is of no clinical relevance.
3. The treatment of truly post-phlebitic disease remains unsatisfactory. Such cases are difficult to identify with certainty and they behave in an unpredictable fashion. Many investigators tend to ignore them as a separate group. Perforator ligation plays no part in the management and what evidence there is suggests that saphenous ligation does not either. The place for skin grafting is unknown. Surgery may be tailored to what might be demonstated to be the venous abnormality but it is not to the patient's need.
4. On the basis of the above the place for perforator ligation seems limited. There may possibly be a small group in whom primary perforator reflux is the only demonstrable abnormality, but in reality these patients are rare and in fact may be truly post-phlebitic. In that case perforator ligation would not be expected to confer benefit. There may be another group with primary deep incompetence in whom ulceration persists in spite of saphenous ligation, where perforator interruption would be logical. If both these procedures fail then valve repair would be the next logical step. All these issues remain unclear.

References

1. Beebe HG, Bergan JJ, Bergqvist D, et al. Classification and grading of chronic venous disease in the lower limbs: a consensus statement. Eur J Vasc Endovasc Surg 1996;12:482–486.

2. Callam MJ, Ruckley CV, Harper DR, Dale JJ. Chronic ulceration of the leg: extent of the problem and provision of care. BMJ 1985;290:1855–1856.
3. Nelzen O, Bergqvist D, Linhagen A. Venous and non-venous ulcers: clinical history and appearance in a population study. Br J Surg 1994;81:182–187.
4. Nelzen O, Bergqvist D, Linhagen A. Leg ulcer aetiology: a cross sectional population study. J Vasc Surg 1993;10:345–350.
5. Browse NL, Clemenson G, Lea Thomas M. Is the post-phlebitic leg always post-phlebitic? Relation between phlebographic appearances of deep vein thrombosis and late sequelae. BMJ 1980;281:1167–1170.
6. Milne AA, Stonebridge PA, Bradbury AW, Ruckley CV. Venous function and clinical outcome following deep vein thrombosis. Br J Surg 1994;81:847–849.
7. Caprini JA, Arcelus JI, Hoffman KN, et al. Venous duplex imaging follow-up of acute symptomatic deep vein thrombosis of the leg. J Vasc Surg 1995;21:472–476.
8. Darke SG. Chronic venous insufficiency: should the long saphenous vein be stripped? In: Barros D'Sa AAB, Bell PRF, Darke SG, Harris PL, editors. Vascular surgery: current questions. London: Butterworth Heinemann, 1991.
9. Darke SG. What is the evidence for regrowth varicose veins? In: Greenhalgh RM, Fowkes FGR, editors. Trials and tribulations of vascular surgery. Philadelphia: WB Saunders, 1996:385–394.
10. Yong Y, Royle J. Recurrent varicose veins after short saphenous vein surgery: a duplex ultrasound study. Cardiovasc Surg 1996;4:364–367.
11. Darke SG. Recurrent varicose veins and short saphenous insufficiency: evaluation and treatment. In: Bergan JJ, Yao JST, editors. Venous disorders. Philadelphia: WB Saunders, 1991.
12. Pierik EGJ, van Urk H, Hop WCJ, Wittens CHA. Endoscopic versus open subfascial division of incompetent perforating veins in the treatment of venous leg ulcer: a randomised trial. J Vasc Surg 1997;26:1049–1054.
13. Eriksson I, Almgren B, Nordgren L. Late results after venous valve repair. Inter Angio 1985;4:413–417.
14. Darke SG. Venous reconstruction. In: Bell PRF, Jamieson CW, Ruckley CV, editors. The surgical management of vascular disease. Philadelphia: WB Saunders, 1992.
15. McEnroe CS, O'Donnell TF Jr, Mackey WC. Correlation of clinical findings with venous haemodynamics in 386 patients with chronic venous insufficiency. Am J Surg 1988;156:148–152.
16. Hanrahan LM, Araki CT, Rodriguez AA, et al. Distribution of valvular incompetence in patients with venous stasis ulceration. J Vasc Surg 1991;13:805–812.
17. Darke SG, Penfold C. Venous ulceration and saphenous ligation. Eur J Vasc Surg 1992;6:4–9.
18. Shami SK, Sarin S, Cheatle TR, Scurr JH, Coleridge Smith PD. Venous ulcers and the superficial venous system. J Vasc Surg 1993;17:487–490.
19. Lees TA, Lambert D. Patterns of venous reflux in limbs with skin changes associated with chronic venous insufficiency. Br J Surg 1993;80:725–728.
20. Weingarten MS, Branas CC, Czeredarczuk M, Schmidt JD, Wolferth CC Jr. Distribution and quantification of venous reflux in lower extremity chronic venous stasis disease with duplex scanning. J Vasc Surg 1993;18:753–759.
21. van Rij AM, Solomon C, Christie R. Anatomic and physiologic characteristics of venous ulceration. J Vasc Surg 1994;20:759–764.
22. Darke SG. Outcome of saphenous ligation for venous ulceration with and without deep incompetence. (In preparation).
23. Scriven JM, Hartshorne T, Bell PRF, Naylor AR, London NJM. Single visit venous ulcer assessment clinic: the first year. Br J Surg 1997;84:334–336.
24. Cockett FB, Elgan Jones D. The ankle blow out syndrome: a new approach to the varicose ulcer problem. Lancet 1953;1:1–17.
25. Dodd H, Cockett FB. The pathology and surgery of the veins of the lower limb. Edinburgh: Livingstone, 1956
26. Cockett FB. The pathology and treatment of venous ulcers of the leg. Br J Surg 1955;43:260–278.
27. Cranley JJ, Krauss RJ, Strasser ES. Chronic venous insufficiency of the lower extremity. Surgery 1961;49:48–58.
28. De Palma RG. Surgical treatment for venous stasis. Surgery 1975;76:910–915.
29. Dodd H, Calo AR, Mistry M, Rushford A. Ligation of ankle communicating veins in the treatment of the venous ulcer syndrome of the leg. Lancet 1957;2:1249–1252.
30. Linton RR, Hardy JB. Post-thrombotic syndrome of the lower extremity: treatment by interruption of the superficial femoral vein and ligation and stripping of the long and short saphenous veins. Surgery 1948;24:452–432.

31. Linton RR. The post-thrombotic ulceration of the lower extremity: its etiology and surgical treatment. Ann Surg 1953;138:415–432.
32. Negus D, Friegood A. The effective management of venous ulceration. Br J Surg 1983;70:623–627.
33. Negus D. Prevention and treatment of venous ulceration. Ann R Coll Surg Engl 1985;67:144–148.
34. Wittens CHA, Pierik RGJ, Van Urk H. The surgical treatment of incompetent perforating veins. Eur J Endovasc Surg 1993;9:19–23.
35. Zukowski AJ, Nicolaides AN, Szendrog G, Irvine A, et al. Haemodynamic significance of incompetent calf perforating veins. Br J Surg 1991;78:625–629.
36. Sarin S, Scurr JH, Coleridge-Smith PD. Medial calf perforators in venous disease; the significance of outward flow. J Vasc Surg 1992;16:40–46.
37. Recek C. A critical appraisal of the role of ankle perforators for the genesis of venous ulcers in the lower leg. J Cardiovasc Surg 1971;12:45–49.
38. Hoare MC, Nicolaides MS, Miles CR, et al. The role of primary varicose veins in venous ulceration. Surgery. 1982;92:450–453.
39. Sethia KK, Darke SG. Long saphenous incompetence as a cause of venous ulceration. Br J Surg 1984;71:754–755.
40. Bass A, Chayen D, Weimann EE, Ziss M. Lateral venous ulcer and short saphenous vein insufficiency. J Vasc Surg 1997;25:654–657.
41. Burnand KG, Lea Thomas M, O'Donnell TF, Browse NL. The relationship between postphlebitic changes in the deep veins and results of surgical treatment of venous ulcers. Lancet 1976;1:936–938.
42. Bradbury AW, Stonebridge PA, Callam MJ, Ruckley CV, Allan PL. Foot volumetry and duplex ultrasonography after saphenous and subfascial perforating vein ligation for recurrent venous ulceration. Br J Surg 1993;80:845–848.

Section IV

Priorities for Treatment

15 Medical Treatment for Venous Diseases

H.A.M. Neumann

Introduction

Chronic venous insufficiency (CVI) is a very common disease [1]. Different skin changes, such as erythema, pigmentation, white atrophy and a corona phlebectatica (ankle flare) can be detected in the course of the disease. Brown-coloured indurated patches, known as lipodermatosclerosis, are seen in long-standing cases [2]. Finally, a venous leg ulcer will occur in the end stage.

During the past decade, more attention has been given to the important relationship between the macro- and microcirculation in CVI. In the venous system of the lower leg of CVI patients there exists some degree of venous reflux, which leads to a higher walking venous pressure (WVP). This high WVP is transmitted to the microvascular system of the skin, leading to dilatation and a tortuous course of the capillaries. Due to the high capillary pressure the inter-endothelial spaces widen and an abnormally high capillary filtration rate induces an accumulation of water and other plasma components in the interstitium [3]. This leads to oedema and later to dermal backflow of lymphatic fluid. Skin biopsies of CVI skin lesions show an apparent proliferation of capillaries (Fig. 15.1) and a so called peri-capillary halo. The total number of capillaries is actually reduced but, in histological sections, the tortuous loops give the impression of a capillary increase [4].

Microcirculation plays an important role in the total vascular system. However until a few years ago the microcirculation was underestimated in angiology. This was mainly due to the fact that good investigative instruments were lacking. In the past decades several non-invasive techniques have become available for this purpose [5].

The skin microcirculation can be divided into two major parts: the nutritional flow and the thermoregulatory flow. The capillary loops, which run from just under the epidermis into the dermal papillae, are the nutritional capillaries. Flow in this part is only 15% of the total microcirculatory flow. The deeper capillaries have as their main function regulation of the body temperature (thermoregulation). Flow here is 85% of the total flow. As not all techniques can penetrate to both parts of the microcirculation, a combination of tests has often to be used.

Compression therapy is regarded as the major therapeutic modality for CVI patients [6]. It is widely known that – with correction of venous insufficiency by compression therapy and other routine conservative measures – the vast majority of venous ulcers can be healed without major problems within 2–3 months [7]. However, in a study of 600 patients with chronic leg ulcers, the median duration of ulcers was found to be 9 months and 20% had not healed after 2 years. The vast

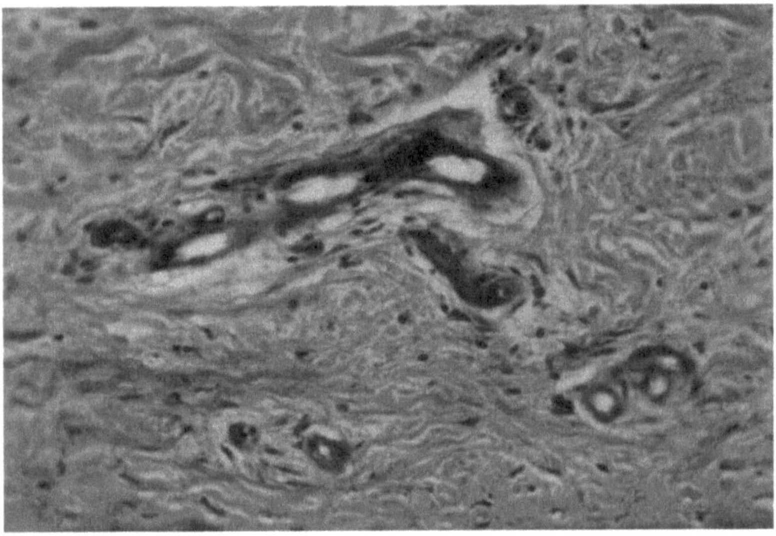

Fig. 15.1. Skin biopsy of a CVI lesion shows an apparent proliferation of capillaries. *(See also Plate III)*

majority of patients had had recurrences, 66% having episodes of ulceration for more than 5 years [8].

A large number of patients are also treated with drugs. Medical treatment may be used as monotherapy or adjuvant therapy. Most of the drugs used act on the microcirculation. Felix [9] has reviewed the veno-active drugs, which may influence venous diseases in one of two ways. The first is to affect the veins directly by activating the muscles of the venous wall. The veins thus contract, reducing their diameter, with the result that the valves become competent again. Consequently reflux diminishes and venous circulation can become normal. The second and most important target for veno-active drugs is the microcirculation. As all clinical signs of CVI are correlated with an altered microcirculation, this part of the circulation seems to be a good target for medical treatment. The major so-called veno-active drugs will be reviewed in this article.

Available Veno-active Drugs

Dihydroergotamine (Ergotamines or Secale-alkaloid Derivatives)

Dihydroergotamine (DHE) has long been known as a veno-active drug [10] that reduces the venous volume of the leg. In a double-masked, crossover, prospective, randomised trial of 20 patients with primary varicose veins, Bjerle et al. [11] showed that oral treatment with 10 mg DHE caused a reduction in venous pressure by 10% and venous reflux by 17%. Although this is a rational treatment and such drugs were used in the past, their use in daily practice is limited. This is due to the small therapeutic scale: the dose of good effect is too close to that producing intoxication (ergotism). Thus, intoxication occurs frequently. Until now no drugs have been available with a selective effect on the muscles of the veins. All other drugs used are employed for their effect on the microcirculation.

Oedema-protective Drugs in the Treatment of CVI [12,13]

Most of the drugs advocated for the medical treatment of CVI, so-called veno-active drugs, have specific effects on the microcirculation. The first sign of decompensation in patients with CVI is oedema. By influencing the capillary filtration of the microcirculation of the legs, oedema will diminish. For that reason, these drugs are often named oedema-protective drugs. Protection against oedema seems a rational goal in the treatment of CVI. Rutosides, and especially hydroxyethylrutosides (HR) are widely used. Diosmin and horse chestnut extract have been used also. Recently, these drugs were reviewed by Diehm [13]. As CVI is an ongoing disease and no consensus exists about the best evaluative technique, studies are not always easy to compare. Experimental studies have proved that the flavonoid HR will reduce the size of expanded inter-endothelial pores [14,15]. Clinical studies have also shown that HR can reduce transvascular leakage of ^{125}I-albumin [16], capillary filtration rate [17,18] and oedema [19,20] in patients with CVI. Drugs such as HR are often described as oedema-protective drugs in the literature. Oedema-protective drugs mainly decrease the capillary filtration [20]. This effect is based on a reduction of the microvascular permeability and thus leads to a reduction in oedema [21]. As oedema is the most important clinical sign of decompensation of the microcirculation in CVI, many regard this effect as important. This legitimises the use of these drugs in CVI. As HR is the most studied drug in the group of oedema-protective drugs, we will discuss its effects extensively.

Wadworth and Faulds [21] studied in detail the pharmacology and therapeutic efficacy of HR in venous insufficiency and related disorders. Venous blood partial oxygen pressure (pO_2) oxygen content and oxygen saturation were lower, and tissue oxygen extraction was higher, in legs of patients with CVI than in the legs of healthy volunteers [22]. Several investigators demonstrated that HR improves these parameters (Table 15.1). For example, oral HR (1–2 g/day for 4 weeks) in patients with CVI increased leg venous pO_2 by 35% and oxygen content by 30%, decreased leg tissue oxygen extraction by 34% (all $p \leq 0.01$ versus baseline) [22], and improved venous refilling time and transcutaneous pO_2 (16%; $p = 0.001$ versus pretreatment) [23]. Venous refilling time also improved markedly in patients with varicose veins with or without CVI during days 10–21 of treatment with HR 1–3 g/day for 3 weeks [24]. Administration of HR (1 g/day

Table 15.1. Overall vascular effects of hydroxyethylrutosides in the legs of patients with chronic venous insufficiency [18,22,23,25,26]

Pharmacodynamic parameter	In patients with CVI (vs healthy volunteers)	Effect of HR in patients with CVI*
Capillary filtration rate	Increase	Decrease
Venous blood pO_2	Decrease	Increase
Transcutaneous pO_2	Decrease	Increase
Transcutaneous pCO_2	Increase	Decrease
Resting skin blood flow	Increase	Decrease
Venoarteriolar response	Decrase	Increase
Venous refill time	Decrease	Increase

HR, hydroxyethylrutosides; pCO_2, partial carbon dioxide pressure; pO_2, partial oxygen pressure.
*Effects were significant ($p < 0.05$) versus placebo or pretreatment levels.

for 4 weeks) improved transcutaneous oxygen levels in the skin of the ulcer-bearing area of patients with CVI ($p = 0.02$ versus placebo-treated patients) [25]. In addition, a significant reduction in transcutaneous partial carbon dioxide pressure (pCO_2, −11%) and basal skin flow (−27%), and significant increases in transcutaneous pO_2 (13%) and venoarteriolar response (49%, all $p \leq 0.05$ versus baseline), were observed after 6 weeks' therapy with HR 1 g twice a day in patients with venous hypertension with associated skin alterations and ankle oedema [26]. A further study showed that these changes in microvascular perfusion were maintained for 6 months. Treatment with HR also increased lower limb transcutaneous pO_2 by 8%, and peak post-occlusive response by 100% [27].

In patients with CVI, HR 0.6–1.2 g/day for up to 6 months significantly improves objective and subjective measures of lower limb venous insufficiency. In most placebo-controlled studies the improvements in leg volume, calf and/or ankle circumference, and relief from symptoms of pain, tired legs, night cramps and restless legs achieved during HR therapy were significantly greater than those reported during placebo therapy. Overall, 73–100% of patients had some improvements during HR therapy and 25–90% responded to placebo treatment. Response rates (percentage of patients with improvements) for individual symptoms during HR therapy ranged from 54% to 82% for pain, 35% to 53% for restless legs, 64% to 68% for tired "heavy" legs and 59% to 91% for cramps. Improvements in signs and symptoms of venous insufficiency (including cramps, irritation, swelling and pain) and reductions in accumulation of extravascular fluid correlated with improvements in microcirculatory parameters. Reduction in ankle circumference, and improvements in symptoms of pain, night cramps and paraesthesia, was achieved in patients with varicosis of pregnancy treated with HR 0.3–1.8 g/day [21].

In a total of 344 patients with venous ulcers healed within the preceding year, the resultant plotting of regression lines for the rate of recurrence (%) of ulcers in each group at each visit showed a significant difference between the HR group and the placebo group ($p < 0.03$). Thus, the ulcer recurrence rate was progressively decreased in the HR group and increased in the placebo group. The difference in recurrence rate between the two groups became significant after 20 months [28]. This indicates the need for prolonged – maybe lifetime – treatment.

Anabolic Steroids

Fibrin is very often found around the capillaries. Browse and Burnand developed from this finding the "fibrin cuff" theory [2,29,30]. In combination with a finding of low $TcPO_2$ values, the theory was that the fibrin cuffs acted as a barrier to oxygen. Michel proved in a theoretical model [31], which was later established in a clinical study, that fibrin cannot act as a barrier to oxygen [29]. Stanozolol is the most commonly used anabolic steroid in phlebology. It is a modified anabolic steroid, which enhances deficient fibrinolysis and has been shown to be useful in reducing the area of lipodermatosclerosis when combined with elastic compression [32]. Stanozolol is also used for the treatment of leg ulcers [33,34]. Treatment with elastic stockings and stanozolol has not been proved to be beneficial in preventing leg ulcer recurrence [35]. Although this drug is not widely accepted, it seems to be interesting enough to explore the possibilities of fibrinolytic enhancement for venous diseases more extensively [36,37]. The special effect of stanozolol in relief of pain, as well as in healing of leg ulcers caused by cryofibrinogenaemia, is interesting [38].

Prostaglandin

Prostaglandin E_1 has been widely used in the treatment of peripheral vascular disease. Its properties include vasodilatation inhibition or platelet aggregration and inhibition of neutrophil activation. Rudofsky [39], in a study (double-masked, placebo-controlled) of 44 patients with venous ulceration, found a significant beneficial effect of prostaglandin E_1. It is, however, an intravenous therapy and rather expensive, which limits its application in daily practice.

Methylxanthines

Pentoxifylline has been used for many years in the treatment of peripheral arterial occlusive disease [40]. Its effects include increasing red cell deformability with resultant improvement in oxygen delivery to tissue, reduced white cell aggregation and activation, and mild fibrinolytic activities. These effect could be helpful in the treatment of venous disease.

Weitgasser [4] was the first to report a placebo-controlled double-masked study of 59 patients with venous ulceration. Twenty-six of the 30 patients on active treatment showed improvement over the study period in contrast to 13 of the 29 patients on placebo. Angelides et al. [42] showed partial or complete healing in 8 of 10 patients with definite venous ulceration following 6 weeks of treatment with pentoxifylline. A multicentre prospective double-masked placebo-controlled study in patients with refractory venous ulceration was undertaken [43] in which 80 patients were randomised to treatment with placebo or pentoxifylline in addition to conventional compression therapy. After 6 months, 23 of the 38 patients receiving pentoxifylline had complete ulcer healing in contrast to 2 of the 42 patients receiving placebo.

Flunarizine

In a placebo-controlled double-masked study of 139 patients suffering from varicose veins combined with a range of subjective symptoms, flunarizine was statistically significantly superior to placebo in improving symptomatology, and reducing the circumference of swollen legs and ankles [44]. However, the selection criteria were oriented more towards varicose veins than to CVI.

Aspirin

Aspirin was recently introduced for the treatment of venous leg ulcers. Treatment with 300 mg/day aspirin resulted in a significant reduction in healing time [45,46]. Capillaroscopy has proved that microthrombi play a role in the aetiology of severe CVI [47], so it seems possible that these microthrombi are of clinical importance in the aetiology of venous leg ulcers. Coagulation-preventing medication could be of help according to this hypothesis, supported by the positive results of aspirin therapy.

Discussion

Treatment of CVI is still far from ideal. In cases where no permanent correction of the high ambulatory venous pressure is possible, compression therapy will still be the cornerstone of treatment [48].

Medical treatment has a small place as monotherapy and certainly a place as an adjuvant treatment. Three major aims can be pursued:

1. *Reduction of symptoms.* Many patients with CVI have complaints of heavy and swollen legs in the evening, aching pain in the lower legs, night cramps, restless or fidgety legs and the sensation of pins and needles. These complaints are difficult to evaluate. Pulvertaft [49] showed a high placebo effect; though after treatment he found a significant reduction in these complaints. Pulvertaft rightly advises careful patient selection to ensure that patients with the correct diagnosis and symptoms of sufficient severity are admitted to this type of clinical trial [49].
2. *Oedema protection.* Placebo-controlled clinical trials have shown that drugs such as HR, diosmin, horse chestnut extract and heptaminol [50] reduce oedema and improve signs and symptoms of CVI [9,13,21,37]. Clinical efficacy can be measured objectively: oedema by electro-optical volumetry, oxygen by $tcPO_2$, venous refill time by photoplethysmography, and CFR by strain gauge plethysmography/air plethysmography. The effect of preventing ulcer breakdown is less clear [28]. The resultant effect on the prevention of recurrences of venous ulcers, although not striking, was significant in those patients. Combined treatment of veno-active drugs and compression therapy (medical elastic compression stockings) shows greater clinical benefits than either treatment alone [23]. These drugs are well tolerated as shown in clinical trials and therapeutic use.
3. *Ulcer treatment.* Although venous leg ulcers will never be treated alone, drugs can be helpful in speeding up the healing process. In particular the effect of aspirin needs more attention and future investigation.

Although ergotamine is from a theoretical point of view an excellent drug for the treatment of primary venous insufficiency, I would not recommend it due to the high risk of intoxication (ergotism). Prostaglandin is promising, but due to the necessity of intravenous administration it cannot be used widely in so common a disease as CVI.

The drugs that are an appropriate option in the management of CVI are the flavonoids. HR especially has been studied extensively. An excellent review by Wadworth and Faulds [21] brings all the effects together. The observation that HR is absorbed by the vascular wall of the venous system is interesting [51]. The place for stanozolol seems to be limited. Unfortunately, a good comparative study between stanozolol and HR is lacking. More information is needed about the place of pentoxifylline and aspirin, especially in the treatment of venous leg ulcers.

From clinical data and the many studies carried out, we can conclude that venotropic drugs are effective but that their therapeutic power is low. This means a reduction of signs and symptoms is obtained but no total healing. It is this discrepancy between the hard data of many clinical trials and the more or less adjuvant effect of veno-active drugs which makes practitioners doubt the value of prescribing this type of drug. On the other hand, as CVI is a chronic disease which ends finally in a leg ulcer, a drug that can slow this process is helpful. The cost of this treatment compared with the cost of leg ulcer treatment is relatively low. Thus a long-term study which also takes into account the quality of life and the cost of treatment is required.

At present we can conclude that the most appropriate veno-active drugs are from the flavonoid group, such as HR. We can use them in the early phases of CVI as monotherapy for oedema prevention and later on in combination with compression therapy as adjuvant therapy to slow down the disease process.

References

1. Widmer LK, Stähelin HB. Peripheral venous disorders: prevalence and socio-medical importance. Observations in 4529 apparently healthy persons. Basle study III. Bern: Hans Huber, 1978.
2. Browse NL, Burnand KG. The cause of venous ulceration. Lancet 1982;2:243–245.
3. Wenner A, Leu HJ, Spycher M, Brunner U. Ultrastructural changes of capillaries in chronic venous insufficiency. Exp Cell Biol 1980;48:1–14.
4. Fagrell B. Microcirculatory disturbances: the final cause for venous leg ulcers? Vasa 1982;11:101–103.
5. Neumann HAM. Measurement of microcirculation. In: Altmeyer X, et al., editors. Wound healing and skin physiology. Berlin Heidelberg New York: Springer, 1995:115–126.
6. Partsch H. Compression therapy of the legs: a review. J Dermatol Surg Oncol 1991;17:799–805.
7. Haeger K. X In: Hobbs, JT, editor. Treatment of venous disorders. Lancaster: MTP Press, 1977:272–291.
8. Callam MJ, Harper DR, Dale JJ, Ruckley CV. Chronic ulcers of the leg: clinical history. BMJ 1987;294:1389–1391.
9. Felix W. Spektrum Venenmittel. Arzneimitteltherapie Heute 1986;45.
10. Rieckert H. Die Pharmakodynamik des Dihydroergotamin, eine Studie über die Hämodynamik in hapazitiven Gefäbsystem. In: Pabst HW, Maurer G, editors. Postoperative thromboembolie. Prophylaxe. Stuttgart: Schattauer Verlag 1977:69.
11. Bjerle P, Gjöres JE, Thulesius O, Berlin E. Treatment of venous insufficiency with dihydroergotamine. Vase 1979;8:158–162.
12. Markwardt F. Pharmacology of oedema protective drugs. Phlebology 1996;11:10–15.
13. Diehm C. The role of oedema protective drugs in the treatment of chronic venous insufficiency: a review of evidence based on placebo-controlled clinical trials with regard to efficacy and tolerance. Phlebology 1996;11:23–29.
14. Arturson G. Effects of *O*-(β-hydroxyethyl-)rutosides (HR) on the increased microvascular permeability in experimental skin burns. Acta Chir Scand 1972;138:111–117.
15. Hammersen F. The ultrastructural changes in the microcirculation in experimental oedema: a suitable morphological test-model for the effect of vasoactive drugs. Biorheology 1970;6:343–351.
16. Hishon S, Hunter JO, Rose JD. The effect of hydroxyethylrutosides on albumin escape rate in cirrhosis. In: Hydroxyethylrutosides in vascular disease. Royal Society of Medicine Symposium Series 1981;42:55–59.
17. Roztocil K, Fischer A, Novak P, Razgova L. The effect of *O*-(>b-hydroxyethyl-)rutosides (HR) on the peripheral circulation of patients with chronic venous insufficiency. Eur J Clin Pharmacol 1971;3:243–246.
18. Roztocil K, Prerovsky I, Oliva I. The effect hydroxyethylrutosides on capillary filtration rate in the lower limb of man. Eur J Clin Pharmacol 1977;11:435–438.
19. Balmer A, Limoni C. A double-blind placebo-controlled clinical trial of Venoruton on the symptoms and signs of chronic venous insufficiency: the importance of patient selection. Vasa 1980;9:76–82.
20. Bergqvist D, Hallbrook T, Lindblad B, Lindhagen A. A double-blind trial of *O*-(β-hydroxyethyl)-rutoside in patients with chronic venous insufficiency. Vasa 1981;10:253–260.
21. Wadworth AN, Faulds D. Hydroxyethylrutosides: a review of its pharmacology, and therapeutic efficacy in venous insufficiency and related disorders. Drugs 1992;44:1013–1032.
22. McEwan AJ, McArdle CS. Effect of hydroxyethylrutosides on blood oxygen levels and venous insufficiency symptoms in varicose veins. BMJ 1971;2:138–141.
23. Neumann HAM, Broek MJThB van den. Evaluation of *O*-(β-hydroxyethyl)-rutosides in chronic venous insufficiency by means of non-invasive techniques. Phlebology 1990;5:13–20.
24. Stemmer R, Furderer CR. Posologie de l'*O*-beta hydroxyethylrutoside dans l'insuffisance veineuse chronique. Phlebologie 1986;39:95–1003.
25. Burnand KG, Powell S, Bishop C, Stacey M, Pulvertaft T. Effect of Paroven on skin oxygenation in patients with varicose veins. Phlebology 1989;4:15–22.

26. Belcaro G, Rulo A, Candiani C. Evaluation of the microcirculatory effects of Venoruton in patients with chronic venous hypertension by laser Doppler flowmetry, transcutaneous pO_2 and pCO_2 measurements, leg volumetry and ambulatory venous pressure measurements. Vasa 1989;18:146–151.
27. Quigley FG, Faris IB. A study on the effect of hydroxyethylrutoside on transcutaneous oxygen tension measurements in patients with severe venous insufficiency. Vasc Surg 1991;25:42–47.
28. Neumann HAM, Broek MJThB van den, Crombag NH, et al. Evaluation of *O*-(β-hydroxyethyl-)rutosides in the prevention of the breakdown of venous ulcers: a long-term international multicentre controlled clinical trial. Scripta Phlebol 1996;4:55–63.
29. Neumann HAM, Broek MJThB van den, Boersma IH, Veraart JCJM. Transcutaneous oxygen tension in patients with and without pericapillary fibrin cuffs in chronic venous insufficiency, porphyria cutanea tarda and non-venous leg ulcers. Vasa 1996;25:127–133.
30. Burnand KG, Whimster I, Naidoo A, Browse NL. Pericapillary fibrin in the ulcer-bearing skin of the leg: the cause of lipodermatosclerosis and venous ulceration. Br Med J Clin Res Ed 1982;285:1071–1072.
31. Michel CC. Oxygen diffusion in edematous tissue and through pericapillary cuffs. Phlebology 1990;5:223–230.
32. Neumann HAM, Broek MJThB van den. Stanozolol and the treatment of severe chronic venous insufficiency. Phlebology 1988;3:237–246.
33. Layer GT, Stacey MC, Burnand KG. Stanozolol and the treatment venous ulceration: an interim report. Phlebology 1986;1:197–203.
34. Colgan MP, Moore DJ, Shanik DG. Drug therapy for venous ulcers: new methods of treatment. Phlebology 1992;1:41–43.
35. Stacey MC, Burnand KG, Layer GT, Pattison M. Transcutaneous oxygen tensions in assessing the treatment of healed venous ulcers. Br J Surg 1990;77:1050–1054.
36. McMullin GM, Watkin GT, Coleridge-Smith PD, Scurr JH. Efficacy of fibrinolytic enhancement with stanozolol in the treatment of venous insufficiency. Aust N Z J Surg 1991;61:306–309.
37. Colgan MP, Moore DI, Shanik DG. New approaches in the medical management of venous ulceration. Angiology 1993;44:138–142.
38. Kirsner RS, Eaglstein WH, Katz MH, Kerdel FA, Falanga V. Stanozolol causes rapid pain relief and healing of cutaneous ulcers caused by cryofibrinogenemia. J Am Acad Dermatol 1993;28:71–74.
39. Rudofsky G. Intravenous prostaglandin E_1 in the treatment of venous ulcers: a double-blind, placebo-controlled trial. Vasa 1989;28:39–43.
40. McCollum PT, Kent P, O'Driscoll K, et al. Intravenous pentoxifylline in the treatment of rest pain: a preliminary report. Ann Vasc Surg 1989;3:220–223.
41. Weitgasser H. The use of pentoxifylline ("Trental" 400) in the treatment of leg ulcers: results of a double-blind trial. Pharmatherapeutica 1983;3:143–151.
42. Angelides NS, Weil von der Ahe CA. Effect of oral pentoxifylline therapy on venous lower extremity ulcers due to deep venous incompetence. Angiology 1989;40:752–763.
43. Colgan MP, Dormandy JA, Jones PW, Schraibman IG, Shanik DG, Young RAL. Oxpentifylline treatment of venous ulcers of the leg. BMJ 1990;300:972–975.
44. Roeckaerts F, Morias J, Platteau K, et al. The efficacy of flunarizine in venous insufficiency: a double-blind placebo-controlled study. Curr Ther Res 1979;26:363.
45. Ibbotson SH, Layton AM, Davies JA, Goodfield MJ. The effect of aspirin on haemostatic activity in the treatment of chronic venous leg ulceration. Br J Dermatol 1995;132:422–426.
46. Layton AM, Ibbotson SH, Davies JA, et al. Randomised trial of oral aspirin for chronic venous leg ulcers. Lancet 1994;344:164–165.
47. Leu AJ, Leu HJ, Franzeck UK, Bollinger A. Microvascular changes in chronic venous insufficiency: a review. Cardiovasc Surg 1995;3:237–245.
48. Neumann HAM, Tazelaar DJ. Compression therapy. In: Bergan JJ, Goldman MP, editors. Varicose veins and telangiectasias: diagnosis and treatment. St Louis: Quality Medical Publishing, 1993:103–122.
49. Pulvertaft TB. General practice treatment of symptoms of venous insufficiency with oxerutins: results of a 660 patient multicentre study in the UK. Vasa 1983;12:373–376.
50. Schmidt C, Gavoille R, Perez P, Schmitt J. Double-blind plethysmographic study of venous effects of heptaminol adenosine phosphate in patients with primary varicose veins. Eur J Clin Pharmacol 1989;37:37–40.
51. Neumann HAM, Carlsson K, Brom GHM. The uptake and localisation of *O*-(β-hydroxyethyl-)rutosides in the venous wall, measured by laser scanning microscopy. Eur J Clin Pharmacol 1992;26:20–27.

16 Telangiectasia: Is Treatment Worthwhile and Who Should Pay?

Awf Quaba

Introduction

The term telangiectasia, literally "end vessel dilatation", was first used in 1807 by Von Graf to describe a superficial vessel of the skin that is visible to the human eye [1]. These vessels usually measure 0.1–2 mm in diameter and may represent expanded capillary, venule or arteriole. Histological examination shows a single endothelial cell lining in a normal dermal stroma [2]. Being common, these vessels are known by many names such as thread veins, spider veins, venous stars and venous flares. Many are asymptomatic, but some patients complain of local aching, heaviness and fatigue. These symptoms are probably caused by the deeper veins.

There is no universally accepted classification of telangiectasia. One classification, based on clinical appearance, groups telangiectasia into simple (linear), arborising, spider and papular [3]. Two common patterns of telangiectasia on the legs are the parallel linear pattern, usually found on the medial thigh and inner knee and the radiating cartwheel pattern, seen most often on the lateral thigh. Arborising telangiectasia, sometimes called essential progressive telangiectasia is caused by intensely red superficial 0.1–0.3 mm vessels that most commonly appear on feet and ankles and spread proximally (Fig. 16.1).

Leg telangiectasia is one of the most common cosmetic concerns in women. Some authors report an incidence of about 40% [4]. It is beyond the scope of this chapter to list all possible causes of leg telangiectasia; however, one or more of the following factors may be implicated in the majority of cases.

(1) *Varicose veins.* Doppler examination [5] and duplex scanning [6] have demonstrated association with feeding reticular veins which are not necessarily part of any truncal varicosities. Venous hypertension could result in the formation of telangiectatic vessels by opening up and dilatation of pre-existing vascular anastomotic channels or the relative anoxia associated with venous hypertension could lead to angiogenesis.

(2) *Hormonal factors.* Pregnancy is the most common physiological condition associated with telangiectasia. Almost 70% of women develop telangiectasia during pregnancy but the majority of these vessels disappear during the first 3 months post-partum. The contraceptive pill has also been implicated. Davis and Duffy [7] reported an apparent association of oestrogen excess states with the development of telangiectatic matting after sclerotherapy for telangiectasia.

(3) *Physical factors.* Ultraviolet rays could induce telangiectasia in individuals with

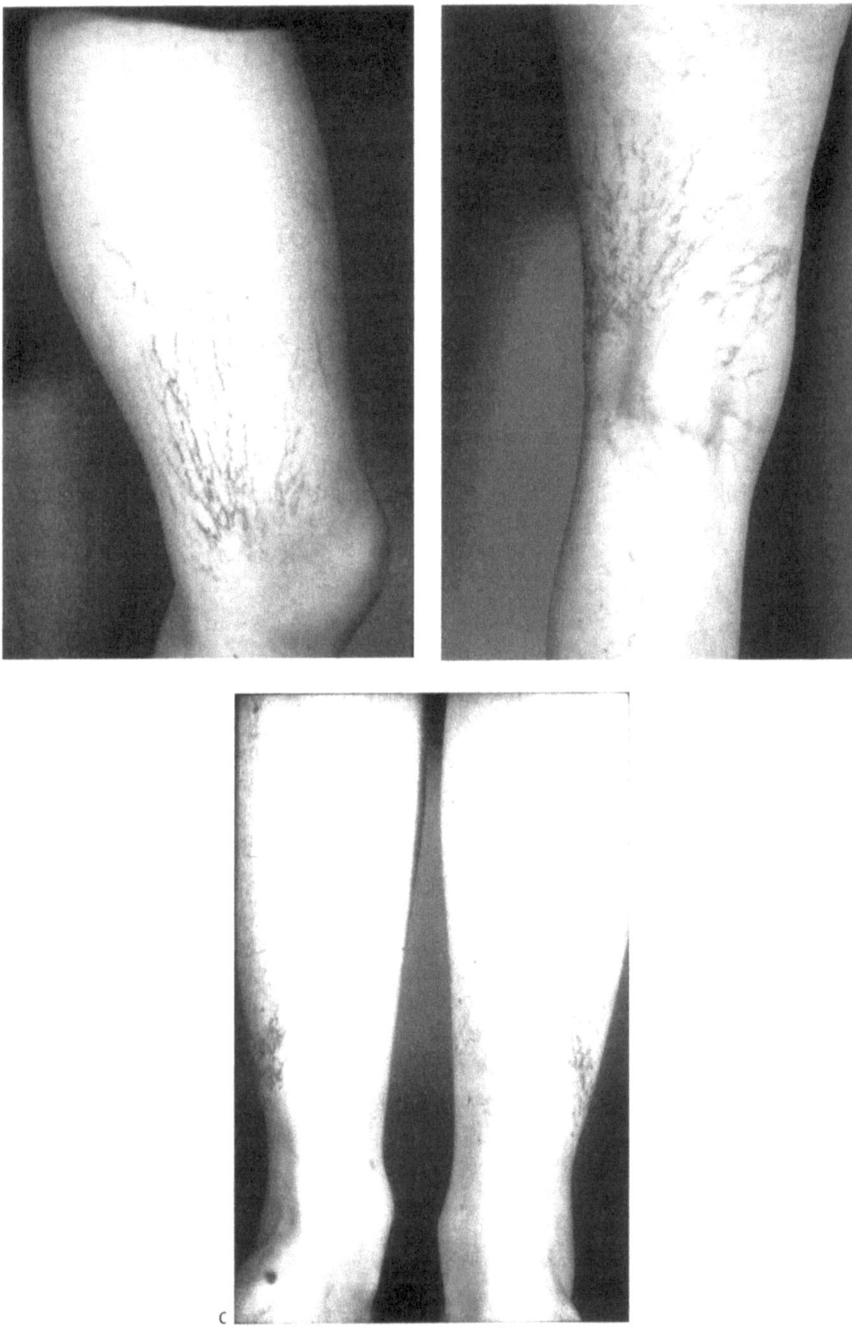

a b c

Fig. 16.1a–c. Examples of telangiectasia. **a** Linear parallel on the inner thigh. This is usually difficult to remove. **b** Linear cartwheel on the posterolateral thigh with reticular veins on the popliteal fossa. **c** Progressive arborising telangiectasia. This starts on the feet and ankles and spreads proximally. It is usually 0.2 mm or less in diameter and responds well to laser. *(See also Plate IV)* fair complexions. Naturally, the face is more susceptible but the legs are not exempt. Contusion injury, especially on the outer aspect of the thighs, is a common mechanism for the development of a localised area of telangiectasia, perhaps through neovascularisation. Also, patients undergoing extensive ligation and stripping of varicose veins may develop telangiectasia around the surgical scars within weeks of surgery, particularly in those who report extensive immediate post-operative bruising.

Therapeutic Options: Overview

Methods for the treatment of leg telangiectasia include electrolysis, microsclerotherapy and laser therapy. Electrolysis could, when employed with extreme care, successfully treat the arteriolar-type spider telangiectasias such as those involving the face, but its role in the management of leg veins is limited and the treatment frequently results in inadequate removal, hypopigmentation and even scarring. Laser and, more recently, non-coherent pulsed light sources, are perceived as being high technology "state-of-the-art" techniques and are sought by the general public because "high-tech" is thought of as safe and better. Unfortunately, on the whole the results of laser treatment of the average patient with leg telangiectasia have been disappointing. Microsclerotherapy remains the mainstay of treatment but it is invasive, time-consuming, technically demanding and not entirely free of side effects. The outcome of the treatment varies a great deal depending on the type of sclerosant used, its concentration, the amount injected per site, the frequency of injections, the pressure and rapidity of the injection and whether or not post-microsclerotherapy compression is used.

Microsclerotherapy

General

Sclerotherapy refers to the introduction of an irritating solution into the lumen of a vessel causing damage to the endothelial lining and subsequent fibrosis. When performed on 0.3–2 mm vessels it is referred to as microsclerotherapy.

Good results can be obtained on slow-filling linear or radiating vessels on the lower extremities (Fig. 16.2). Patients should be advised that the aim of the treatment is to control rather than cure the problem and that new veins could develop at other sites and sometimes at the same site as the injection (telangiectatic matting). More than one session is usually necessary, with some areas requiring several treatments. Nevertheless, some 50% improvement is usually expected after the first session and if this is not observed then a different sclerosing agent may need to be considered. The sessions are usually given at 6–8 weekly intervals. Patients must be advised of the approximate number of the sessions and the duration to complete treatment. Some flexibility, depending on the outcome, is required. Reticular 2–3 mm feeding veins and perforators must be sclerosed first. Pregnancy is a relative contraindication to treatment and the presence of allergic conditions such as asthma may influence the choice of the sclerosing agent. Patients with history of deep vein thrombosis, superficial thrombophlebitis and leg ulceration require proper evaluation prior to microsclerotherapy. Extra care is required in patients with ischaemic legs and diabetic neuropathy as well as in patients with a history of blood-borne disease.

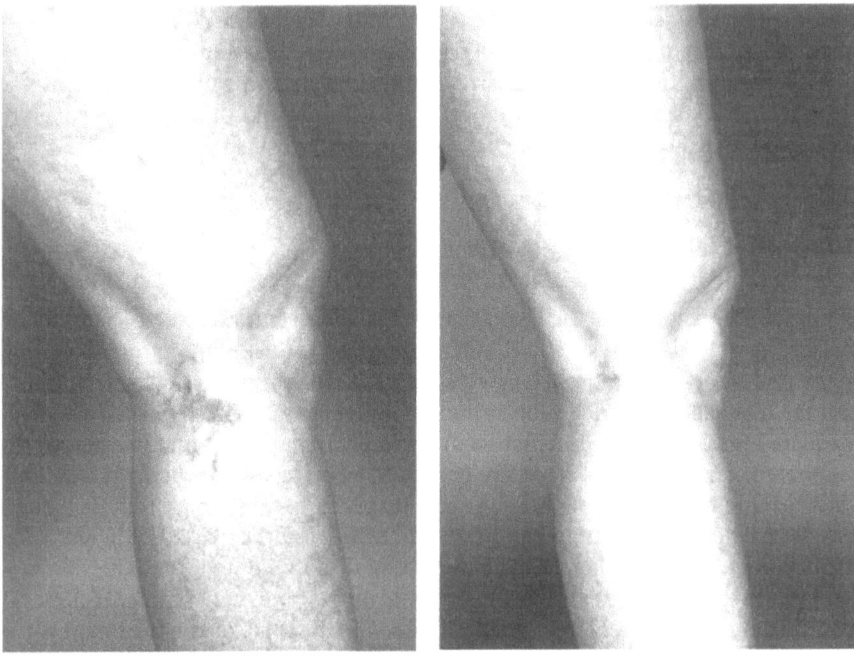

a b

Fig. 16.2a,b. Average result of microsclerotherapy after two sessions using 30% hypertonic saline. Total volume per session did not exceed 0.4 ml. *(See also Plate V)*

Types of Sclerosing Solutions

Some practitioners use one agent exclusively for microsclerotherapy. Others are prepared to try more than one agent depending on the clinical response. The ideal solution should be painless, inexpensive, approved and available, non-allergenic and non-toxic. The available agents can be divided into three groups:

Detergent Solutions

Examples of detergent solutions are sodium tetradecyl sulphate (STS), ethanolamine oleate and polidocanol (POL). These agents cause endothelial damage by interfering with cell surface lipids. Strong detergent sclerosants have a low safety margin [8].

Osmotic Solutions

Hypertonic saline or hypertonic glucose produces dehydration of the endothelial cells through osmosis, resulting in damage which is proportional to the concentration of the agent. The advantage of hypertonic saline is its lack of allergenicity, however, like many other agents it will cause skin necrosis if injected perivascularly. Concentrations of 20–30% can be used depending on the vessel diameter. Some authors believe that reducing the concentration to less than 20% may not reduce the effectiveness but could reduce complications. However, it is important to remember that any osmotic agent is rapidly diluted in the bloodstream and therefore loses its potency within a short distance of injection. Haemolysis of red blood cells occurs through non-specific osmotic damage leading to release of haemosiderin, which could extravasate leading to post-treatment pigmentation. Sadick [9] found that the addition of heparin to hypertonic saline provided no benefit in microsclerotherapy. Two millilitres of 30% hypertonic saline can be diluted with 0.5 ml of 2% lidocaine and this amount is sufficient to treat quite extensive areas. The lidocaine is helpful in reducing the transient pain and muscle cramping experienced in patients undergoing microsclerotherapy with hypertonic saline.

Chemical Solutions

Chromated glycerine, marketed in Europe under the trade name Scleremo (72% chromated glycerine), is a very mild agent and allergic reactions are very rare.

Technique and Aftercare

Microsclerotherapy is performed with the patient in the supine position. The skin is wiped with alcohol, making the telangiectasia more visible because of a change in the index of refraction of the skin. Magnification (surgical loupes ×3.5) is essential for the accurate placement of the sclerosing agent within the 0.3–2 mm vessels. Half inch 30 gauge needles 0.3 mm in external diameter are used for the injection. The narrower point of the bevel permits cannulation of vessels more than 0.1 mm in diameter. These needles should be changed after 8–10 injections. Disposable syringes, preferably 2–2.5 ml, are recommended as they fit well in the palm and can be easily manipulated. Higher injection pressures can be generated when 1 ml insulin syringes are used but with increasing risk of extravasation. With magnification and adequate lighting, the 30 gauge needle, carefully bent to a 30°–40° angle, can easily be placed within the vessel lumen and the penetration of the vessel is "felt". The most common mistake is to place the tip of the needle deep to the vessel. It is recommended to stop the injection of a particular site once an area of 1–2 cm is emptied of blood (Fig. 16.3), although occasionally quite dramatic blanching [9,10] can take place when a fast-flowing spider vein with interconnecting arborising patch is injected. It is essential to remember that high injection pressure and the injection of large volumes per site could result in extravasation. A volume of sclerosing agent that could easily travel undiluted to the deep venous system should not be injected at any one particular site [11]. The injection of more than 0.3 ml per site of hypertonic saline usually results in pain and cramping, particularly when ankles or lower legs are injected. The same area should not be treated more often than every 6 weeks.

There is no consensus regarding the type of the sclerosing agents and the optimal concentration of the solutions used. Carlin and Ratz [12] tested polidocanol 0.25%, STS 0.5% and hypertonic saline 20% in the treatment of leg telangiectasia and found that whereas hypertonic saline and STS gave quicker clearing of telangiectasia with fewer injections the overall level of improvement was identical for all agents. In general, the smaller the diameter of the telangiectasia the less the need to use high concentrations of sclerosant. Slow injection allows a mild sclerosing agent to stay in contact with the vessel wall for a longer period of time. In fact, vessels will remain blanched (filled with the sclerosing solution) if the plunger of the syringe is held with almost zero force while the needle remains motionless. Inadvertent extravasation should be immediately diluted by injecting normal saline or local anaesthetic followed by massage.

The patient with cosmetic telangiectasia is not keen on expensive, uncomfortable and inconvenient post-sclerotherapy protocols. The majority of patients are advised that they should not alter their activity one way or the other and leave after a session of treatment without dressings or compressions. However, graduated compression

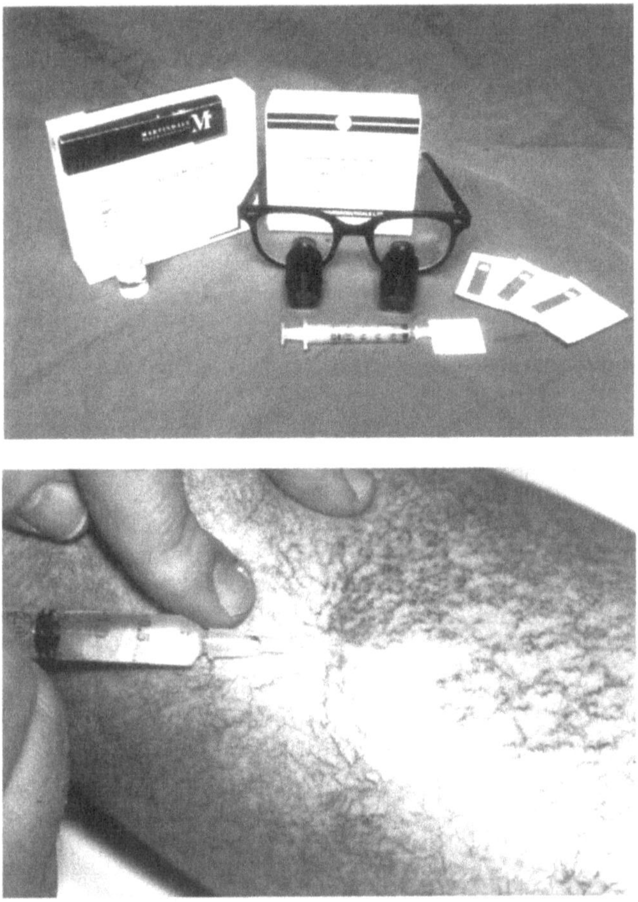

a

b

Fig. 16.3. **a** Simple and relatively inexpensive equipment required for microsclerotherapy (see Appendix A). **b** Technique of injection. It is recommended to stop the injection of a particular site once an area 1–2 cm is emptied of blood. To increase the contact of the sclerosant with the endothelial wall, the plunger of the syringe can be held with almost zero force while the needle remains motionless. *(See also Plate VI)*

stocking for 72 h after microsclerotherapy might benefit some patients with distal leg telangiectasia, especially when there is a history of hyperpigmentation, or minor thrombophlebitis following previous injections. A localised pressure dressing (cotton or foam pad taped directly on the injection site) could be used when larger 1–2 mm veins are injected.

Complications

Microsclerotherapy carries with it a number of potential complications such as perivascular cutaneous pigmentation, flare of new telangiectasias, oedema of the injected site, pain and localised hirsutism. Localised cutaneous necrosis, systemic allergic reactions, thrombophlebitis and deep vein thrombosis are serious but fortunately very rare complications.

Hyperpigmentation

Hyperpigmentation depends not only on the type of the agent but also on its concentration and the technique used. The immediate cause of pigmentation is excessive haemosiderin deposition rather than increased melanocytic activity [13]. The following factors are believed to affect the risk of pigmentation:

1. High pressure used to inject the sclerosing agent results in extravasation of red blood cells.
2. STS causes more pigmentation than hypertonic saline.
3. Distal and blue telangiectasias are more susceptible than proximal 0.2–0.5 mm vessels.
4. Patients with saturated serum iron level and histamine hypersensitivity may have an innate predisposition to pigmentation [14].

Pigmentation often lasts 6–12 months. Rarely, the use of pulsed dye laser at 510 nm or Q-switched laser at 532 nm stimulates haemosiderin fragmentation and absorption.

Telangiectatic Matting (Flares, Distal Angioplasia)

Telangiectatic matting is the new appearance of a previously unnoticed network of bright red, fine capillaries less than 0.2 mm in diameter at the injection sites (Fig. 16.4a,b). More frequently seen on the thighs and reported in approximately 16% of cases [15], this could follow angiogenesis or dilatation of existing subclinical vessels. Predisposing factors include obesity and the use of oestrogen-containing hormones. Injection under pressure leading to initial subclinical extravasation of the sclerosing agent could be a predisposing factor. Therefore, the injection blanch should be limited to no more than 2 cm. It is disconcerting for the practitioner to produce new areas of telangiectasia but it is important to remember that matting usually resolves spontaneously over 3–12 months. Occasionally, laser therapy may help in resistant cases, but repeat sclerotherapy to the site of matting should be avoided.

Cutaneous necrosis

Cutaneous necrosis is uncommon but could follow extravasation or perivascular injections. STS is more toxic than hypertonic saline which in turn is more toxic than polidocanol. Polidocanol is so mild that in concentrations of 0.25–0.5% deliberate perivascular injections have been used to eradicate narrow-diameter telangiectasia. Inadvertent extravasation should be diluted with copious amounts of normal saline or lidocaine with or without hyaluronidase. A 0.5 cm eschar may form in 10 days and takes 6–8 weeks to separate and heal by secondary intention, leaving a small BCG-like hypopigmented scar. Patients should be warned about this possibility.

Laser and Other Pulsed Light Sources

Apart from its "high-tech" appeal, laser is seen as a non-invasive and less painful method of treatment, particularly for patients with needle phobia. There is no risk of allergic reactions or telangiectatic matting but hyperpigmentation is all too common. Most

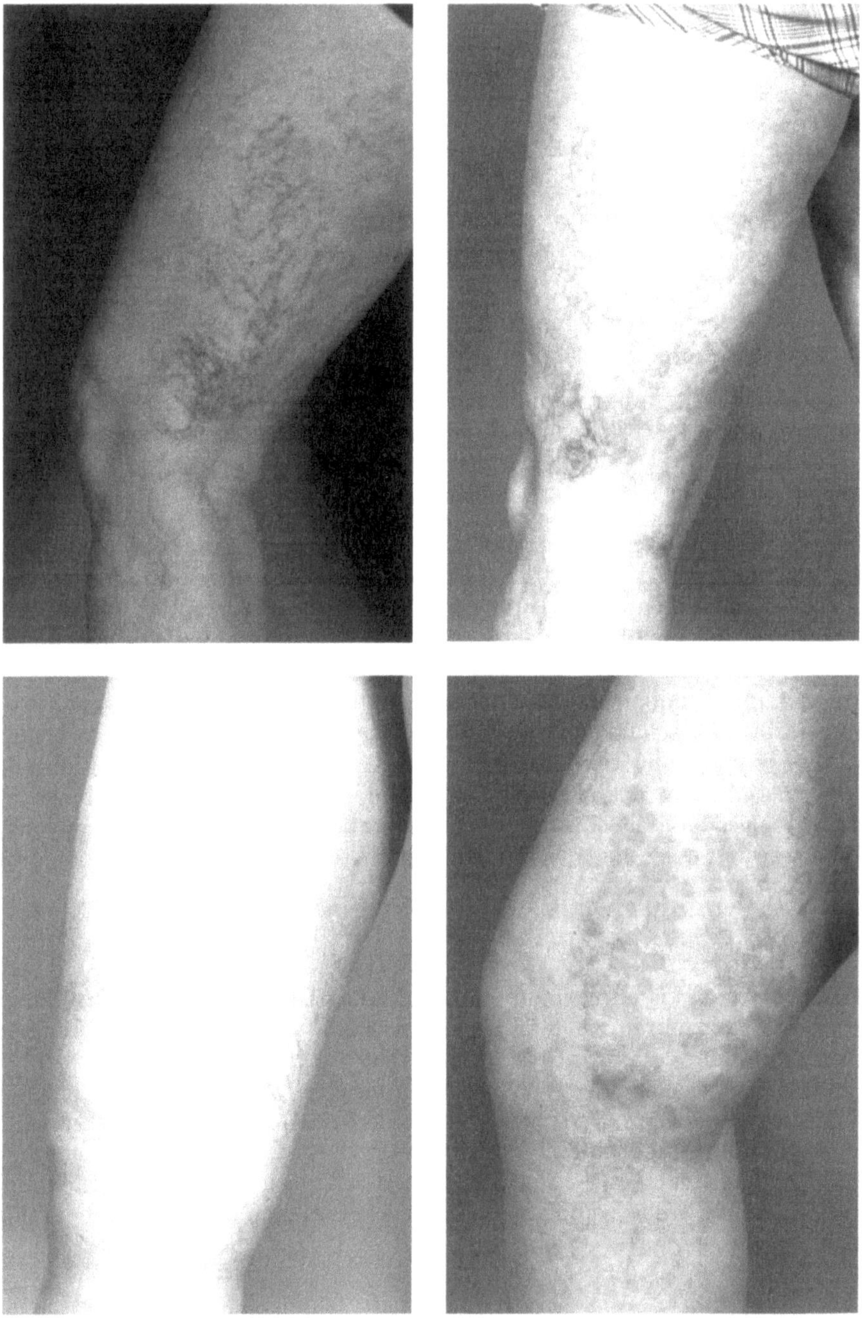

Fig. 16.4a–d. Complications of treatment of leg telangiectasia. **a,b** Telangiectatic matting and some pigmentation following three sessions of microsclerotherapy using 22% hypertonic saline (0.5–2 mm vessels). **c,d** Extensive pigmentation following 585 nm pulsed dye laser (7 mm spot) to inner thigh telangiectasia less than 0.5 mm in diameter. The pigmentation took several months to resolve. *(See also Plate VII)*

lasers work through the principle of selective photothermolysis and therefore the risk of scarring is negligible. Laser parameters can be prescribed by the clinician and the treatment easily carried out by laser nurse practitioners. The two main limiting factors are a low success rate and the expensive capital outlay required to purchase a laser machine. Many types of lasers have been used to treat telangiectasia: argon, pulsed dye and the frequency doubled Nd:YAG. In addition, a new non-coherent intense pulsed light source is being promoted as a method of coagulating reticular veins up to 3 mm in diameter (Appendix B).

Argon Laser

The blue/green light of the argon laser at 488 and 514 nm is theoretically suited for treating telangiectasia but it is only partially vessel-selective with significant epidermal melanin absorption, leading to temporary hyperpigmentation and a more permanent hypopigmentation. Also, the non-specific thermal damage of the dermis could lead to atrophic or hypertrophic scarring. Argon laser is painful and the treatment could result in blistering and scab formation [15].

Pulsed Dye Lasers

The role of the pulsed dye lasers (PDL) in the treatment of capillary vascular malformations and facial telangiectasia is now well established. The first-generation PDL at 577 nm has effective penetration of only 0.5 mm from the dermal–epidermal junction and is not suitable for leg telangiectasia [16]. In the early 1990s, this author used the flash lamp PDL (585 nm, 6–8.5 J/cm^2, 450 μ and 5–7 mm spot) to treat a large variety of thread veins and found it helpful only in vessels measuring less than 0.2–0.3 mm in diameter. This laser is tolerated well by patients but produces immediate purpura that lasts 2–3 weeks to be followed in 30–40% of patients by hyperpigmentation which lasts several months (Fig. 16.4c,d). Patients with dark or tanned skin cannot be treated. A new generation of PDL with a longer wavelength (595 nm), elliptical-shaped spot and longer pulse duration (1500 μ) is being marketed as ScleroPLUS (Candela Corporation). Energy densities twice those generally considered safe for vascular lesion treatment were used with epidermal cooling [17] and modest results were reported, although these have not been substantiated by the author's experience.

Frequency Doubled Nd:YAG Laser

The frequency doubled Nd:YAG laser is a solid state laser that emits green light at 532 nm, which coincides with one of the peaks of absorption of oxyhaemoglobin. But at 532 nm melanin absorption is stronger than at the longer wavelength of the PDL, possibly resulting in more epidermal injury. This may limit the energy density than can be safely used without excessive damage to the epidermis. Examples of this laser include the Coherent Versapulse and Laserscope Aura systems. The treatment is well tolerated and does not result in purpura but only temporary erythema. Long-term favourable results are yet to be reported.

Intense Non-coherent Pulsed Light

Evidence has been accumulating that the monochromatic nature of laser light is not essential for obtaining selective photothermolysis. Recently, a high-energy gas discharge lamp has become available (Photoderm VL) that produces non-coherent pulsed broad spectrum (600–900 nm) light with energy densities of 20–80 J/cm^2 over 5–20 ms. This has been demonstrated to coagulate vessels up to 3 mm in diameter 2 mm below the epidermis. There is no vessel rupture and therefore no purpura. This light could be delivered through a foot print, which permits exposure of larger sections of the telangiectatic vessels. Clear coupling gel is placed on the skin as a thin layer between the light guide and epidermis. The gel acts as a heat sink absorbing reflected light and therefore minimising damage to the epidermis. Initial reports [18] are encouraging but further studies are necessary to establish the role of this novel approach in the treatment of vascular lesions.

Combination of Laser and Sclerotherapy

PDL–microsclerotherapy treatment does not offer any advantage over PDL treatment alone and may result in a higher rate of complications. However, microsclerotherapy may be used to treat feeding reticular veins before laser treatment can be considered.

Fibre-Guided Laser Coagulation

Fibre-guided laser coagulation was reported by Trelles et al. (International Society of Cosmetic Laser Surgeons, Palm Desert, California, February 1993). A vessel is canulated with a 0.8 × 40 mm hypodermic needle and 200 μ optical fibre is passed through the needle into the vein. After that, pulses of laser light adjusted to coagulate the vessels are delivered while the overlying skin is cooled with ethyl chloride. Some 60% of treated patients were satisfied with the results 5% developing depressed or pigmented scars. This is an unnecessarily complicated and time-consuming approach and the results are no better than those reported for microsclerotherapy.

Is Treatment Worthwhile and Who Should Pay?

There is a great demand for the removal of leg telangiectasia that is fuelled by intensive targeted advertising, summer holidays and fashion. Women, reluctant to seek help from discouraging if not dismissive General Practitioners, are exposed to exploitation by unscrupulous operators and some waste thousands of pounds on treatments and creams which are barely effective.

Plastic surgeons, dermatologists and vascular surgeons should play a more active role in the management of this condition, even after simple clinical or non-invasive diagnostic investigation has excluded incompetence of the superficial venous system. There is no doubt that with careful selection, adequate counselling and realistic expectations, good results could be obtained in the majority of patients. Microsclerotherapy, the mainstay in the management of leg telangiectasia, is a consulting room procedure requiring relatively little specialised equipment (Appendix A). The technique is not difficult to learn and, with attention to basic principles, is free of serious side effects, fulfilling an important criterion of cosmetic treatment. However, it can be time-consuming, with sessions lasting up to 30 min. However, because of the nature of the procedure and the inexpensive consumables the cost could be contained (Minor 1–5 per session, Bupa scale). Patients should be advised of the average number of sessions required to produce a clinically satisfactory response, to budget for the full course of the treatment. Also, the possibility of recurrence or appearance of new veins in years to come should be borne in mind. The cost of laser treatment has come down significantly over the last 5 years following intense competition. Although laser treatment can be carried out by nurse practitioners the cost of a session of treatment remains as high as that of microsclerotherapy, reflecting the capital (£40 000–£80 000) or lease cost of laser machines.

Treatment of leg telangiectasia should be self-funded in the majority of cases. Private medical insurance companies consider the treatment cosmetic and rarely consider the costs reimbursable. A small proportion of patients may be eligible for NHS treatment despite the fact that most cosmetic interventions are being excluded by NHS purchasers. Possible candidates for NHS treatment are:

1. Patients with very extensive leg telangiectasia which is considered cosmetically disabling causing the patient unacceptable restriction of social and sporting activities (Fig. 16.5).

a 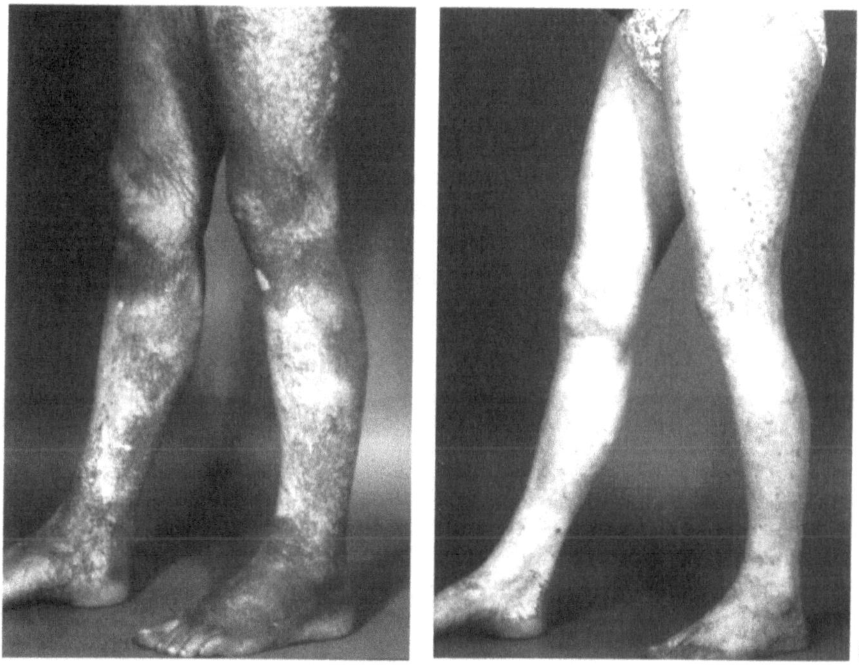 b

Fig. 16.5a,b. An extreme example of arborising ascending telangiectasia. This patient was eligible for NHS treatment and satisfactory fading was achieved following multiple PDL (585 nm) sessions combined with occasional microsclerotherapy for the larger vessels. The residual pigmentation on the thigh will fade with time. *(See also Plate VIII)*

2. Women who perceive telangiectasia as a complication of surgery for varicose veins, especially when there is chronological and topographical corroboration of their perception.
3. When the telangiectasia is associated with discomfort, particularly in the presence of reticular veins and incompetent perforators. However, it is unfortunate that discomfort could be used as a pretext by some patients for obtaining free cosmetic treatment.

Appendices

Appendix A. Equipment for Microsclerotherapy

Sclerosing Agents

1. Sterile sodium chloride concentrate BP 3 g in 10 ml (30% w/v) 10 × 10 ampoules. Martindale Pharmaceuticals Ltd., Bampton Road, Haroldhill, Rumford, Essex RM3 8UG, UK.
2. Sclerovein (polidocanol – a.k.a. athoxysclerol). Vascular Products, Inc., 35 King Street, Bristol BS1, UK.
3. Fibro-Vein (sodium tetradecyl sulphate). STD Pharmaceuticals, Fields Yard, Plough Lane, Hereford HR2 0EL, UK.

Foam Pads

STD Pharmaceuticals, Fields Yard, Plough Lane, Hereford HR2 0EL, UK.

Needles

30 G, box of 100. Becton Dickinson UK Ltd., Between Towns Road, Cowley, Oxford OX4 3LY, UK.

Surgical loupes

Designs for vision ×3.5 loupes with a working distance of 3.5 cm.
CLS Medical, Wingrove House, Ponteland Road, Newcastle upon Tyne NE5 3AJ, UK.

Appendix B. Lasers of Use in the Treatment of Telangiectasia

1. ScleroPLUS (Candela Corporation) with Candela Dynamic Cooling Device (585–600 nm, 1500 μ). Cross Medical Ltd, 8 Chase Road, Park Royal, London NW10 6QD, UK.
2. Versapulse (3 lasers in 1: vascular, pigmented and tattoo). The vascular laser is frequency doubled Nd:YAG 532 nm. Coherent (UK) Ltd., Cambridge Science Park, Milton Road, Cambridge CB4 4FR, UK.
3. Laserscope Aura (KTP/532 nm). Laserscope, Raglan House, Llantarnan Park, Cwmbran, Gwent NP44 3AX, UK.
4. Photoderm VL/PL. ESC Medical Systems Ltd., Yokneam Industrial Park, Yokneam 20692, Israel.

References

1. Merlen JF. Red telangiectasias, blue telangiectasias. Soc Franc Phlebol 1970;22:167.
2. Alngren B, Eriksson I. Valvular incompetence in superficial, deep and perforator veins of the limbs with varicose veins. Acta Chir Scand 1990;156:69.
3. Redisch W, Pelzer RH. Localised vascular dilatation of the human skin: capillary microscopy and related studies. Am Heart J 1949;37:106.
4. Engel A, Johnson ML Haynes SG. Health effects of sunlight exposure in the United States: results from the first National Health and Nutrition Examinations Survey, 1971–1974. Arch Dermatol 1988;124:72.
5. Weiss RA, Weiss MA. Doppler ultrasound findings in reticular veins of the thigh subdermic lateral venous system and implications for sclerotherapy. J Dermatol Surg Oncol 1993;19:947.
6. Salles-Cunha SX. Telangiectasias: classification of feeder vessels with colour flow. Radiology 1993;186:615.
7. Davis LT, Duffy DM. Determination of incidence and risk factors for post-sclerotherapy telangiectatic matting of the lower extremity: a retrospective analysis. J Dermatol Surg Oncol 1990;16:327.
8. Imhoff E, Stemmer R. Classification and mechanism of action of sclerosing agents. Soc Franc Phlebol 1969;22:143.
9. Sadik NS. Sclerotherapy of varicose and telangiectatic leg veins: minimal sclerosant concentration of hypertonic saline and its relationship to vessel diameter. J Dermatol Surg Oncol 1991;17:65.
10. Ouvry P, Davy A. Le traitement sclerosant des telangiectasies des membres inférieurs. Phlebologie 1982;35:349.
11. Goldman MP. Sclerotherapy, 2nd ed. St Louis: Mosby. 1995.
12. Carlin MC, Ratz JL Treatment of telangiectasia: Comparison of sclerosing agents. J Dermatol Surg Oncol 1987;13:1181.
13. Goldman MP, Kaplan RP, Duffy DM. Post-sclerotherapy hyperpigmentation: a histologic evaluation. J Dermatol Surg Oncol 1987;13:547.
14. Thibault P, Wlodarczyk J. Post-sclerotherapy hyperpigmentation: the role of serum iron levels and the effectiveness of treatment with the copper vapor laser. J Dermatol Surg Oncol 1992;18:47.
15. Davis LT, Duffy DM. Determination of incidence and risk factors for post-sclerotherapy telangiectatic matting of the lower extremity: a retrospective analysis. J Dermatol Surg Oncol 1990;16:327.
16. Dickson JA, Gilbertson JJ. Cutaneous laser therapy. In: High tech medicine (special issue). West J Med 1985;143:758.
17. Polla LL, et al. Tunable pulsed dye laser for the treatment of benign cutaneous vascular ectasia. Dermatologica 1987;174:11.
18. Hsia J, Lowery JA, Zelickson B. Treatment of leg telangiectasia using a long-pulse dye laser at 595 mm. Lasers Surg Med 1997;20:1.
19. Goldman MP, Eckhouse S. Photothermal scleroses of leg veins. Dermatol Surg 1996;22:323.

17 Which Patients Should Be Selected For Venous Surgery?

C.R.R. Corbett

Introduction

This chapter considers which patients should be selected for venous surgery. If, like the author, one is an enthusiast for operating on varicose veins there are very few patients who are not suitable for consideration provided that is what the patient wants. It is more a question of identifying the small group who are unsuitable. When considering which patients with venous ulcers might benefit, there is less certainty.

There are now some threats to the freedom of the surgeon to advise operation in patients with varicose veins within the UK National Health Service (NHS). There has always been some rationing imposed by long waiting lists, but provided the patient was willing to wait it would be done. Formerly the waiting time could have been as much as 5 years, but there is now a general requirement not to exceed 18 months. This could change. Some Health Authorities have considered not funding varicose vein surgery, or at least restricting it to those with more severe disease. In the private sector, insurers have traditionally taken the view that they do not provide cover for varicose veins that are purely cosmetic, and there is evidence now of more rigorous enforcement.

Surgeons are now asked to provide evidence that their operations can improve the natural history of disease. The problem is that we have very little evidence to support the case. Partly this is because formerly there was no need to argue the case, it was enough that the patient wanted the operation. A greater obstacle is the difficulty in obtaining reliable information about a chronic disease which can last from the second decade until death. It is the opposite to arterial surgery, in which the end points are easy to measure and most events occur in the last decade. For venous disease more longitudinal studies are required with follow-up of both operated and non-operated patients over extended periods. This requires great patience on the part of investigators and considerable resources. Patients lose interest or move and are lost to follow-up.

This chapter looks at the indications for venous surgery, and how these might be curtailed by financial restrictions. We examine what is known about the clinical history of varicose veins, in both operated and non-operated patients.

Selection of Patients for Operation

Most UK surgeons with an interest in venous surgery tend to favour surgery over sclerotherapy. This surgical bias is reinforced by the large randomised comparison of surgery and sclerotherapy, published by Hobbs in 1974 [1], which suggested that although sclerotherapy could be superior at 1 year, by 5 years the success rate was much higher in the surgical group. This applied particularly to patients in whom there was incompetence involving the long and short saphenous trunks. One of the great problems in trying to compare the two forms of treatment is that the respective experts are usually different types of practitioners working in different institutions, and multicentre investigations in this field are difficult to control. Sclerotherapy has always been more popular in continental Europe and has gained in popularity in North America [2]. Sclerotherapy is considered in Chapter 12 and this chapter deals with the surgical options. Reference is made to our own series of 1123 patients operated on at this institution over approximately 12 years. The case notes of all these patients have been carefully checked. A small proportion of these patients have been followed-up at intervals from 1 to 8 years after operation.

Factors Influencing the Decision to Operate

Sex

In an extensive review Callum [3] showed that females predominate in most epidemiological studies. He suggested that in an unselected western adult population visible varicose veins would be found in 20–25% of women and 10–15% of men. Women who are affected are more likely to undergo operation than affected men. In Finland, Sisto et al. [4] reported that 53% of affected women had received surgical treatment but only 29% of affected men. In our own series of 1123 patients the female to male ratio was 2.4:1. However, sex had no influence on whether to operate or not. We have no evidence that sex influences the long-term outcome, but Davies et al. [5] noted that women were more ready to express dissatisfaction.

Age

The average age of our patients, at operation, remains close to 50 years (50.26 years), with the range from 16 to 84 years. In the young it is sensible to advise deferring operation for a few years, particularly in women who have not yet borne children, but equally they may have considerable symptoms and the cosmetic embarrassment is greatest at this age. It is reasonable to operate but at the same time to warn the individual that further operations are likely to be necessary. Patients with most operations over a lifetime have usually had their first operation in their teens or early twenties. At the other extreme it is reasonable to exclude from surgical treatment patients over the age of 70 if their symptoms are mild. However, if they have considerable symptoms or complications, and are fit, then operation should be considered. Our eldest patient aged 84 years was very grateful for operation because bruising from the varicose veins was interfering with her continued ability to enjoy horse riding. Most of the surgery in the elderly is for venous ulceration and the indications are discussed below.

Obesity

Surgeons point the accusing finger at the obese patient, blaming obesity for the varicosities. Particularly this is so when the patient has recurrence and the surgeon sees that an earlier operation has failed. Callum [3] pointed out that the epidemiological evidence is conflicting and suggested that obesity promotes varicose veins rather than being a primary risk factor. Obesity would appear to promote the symptom of aching discomfort. Sisto et al. [4] found a positive association between varicose veins and obesity, while pointing to the importance of height as an independent determinant of varicose veins in women. In a detailed follow-up study of 67 post-operative patients we found no evidence that obese patients developed more recurrence [6]. Consideration must be given to the anaesthetic risk and increased surgical risks in obese patients, and so the surgeon often refers such patients to the dietitian rather than add another name to the waiting list. Some patients succeed in losing weight but more return after an interval with increased symptoms and increased weight. Lipodermatosclerosis may develop with the risk of ulceration. The surgeon then wonders whether operating might be preferable to having the patient return with a difficult ulcer.

Pregnancy

It is generally accepted that childbearing increases the risk of developing varicose veins [3] and the risk is increased with multiple pregnancies. For this reason women are often advised to defer surgical treatment until their family is complete. This is not always practical, particularly with many career women now deferring their first pregnancy until well into their thirties. Nor is it uncommon for a woman who has had two children to complain about her varicose veins whilst being unsure as to whether she wishes further pregnancies. Varicosities appearing during pregnancy may regress after delivery, but this happens less with successive pregnancies. Sometimes women are referred during pregnancy with extensive and distressing telangectasias over the lower limbs. Reassurance is appropriate as the flares usually regress in an equally dramatic manner after delivery.

Family History

Clinicians consider family history to be important but, as Callum [3] points out, reliable epidemiological evidence is scanty. Family history does not influence the selection for surgery but if the patient reports that her forebears experienced endless recurrence after numerous operations, the cautious surgeon would warn that she will not necessarily fare better.

Risk of Deep Vein Thrombosis

Various factors such as a previous deep vein thrombosis (DVT), usage of the oral contraceptive pill (OCP), hormone replacement therapy (HRT), obesity and increasing age are widely regarded as risk factors for DVT after varicose vein surgery. We have investigated this in our own patients and found no increased risk from the OCP or HRT. Indeed, the female incidence of post-operative DVT was only 1 in 830 (0.12%) and the 66-year old affected woman was not on HRT. Instead we found that the greatest risk factor was male sex, with 5 of 355 (1.4%) affected. Hence the incidence in men was 12 times that in women (χ^2 with Yates' correction = 5.83, $p = 0.02$).

Despite concerns the overall risk of DVT after varicose vein surgery is undoubtedly low, being in the region of 0.15–0.5% [7,8], and so we do not advise against operation in a high-risk individual but instead give low-molecular weight-heparin, starting the day before operation and continuing for a week afterwards.

A clear distinction needs to be drawn between patients with primary varicose veins who happen to have had a DVT and are then referred to a surgeon for treatment, and those who have had one or more thromboses and then present to the surgeon with secondary varicose veins and symptoms of the post-phlebitic limb.

Co-morbidity

The vast majority of patients having varicose vein surgery are fit. In a study of patients operated within the NHS in the course of 1 year, using the grading system of the American Society of Anesthesiologists, we found 78% were ASA grade 1, 21% grade 2 and only 1% were grade 3. Most patients with complicated varicose veins who are ASA grade 3 can be managed with compression hosiery or sclerotherapy. Difficulties only arise where operation needs to be considered in patients with venous ulceration. Often the problem is severe reflux in the saphenofemoral junction and long saphenous vein and operation under local anaesthesia is appropriate. We strip the long saphenous vein as well carrying out flush saphenofemoral ligation. This is well tolerated by the elderly, but there may be major problems. In a series of 1123 patients there has been one fatality which occurred in a 76-year-old man operated on for a venous ulcer resistant to conservative management. Death occurred 36 h post-operatively due to an acute myocardial infarction.

Occupation

As Callum [3] points out the epidemiological evidence regarding the influence of occupation on varicose veins is conflicting and lacks statistical validity. It has no real influence in advising an individual about operation. Patients may report increased symptoms when changing from a sitting to a standing occupation, and conversely others report improvement when changing to a sitting occupation. Not many individuals are able to change their job to ease symptoms so this seldom has any bearing on avoiding operation.

Are the Symptoms Right?

Patients are referred by their General Practitioners with all manner of aches and pains in the lower limbs. The symptoms may draw attention to the varices, but the latter are not necessarily the cause of the symptoms. Varicose veins and osteoarthritis of the knee commonly coexist and Sisto et al. [4] showed a statistically significant association. Where there is doubt it is sensible to prescribe compression hosiery and ask the patient to return after 3 months. If the patient finds stockings helpful, operation is worth considering. If the converse applies then it is unlikely that operation will help. Where there is continuing doubt it is reasonable to operate but warn the patient that relief is not guaranteed.

Day Case or Inpatient, Local or General Anaesthesia?

Having decided on operation a decision must be reached in the outpatient clinic about the means. The decision should not be deferred until later. This topic is considered in Chapter 22. A dramatic increase has occurred in day surgery and a smaller but significant increase in the use of local anaesthesia. We carried out a detailed analysis of all 136 patients operated on under the NHS in 1995/6, finding that 76% had been successfully managed as day cases. Six years earlier there had been no day cases at all. Likewise the proportion having operation under local anaesthesia had risen from 0 to 25%.

More patients could be treated under local anaesthesia if those with bilateral disease had each leg done separately. This is a great inconvenience to patients as most prefer a single operation to reduce social and economic upheaval. Therefore general anaesthesia is appropriate in most bilateral cases.

It is worth giving the patient an information sheet prior to operation. A few will reflect on the drawbacks of surgery and withdraw. As waiting times in the NHS are currently around 18 months the information sheet has to be issued when the patient attends the pre-operative assessment clinic, a week or so before operation.

Analysis of Presenting Symptoms

The stimulus to carry out analysis of our patients was a letter from our main purchasing authority which indicated that there could be a restriction to funding for the milder forms of venous disease. Earlier there had been national publicity about the curtailment of varicose vein surgery under the NHS in Berkshire. In the end this did not materialise and, interestingly, despite the publicity, no discussion took place with the surgeons (R.B. Galland, 1998, personal communication). We, at least, received warning, and so it seemed prudent to collect accurate information, the better to argue the case for patients with deserving symptoms.

We set out to analyse the symptoms of all new patients attending over the course of 1 year, but the data currently relate to 36 weeks. It seemed appropriate to use the CEAP classification [9] which is discussed in Chapter 7. Briefly class 0 signifies no venous disease present, class 1 telangectasias and reticular veins, class 2 varicose veins, class 3 oedema, class 4 patients with skin changes, class 5 patients with healed ulcers and class 6 those with active ulcers. There are some drawbacks. We have difficulty with CEAP class 3 for patients with oedema. A large proportion of patients in class 2 (varicose veins) have oedema at times, but not at others. We are not sure whether mild oedema at the end of the day justifies moving the patient from class 2 to class 3. Consequently in our analysis few patients are in class 3. Superficial venous thrombosis is not considered in the CEAP clinical classification, presumably because it is an acute event and the classification deals with chronic disease, but we regard recurrent attacks as a strong indication for operation, as a cure can be more or less guaranteed. These patients have arbitrarily been placed in class 4.

Table 17.1 summarises the clinical classification at the time of presentation. We have included in class 0 patients who were referred for an opinion but in whom it was concluded there were no visible or palpable signs of venous disease. In some cases an alternative explanation was found and in others no diagnosis was reached. In this group are two patients only with ischaemic ulceration. Most referral letters from local General Practitioners now include ankle Doppler pressure measurements, and so

Table 17.1. Analysis of presenting symptoms in 193 patients, by CEAP classification, and by age and sex

	CEAP class							
	0	1	2	3	4	5	6	Total
Number	16	1	88	8	31	5	44	193
Females	12	1	63	5	21	5	25	132
Males	4	0	25	3	10	0	19	61
Average age (range)	57	29	47	62	61	73	76	58(19–94)

patients with low pressures indicating ischaemic ulceration are seen more quickly in a separate clinic. Seven patients were judged to have mixed arterial and venous ulceration and these are in the CEAP class 6. The whole population divides neatly into two: half with mild to moderate disease (classes 1–2, 89/177) and the other half with severe disease (classes 3–6, 88/177).

Analysis of Planned Management

Table 17.2 summarises management in each of the groups according to the CEAP classification. This is not a final analysis because some patients with uncomplicated varicose veins (class 2) who were initially undecided may later opt for sclerotherapy or surgery, while some in class 5 or 6 may later come to surgery to try to prevent recurrence or to try to heal an ulcer unresponsive to compression bandaging.

The Range of Surgical Options

The range of surgical options are considered in detail in other chapters. We state our preferences in order to explain Table 17.2. In patients with localised tributary incompetence, some have sclerotherapy but multiple phlebectomy under local anaesthesia is a useful option. Where there is proximal incompetence we carry out appropriate ligation and stripping, and in recurrent cases rectify the problems as shown by duplex imaging. In primary operations we are unconvinced that ligating incompetent calf perforating veins will reduce recurrence. In recurrent disease we do ligate incompetent calf perforating veins if they seem to make a significant contribution, but consider an incorrectly ligated junction and the unstripped long saphenous vein to be more important In more severe disease (classes 3–6) we strive to identify patients with incompetence confined to the superficial veins but consider operation in those with

Table 17.2. Analysis of intended management, according to CEAP classification, in 193 patients

	CEAP class							
	0	1	2	3	4	5	6	Total
Advice	5	1	12	0	2	0	0	20
Review	2	0	1	0	0	0	0	3
Stockings	7	0	1	4	11	2	0	25
Bandaging	1	0	0	0	0	0	35	36
Sclerotherapy	0	0	10	0	0	1	1	12
Operation	1	0	64	4	18	2	8	97
Total	16	1	88	8	31	5	44	193

Among 16 patients classed as CEAP 0, one had an ulcerated basal cell carcinoma which was excised (she also had varicose veins which required no treatment), and another was obese with a leg ulcer of uncertain cause, and was bandaged.

severe superficial, and limited, deep venous incompetence. We are not enthusiastic about operating on those with extensive deep venous incompetence. Our experience of subfascial endoscopic perforator surgery (SEPS) is limited and we remain unconvinced about its role. Skin grafting is used in a minority of venous ulcers. Patients with mixed arterial and venous disease are a difficult group who are not considered here.

Priorities for Treatment

If funding for the treatment of chronic venous disease is to be restricted then priorities have to be set. Patients in class 0 are not considered further. The telangectasias and reticular veins of class 1 patients have to be regarded as a cosmetic problem, although it is argued that they cause aching discomfort [10]. The main difficulty is with class 2. This is the largest group, comprising 50% (88/177) of those with venous disease, and within it there is a wide range of symptoms from minimal discomfort to distressing aching discomfort interfering with work and ordinary activities. Class 3 is more deserving but we have only placed 5% (8/177) in this category. Class 4 is a deserving group in whom there is high expectation that operation will prevent ulceration. We have added to this group those patients with recurrent superficial thrombophlebitis and included those with skin changes that have led to haemorrhage. Patients in classes 5 and 6 are the most deserving for the receipt of funding for surgical intervention. The problem lies in selecting those who are likely to benefit, and in our series the proportion is small: only 8 of 44 (18%) with venous ulceration were offered operation.

If funding for operation is only available for patients in CEAP classes 3–6, 32 of 96 operative cases (33%) are eligible, while 64 of 96 (67%) cases in class 2 become ineligible.

The cost of duplex scanning is worth mentioning. Our service is on contract at £30 per scan, making the calculation easy. Overall, duplex scanning was used in 102 of 193 (53%) of patients. In round terms our annual cost of scans was £3000 and we saved a useful £3000 by not scanning all the patients.

The Clinical History of Patients with Varicose Veins

Non-operated Patients

The term clinical history is used to describe what happens after the patient has presented to a doctor. The perspective of the surgeon is slanted by seeing patients with more symptoms, or those who complain more, because the General Practitioner acts as a filter. Many patients have large varicosities for most of their adult life, experience minimal symptoms and never develop a venous ulcer. In terms of providing services to a population there are two important considerations: the proportion of patients who are likely to require surgery for symptoms, and whether varicose vein surgery plays any part in preventing ulceration in old age. In the study by Sisto et al. [4] in Finland 29% of men and 53% of women with diagnosed varicose veins had previously undergone operation. Another Finnish study [10] suggested a rate of 220 operations per annum per 100 000 population. This is a more generous rate than the suggested UK requirement of a "minimum" of 70 per 100 000 [11]. It is unlikely that varicose vein surgery can do much to reduce the later incidence of ulceration because varicose veins are very common and yet venous ulceration is relatively uncommon. Perhaps 15–20% of the adult population have varicose veins [3] but only about 1% have a leg ulcer [12]. At present we do not know whether patients who have had varicose vein surgery are less likely, or perhaps more likely, to develop an ulcer in old age. For patients without skin problems funding has to be justified by evidence of improved symptoms rather than by the prevention of later ulceration. Satisfaction can be demonstrated by questionnaires. These readily show improvement at 6 months [13], but others have reported up to a quarter of NHS patients very dissatisfied with operation in a series extended up to 10 years [5].

By contrast it is relatively easy to justify the provision of funding of varicose vein surgery in those with more severe disease (classes 3–6). The clearest evidence is for those in class 4 with skin complications. It would be unethical to carry out a controlled trial with neither surgery nor compression stockings for patients with lipodermatosclerosis, but it is not uncommon to see such patients who have ignored advice return later with ulceration.

Operated Patients

There are a few reports which give acceptably low recurrence rates after varicose vein surgery – for example that by Rivlin [14] – but this was a personal series not subjected to outside independent assessment. In the UK it would appear that about 20% of all operations for varicose veins are for recurrence [8,15]. Fifty per cent of NHS patients report recurrence [5] and there is never any shortage of patients with recurrent varicose veins presenting themselves for further treatment. The pragmatic view is that treatment helps for a time. Treatment is palliative not curative [16]. The aim of the surgeon is to make the first definitive operation as effective as possible, particularly as we have shown that the results of primary operations are better than the results of operations for recurrence [6]. In another series of 218 patients (322 limbs) we looked in detail at the causes of recurrence. For each limb we made a judgement as to whether the main cause of failure was either a technical error, a diagnostic error, a failure to strip the long saphenous vein if there was no other identified technical or diagnostic error, or simply the progression of disease. The technical errors (137 limbs, 43%) were nearly all inadequate saphenofemoral ligation, diagnostic errors amounted to only 10 limbs (3%), while in 50 limbs (15%) none of the above problems could be identified. This left 125 limbs (39%) in which natural progression of disease was blamed. Bradbury et al. [15] drew similar conclusions about inadequate groin surgery and failure to strip the long saphenous vein.

The best hope of improving the outcome of primary operations is by improving the training and supervision of surgeons in training. Improved diagnosis by duplex scanning of all patients may help, but our findings suggest its contribution would be less than from improving operative technique. The importance of better training and supervision of trainees is now recognised [17]. Any provider of resources should be concerned about this as it has a major influence upon the incidence of recurrence. However, we do not yet have all the evidence. On the one hand there may be a group with difficult disease in whom subsequent operations offer diminishing returns, but alternatively it could be argued that they are a group with severe disease destined to develop ulcers for which everything should be done in the way of prevention.

Much effort has been directed towards finding the place of operation in patients who have healed ulcers or ulcers unresponsive to surgical measures. Burnand et al. [18]

pointed to a clear distinction between patients with normal deep veins on phlebography, who did very well with surgery, healing being maintained in 94%, and the group with phlebological evidence of previous DVT who did extremely badly, all ulcers recurring within 5 years. Negus [19] argued that perforator surgery was effective in patients with damaged deep veins, provided they could be persuaded to wear compression hosiery afterwards. Over 90% of venous ulcers remained healed at 1-6 years and in contrast to the findings of Burnand et al. [18], this was not affected by abnormality of the deep veins. The differences between these reports is unexplained. Darke and Penfold [20] emphasised that in some 40% of patients with venous ulceration the venous reflux is confined to the ankle perforators and saphenous systems. After saphenous surgery without perforator ligation, maintenance of healing for a mean of 3.5 years was reported in 90% of ulcerated limbs. There is, however, suspicion that when the follow-up is continued for longer more relapses are seen, which might weaken the case for funding. Equally those who hold the purse strings should recognise that if a patient with a previously ulcerated limb remains ulcer-free for 3 or 5 years, if not for life, then this is a useful gain.

Conclusion

In this chapter the perspective is from within the NHS, in the UK, but world-wide the same pressures are being exerted upon surgeons to demonstrate the cost-effectiveness of operations. Within the NHS there should be no difficulty in continuing to justify operations for patients in CEAP classes 3-6. The debate centres on CEAP class 2 patients who lack complications. It is not yet clear whether the threat to curtail funding for this group is real or imaginary. In my view any attempt to subdivide the group into those with mild or severe symptoms is difficult and arbitrary because the symptoms are subjective. It is invidious to ask the surgeon to adjudicate.

The present work provides some information on the distribution of severity according to the CEAP classification, confirming that in terms of funding for surgical services class 2 is the important group, making up 67% of the total number of patients put on the waiting list for venous surgery.

References

1. Hobbs JT. Surgery and sclerotherapy in the treatment of varicose veins: a random trial. Arch Surg 1974;109:793-796.
2. Goldman MP. Sclerotherapy treatment for varicose and telangiectatic veins in the United States: past, present and future. J Dermatol Surg Oncol 1990;16:606-607.
3. Callum MJ. Epidemiology of varicose veins. Br J Surg 1994;81:167-173.
4. Sisto T, Reunanen A, Laurikka J, et al. Prevalence and risk factors of varicose veins in lower extremities: mini-Finland health survey. Eur J Surg 1995;161:405-414.
5. Davies AH, Steffen C, Cosgrove C, Wilkins DC. Varicose vein surgery: patient satisfaction. J R Coll Surg Edin 1995;40:298-299.
6. Hafez H, Jarvis S, Harvey A, Corbett R. Get it right first time: the results of primary operations for varicose veins are better than for recurrence. In: Negus D, et al., editors. Phlebology '95. Phlebology 1995; (Suppl 1):400-403.
7. Hagmüller GW. Komplikationen bei der Chirurgie der Varikose. Langenbecks Arch Chir Suppl (Kongressbericht)1992:470-474.
8. Critchley G, Handa A, Maw A, Harvey A, Harvey MR, Corbett CRR. Complications of varicose vein surgery. Ann R Coll Surg 1997;79:105-110.

PLATES

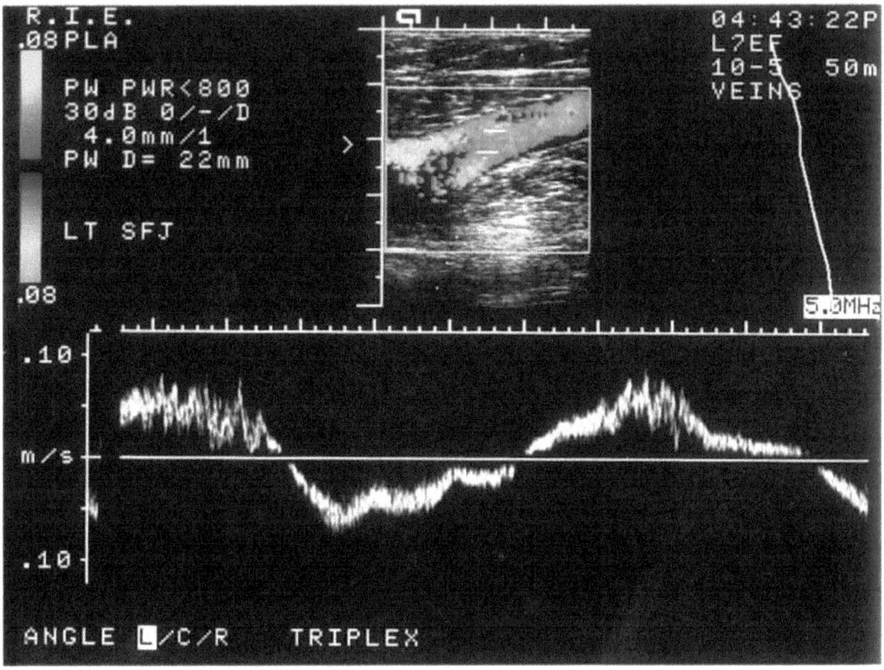

Plate I: Colour Doppler image of an incompetent sapheno-femoral junction and corresponding spectral display. The orange colour indicates flow towards the transducer and the spectral display shows bidirectional flow: flow towards the patient's head is shown below the baseline, whereas reflux with flow back towards the transducer is shown above the baseline.

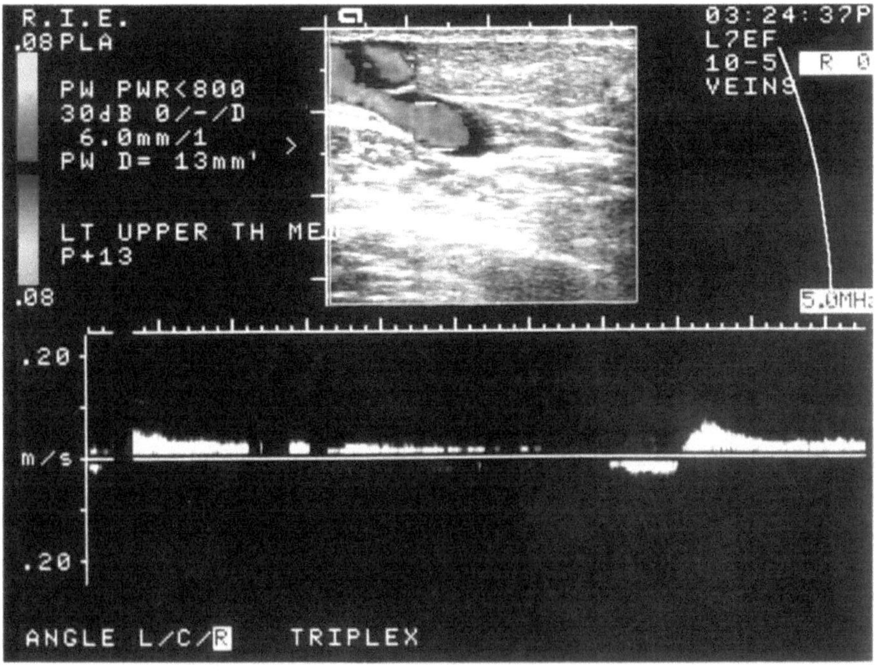

Plate II: Colour Doppler image of an incompetent perforating vein penetrating the fascia in the medial thigh, 13 cm above the patella, showing flow outwards towards the long saphenous vein.

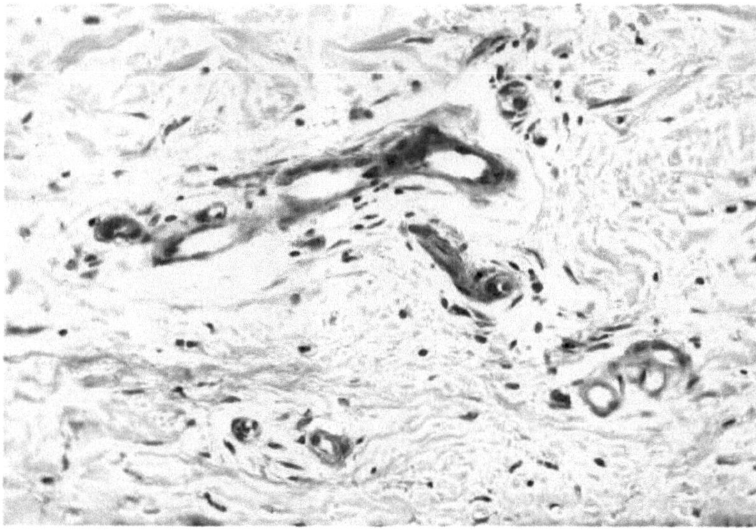

Plate III: Skin biopsy of a CVI lesion shows an apparent proliferation of capillaries.

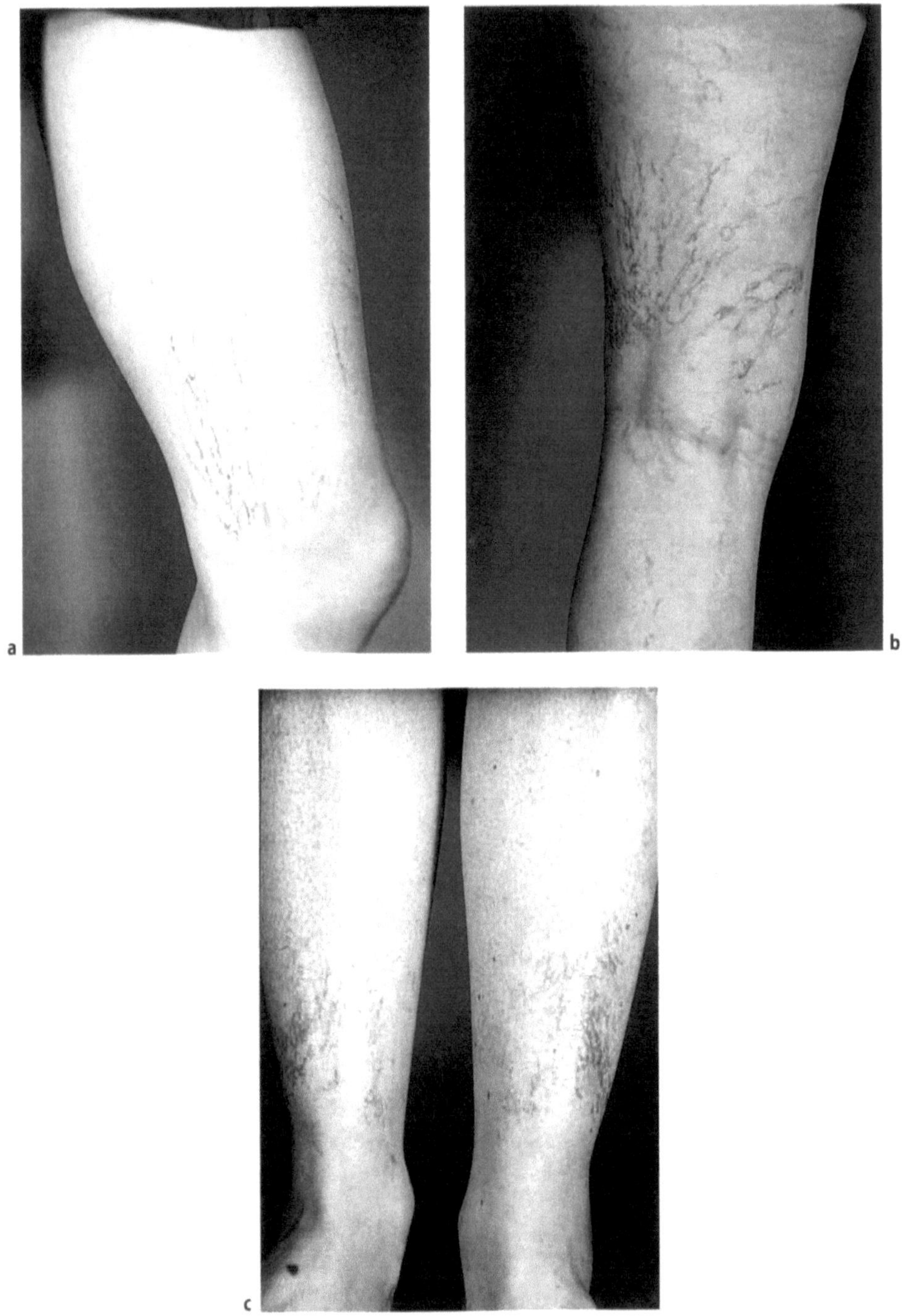

Plate IVa–c: Examples of telangiectasia. **a** Linear parallel on the inner thigh. This is usually difficult to remove. **b** Linear cartwheel on the posterolateral thigh with reticular veins on the popliteal fossa. **c** Progressive arborising telangiectasia. This starts on the feet and ankles and spreads proximally. It is usually 0.2 mm or less in diameter and responds well to laser.

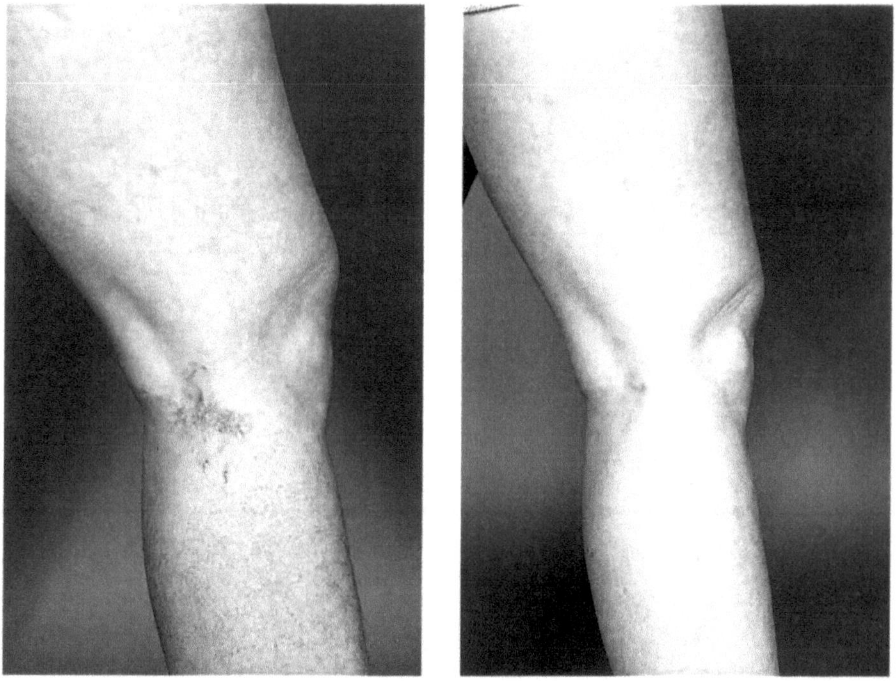

a b

Plate Va, b: Average result of microsclerotherapy after two sessions using 30% hypertonic saline. Total volume per session did not exceed 0.4 ml.

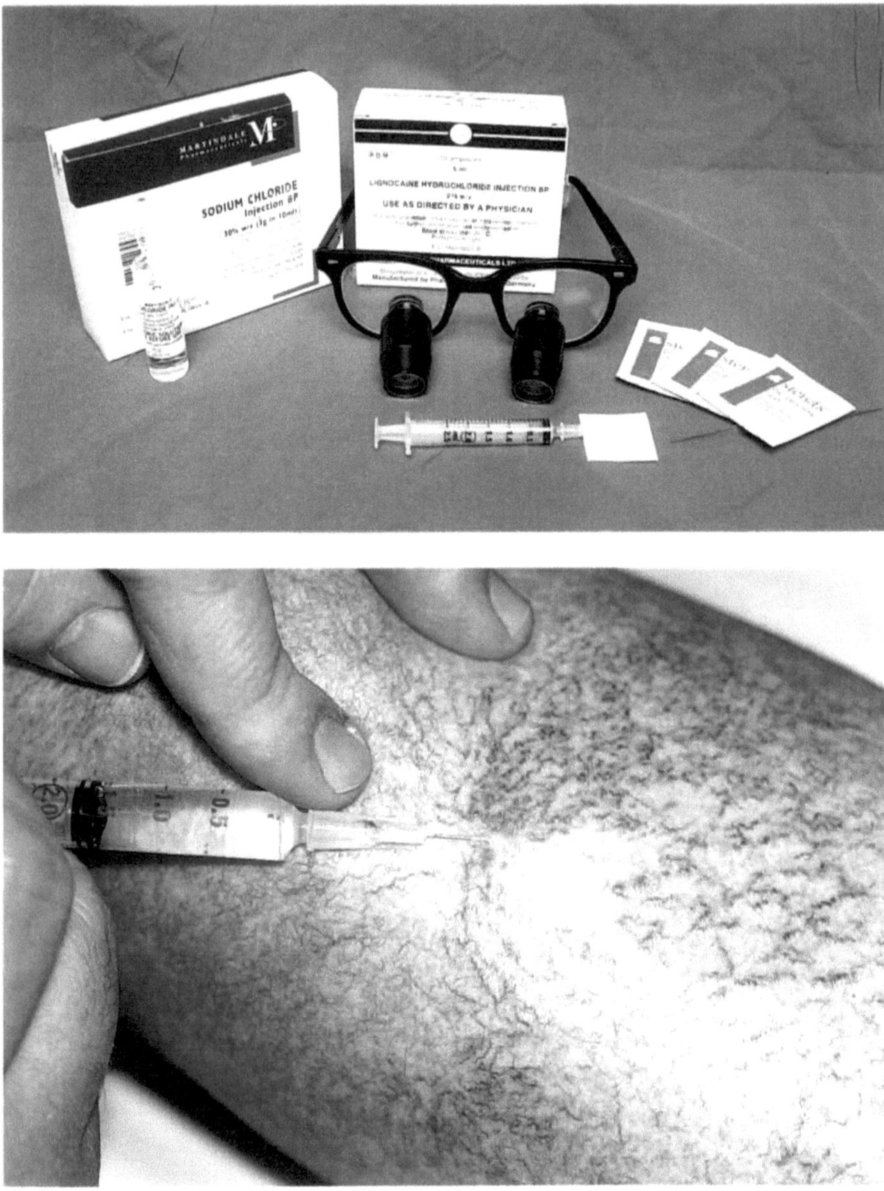

a

b

Plate VIa, b: **a** Simple and relatively inexpensive equipment required for microsclerotherapy (see Appendix A). **b** Technique of injection. It is recommended to stop the injection of a particular site once an area 1–2 cm is emptied of blood. To increase the contact of the sclerosant with the endothelial wall, the plunger of the syringe can be held with almost zero force while the needle remains motionless.

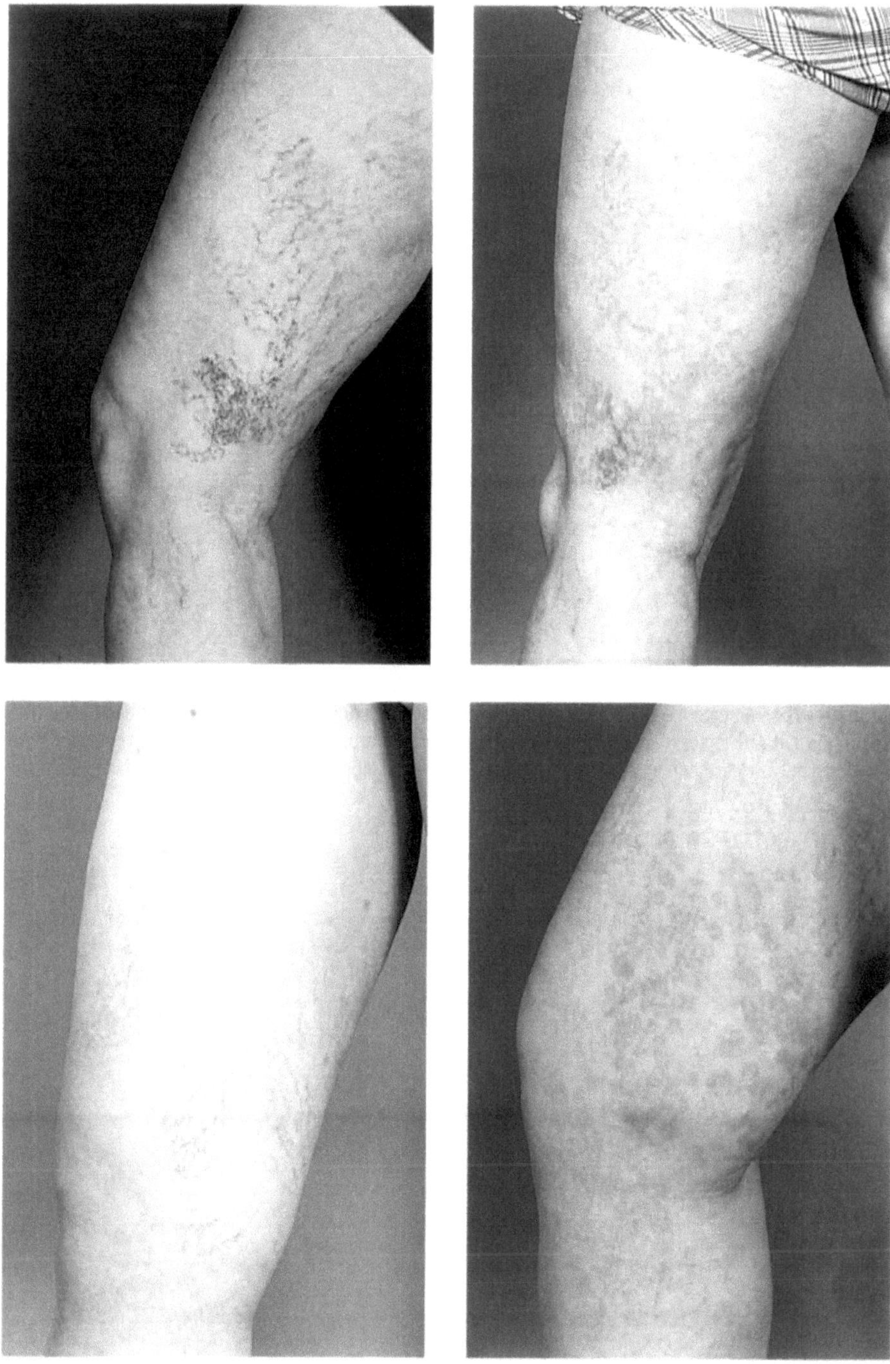

Plate VIIa–d: Complications of treatment of leg telangiectasia. **a,b** Telangiectatic matting and some pigmentation following three sessions of microsclerotherapy using 22% hypertonic saline (0.5–2 mm vessels). **c,d** Extensive pigmentation following 585 nm pulsed dye laser (7 mm spot) to inner thigh telangiectasia less than 0.5 mm in diameter. The pigmentation took several months to resolve.

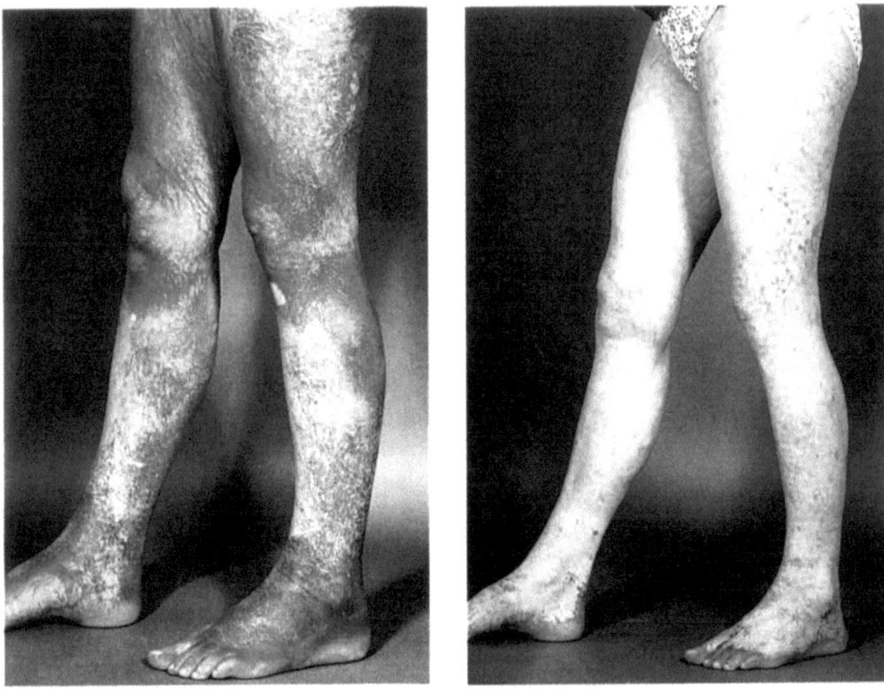

a b

Plate VIIIa, b: An extreme example of arborising ascending telangiectasia. This patient was eligible for NHS treatment and satisfactory fading was achieved following multiple PDL (585 nm) sessions combined with occasional microsclerotherapy for the larger vessels. The residual pigmentation on the thigh will fade with time.

9. Reporting standards in venous disease. Prepared by the Subcommittee on Reporting Standards in Venous Disease, Ad Hoc Committee on Reporting Standards, Society for Vascular Surgery/North American Chapter, International Society for Cardiovascular Surgery. J Vasc Surg 1988;8:172–181.
10. Laurikka J, Sisto T, Auvinen O, Tarkka M, Läärä E, Hakama M. Varicose veins in a Finnish population aged 40–60. J Epidemiol Community Health 1993;47:355–357.
11. Robbins M, Frankel S, Nanchahal K, Coast S, Williams M. DHN Project: Research programme on epidemiologically based needs assessment. Report 9: Varicose vein treatments. Commissioned by the NHS Management Executive, 1992.
12. Callum MJ, Ruckley CV, Harper DR, Dale JJ. Chronic ulceration of the leg: extent of the problem and provision of care. BMJ 1985;290:1855–1856.
13. Baker DM, Turnbull NB, Pearson JCG, Malin GS. How successful is varicose vein surgery? A patient outcome study following varicose vein surgery using the SF-36 Health Assessment Questionnaire. Eur J Vasc Endovasc Surg 1995;9:299–304.
14. Rivlin S. The surgical cure of primary varicose veins. Br J Surg 1975;62:913–917.
15. Bradbury AW, Stonebridge PA, Ruckley CV, Beggs I. Recurrent varicose veins: correlation between preoperative clinical and hand-held Doppler ultrasonographic examination, and anatomical findings at surgery. Br J Surg 1993;80:849–851.
16. Browse NL, Burnand KG, Lea Thomas M. Diseases of the veins: pathology, diagnosis and treatment. London: Arnold, 1988:202.
17. Turton EPL, McKenzie S, Weston MJ, Berridge DC, Scott DJA. Optimising a varicose vein service to reduce recurrence. Ann R Coll Surg Engl 1997;79:451–454.
18. Burnand K, O'Donnell T, Lea Thomas M, Browse NL. Relation between postphlebitic changes in the deep veins and results of surgical treatment of venous ulcers. Lancet 1976;I:936–938.
19. Negus D. Prevention and treatment of venous ulceration. Ann R Coll Surg 1985;67:144–148.
20. Darke SG, Penfold C. Venous ulceration and saphenous ligation. Eur J Vasc Surg 1992;6:4–9.

18 NHS and Independent Provision of Varicose Vein Surgery: a Rational Basis for Case Selection

David D.I. Wright

Introduction

Varicose veins are the "Cinderella" of surgery. This has been the case for many decades; it is no new phenomenon associated with advancing medical inflation and increasing demand on the services as a whole. Over the last 5 or 6 years there have been several attempts to exclude varicose vein treatment from being carried out at the expense of the UK National Health Service (NHS). In the early 1990s one Health Authority wrote to all General Practitioners (GPs) returning all varicose vein patients on the waiting list to their care, asking them to re-refer only if they felt treatment was essential. This, as one could have anticipated, resulted in uproar and the eventual withdrawal of the edict. Another Health Authority, in league with the Trust hospitals and fundholding GPs, agreed to neither provide nor commission any varicose vein treatment. Others have imposed temporary bans on varicose vein treatment while awaiting the arrival of the new financial year. It is therefore quite clear that the management of Health Authorities sees varicose vein surgery as a prime target for exclusion and consequent savings.

Benefits to the NHS from Excluding Varicose Vein Surgery

The most obvious benefit to the NHS of excluding varicose vein surgery is the direct savings from not providing treatment. On average about 40 000 cases are treated each year at an incurred expense of some £500 per case [1] – approximately £20m in total or less than 0.1% of the total NHS budget and presumably that percentage of any one Health Authority's costs. Another benefit would be freeing up surgical time to carry out other procedures. Again this is a relatively small benefit but greatly amplified if only elective surgery is considered. Perhaps a more significant benefit is the numerical effect of removing varicose vein patients from waiting lists, especially when they have been on a list for many months and are approaching the arbitrary 18 month Charter Standard. Finally, one can view the exclusion of varicose vein surgery as a test case for the exclusion of a whole raft of procedures where the medical need and benefit are marginal or have been called into question, such an insertion of grommets, thus narrowing the entire scope of the NHS.

Disadvantages to the NHS of Excluding Varicose Vein Surgery

The disadvantages of excluding varicose vein treatment from the NHS may be considered in both the long and short term. Varicose vein surgery has long been used as an introduction for trainee surgeons to vascular surgery and frequently to running their own list. This is not a practice to which the author subscribes, as it underestimates the complexity of both the anatomy and the potential difficulty of the surgery. The loss of the training value of varicose vein surgery may be of limited importance to the NHS, especially if it does not intend to carry out such surgery in the future.

More serious are the potential problems being stored for the future. Historically, many people went through their adult lives with varicose veins, sometimes supported by various "compression" garments and bandages, only to develop intractable leg ulcers which persisted on and off for tens of years. The estimated cost of this to the NHS is in excess of £2000 p.a. [2] for each leg ulcer, perhaps 40 times the cost of simple vein surgery. This financial approach while perhaps a more influential argument, disregards the benefits to the patient in avoiding the pain, suffering and social isolation occasioned by leg ulcers. However, the full impact of removing varicose vein treatment from the NHS would not be felt for decades, thus making it potentially politically acceptable.

When the Secretary of State for Health was asked recently (March 1998) in the House of Commons whether all treatments would be continued to be available through the NHS, he studiously avoided a direct answer.

In the author's opinion the disadvantages to the NHS of excluding varicose vein surgery far outweigh the benefits. There is, however, a good case to be made for excluding the treatment of simple cosmetic varicose veins from NHS. But how should these be identified and where should any threshold be set?

Is There a Need for Rationing?

In 1986 (a year for which both NHS and private sector data are available) 41 000 varicose vein procedures were carried out in the NHS and a further 13 000 in the private sector [3]. This makes a total of 54 000 operations, of which approximately 20–25% were performed for recurrent varicosities. Completed consultant episodes for varicose veins were 59 835 in 1994/5, suggesting an increasing trend. In epidemiological studies varicose vein disease has been found in 25% of the population over 30 years of age, with a further 5% suffering more severe forms of venous disease [4]. Consequently there is an enormous pool of patients, estimated to be in excess of 5 million in the United Kingdom, with untreated venous disease of all grades. These alarming figures are further supported by the Framingham study [5], which identified an overall incidence of varicose veins of 2% for men and 2.5% for women.

Extrapolating from these data suggests that approximately 250 000 new cases of varicose veins per annum could be anticipated in the UK. Current rates of treatment therefore fall well below that required to keep pace with new cases, let alone deal with any backlog. This is further evidenced by the operation rates in the NHS compared with the private sector. Even after discounting the approximately one-third of patients who fund themselves through the private sector, the rate of surgery amongst those with private insurance is approximately 3 times higher than that in the NHS. It is therefore reasonable to assume that, if unlimited access were provided to venous surgery, demand would rise substantially; also that in the past lack of provision (i.e. long waiting lists), amongst other factors, has suppressed demand.

As rationing of treatment is already happening, albeit on a chaotic basis, can there be any fundamental objection to devising or applying treatment selection criteria?

Which Varicose Veins Should the NHS Treat?

Varicose veins come in all shapes and sizes, from the most trivial thread veins through to gross varicosities and venous ulceration with or without associated deep venous problems. At either end of the spectrum there is little or no argument. It is unlikely that anyone would seriously advocate the treatment of thread veins by a state-funded health service, even though they are frequently more disfiguring than minor to moderate varicose veins. Similarly, there would be almost universal agreement that treatment for gross varicose veins should be provided despite the fact that many of these are reported to be asymptomatic. So, having determined that any universal health service will provide treatment for some varicose veins and venous disorders, the challenge is to establish a rational, fair and easily administered set of parameters that will define the threshold for treatment from the public purse. It is first perhaps necessary to consider the fundamental aims of treatment. These must clearly start with the alleviation or management of symptoms but must also include the arrest of disease progression and the prevention of more serious consequences of venous disease, most specifically venous ulceration. There has been considerable variation in the management of varicose veins over the years. In the UK the current balance of opinion probably favours formal ligation of the source of incompetence and stripping the long saphenous vein, if involved, combined with local avulsions. The results of careful ligation and stripping for major symptoms of aching and itching have been assessed in a consecutive series of 740 patients with over 900 operated limbs. It was found that 97% had complete eradication or improvement of aching and 90% complete eradication or improvement of itching reported to the Venous Forum 1996 [6].

The management of the more extreme consequences of persistent venous disease (lipodermatosclerosis and venous ulceration) remains controversial. However, with careful assessment and selection, rapid healing of long-standing and frequently previously indolent ulcers may be achieved by means of surgery [7].

Methods of Assessing Varicose Veins

Most will be broadly familiar with the range of assessment methods available. Clinical examination has frequently been shown to be unreliable in identifying the source of varicosities [8] and symptoms for apparently similar venous disorders vary enormously. Therefore history and clinical examination plays only a minor role in venous assessment. Hand-held Doppler ultrasound is widely available and is easily applied. Yet, in a recent survey, only 37% of surgeons admitted using Doppler on a regular basis in the assessment of varicose veins [9].

With the exception of detailed anatomical information, Doppler ultrasound may convey as much information about venous reflux as duplex scanning. Both duplex scanning and hand-held Doppler ultrasound may identify the source of incompetence and, perhaps more pertinently, the duration of retrograde flow "reflux time" as a quantitative measure of venous incompetence. Although functional testing of the venous system can be performed by photoplethysmography or direct venous pressure measurement, these are not widely available and only reluctantly applied. Of the methods available only ultrasound provides a non-invasive assessment of both the cause and severity of venous disease. However, as duplex scanning is only available through a limited number of vascular laboratories and radiology departments, the demands on each machine are high for procedures of greater perceived acuity than simple varicose veins. This leaves hand-held Doppler ultrasound and the Doppler reflux time as the prime candidates for screening and selection of patients to be offered venous surgery.

Doppler Reflux Time

The Doppler reflux time is simply defined as: the duration of retrograde flow identified at the highest source of incompetence following a single squeeze and release of the calf (Fig. 18.1). Very short reflux times of less than 0.5 s are considered to be within normal limits [10]. Reflux times longer than this indicate valvular incompetence, the severity of which is inversely proportional to the duration of reflux and correlates with the clinical classification. Hand-held assessment of Doppler reflux time requires a little training and practice but is well within the grasp of trainee surgeons, vascular technicians and trained outpatient nurses. It can be assisted by computerised display of

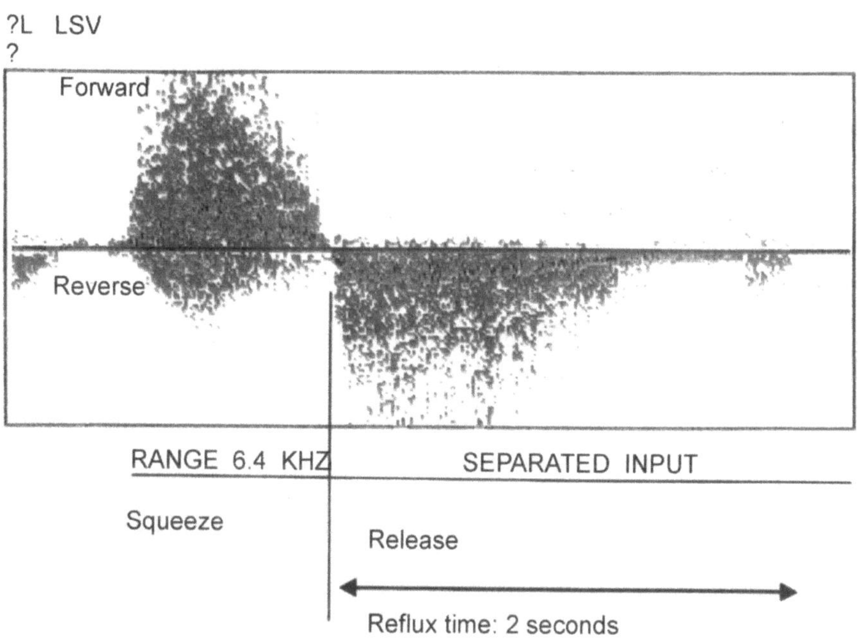

Fig. 18.1. Sonogram of Doppler ultrasound from an incompetent long saphenous vein below the saphenofemoral junction, showing directional blood flow during and after calf squeeze.

directional flow, but an adequately accurate measurement can be made by simple observation of the second hand of a clock.

In previous studies Doppler reflux time correlated well with clinical status of the leg. Despite considerable overlap for simple varicose veins short reflux times < 3 s were almost universal in those with clinical signs of venous insufficiency or leg ulcers [11].

Proposed Selection Criteria

1. Patients should have significant superficial vein incompetence from the saphenofemoral junction, saphenopopliteal junction or a major incompetent perforator in the absence of deep vein incompetence.
2. Having fulfilled one of these criteria they would be sub-classified into "severe", "intermediate" and "trivial" by reflux time:
   (i) Severe venous incompetence (>0.5 ≤ 3 s): vein surgery should be offered to eradicate the source of incompetence and other procedures to remove varicose veins so that the risk of recurrence is minimised.
   (ii) Intermediate incompetence (4–5 s): general advice should be given about minimising venous symptoms, utilisation of support hose and a planned review on an annual or biannual basis.
   (iii) Trivial incompetence (≥ 6 s): no treatment would be offered but general advice as above, with a review only after repeated referral.

Impact of Implementation

An estimate of the impact of implementation of the proposed measures can be inferred by examining the database from Surgicare, an independent provider of venous surgery. The practice draws from an extremely wide referral base and covers patients with venous disease of all severity. Over the past 5 years Surgicare has accumulated a database of over 7000 examinations of patients who have all undergone detailed Doppler examination with the measurement of reflux times where appropriate.

A selected database of limbs examined by Surgicare Doppler Mapping was interrogated. Examinations were performed by either surgeons or trained vascular technicians between November 1992 and July 1997. Data from 3435 patients (870 limbs) were available. Of these, 671 (19.5%) patients had no significant reflux, while the remainder had major incompetence in one leg (1250, 36%) or more frequently both legs (1514, 44%) (Fig. 18.2a). Considering the distribution of incompetence in each limb, 2592 (37.8%) had no major source of incompetence, 3778 (55%) had saphenofemoral incompetence, 1056 (15.4%) had saphenopopliteal incompetence and 556 (8.1%) had both (Fig. 18.2b). The relatively low frequency of saphenous incompetence in this series may reflect the high referral rate for "thread" vein treatment, for which Surgicare has an established reputation. Figure 18.3 plots the frequencies of reflux times for saphenofemoral junction incompetence alone. Figure 18.4 compares reflux time frequencies for saphenofemoral and saphenopopliteal incompetence; they are similarly distributed and differentiation between the two sites is not considered further.

If the decision to offer surgery is based solely on the presence of saphenofemoral

a

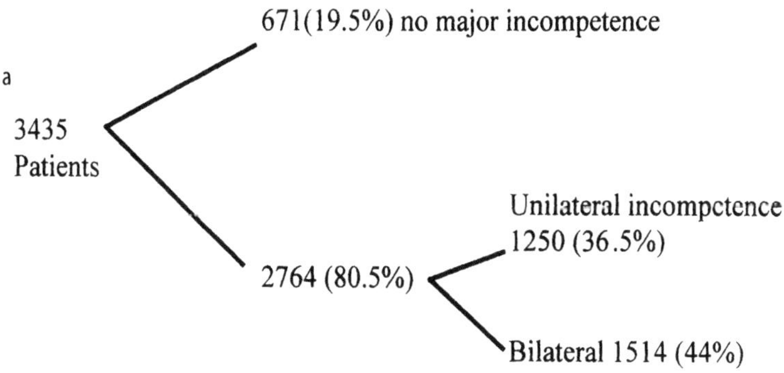

b

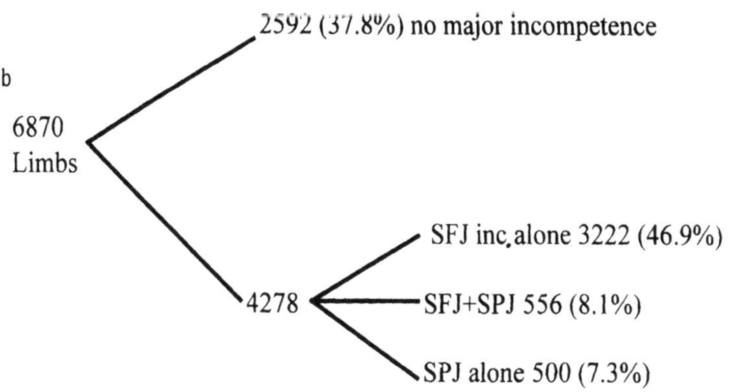

Fig. 18.2. **a** Presence of major vein incompetence in patients examined by systematic continuous wave Doppler ultrasound (Surgicare Doppler Mapping). **b** The distribution of valvular incompetence in the limbs of patients in **a**. SFJ, saphenofemoral incompetence; SPJ, saphenopopliteal incompetence.

or saphenopopliteal incompetence and this criterion is applied unmodified to this series, all but 19.5% of patients would be offered surgical treatment. Further applying the criterion of reflux time to those with saphenofemoral or saphenopopliteal incompetence at the suggested thresholds, 36% of these patients would be classified as "severe" and go forward for surgery, 29% would be considered "intermediate" and offered annual review and the 35% with "trivial" disease would be discharged back to their GP (Fig. 18.5).

Discussion

The management of varicose vein disease and its complications will continue to be needed despite the apparent reluctance of the NHS to fund this area of care. Increasingly treatment will therefore have to be sought from alternative providers; less than a third of patients are at present treated in the independent sector. Unfortunately, despite relatively low "self-pay" fees being available, vein surgery will continue to be beyond the reach of many.

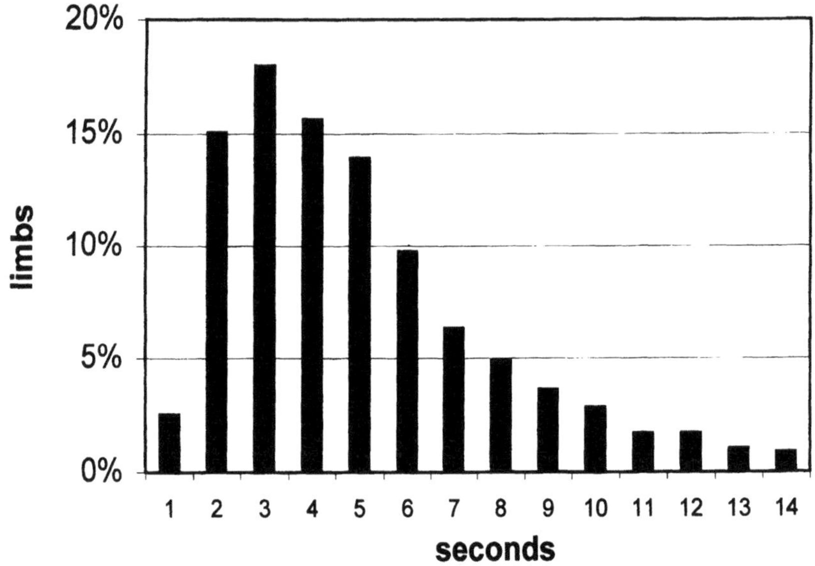

Fig. 18.3. Distribution of reflux times in limbs with varicose veins and saphenofemoral incompetence ($n = 1925$).

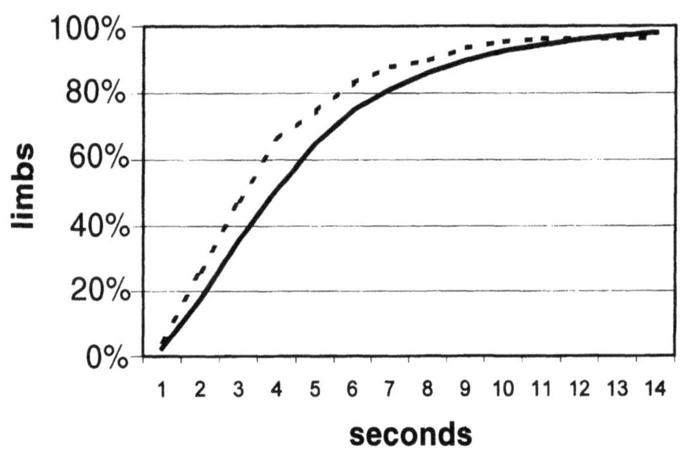

Fig. 18.4. Comparison of the cumulative distribution of reflux time in limbs with saphenofemoral (continuous line) and saphenopopliteal (dashed line) incompetence.

It is therefore perhaps fairer and more rational to establish a set of rules which, if fulfilled, would justify treatment funded by the state. If patients wish to seek treatment for less severe disease, mainly for aesthetic reasons, alternative providers could be sought through the independent sector.

In this chapter a series of criteria have been proposed based on the measurement of reflux time measured by hand-held Doppler which would stratify management. If these tests were accepted they could be carried out within the primary care setting where hand-held Doppler equipment is widely available, and would substantially reduce the number of hospital referrals. Alternatively, assessment could precede any hospital

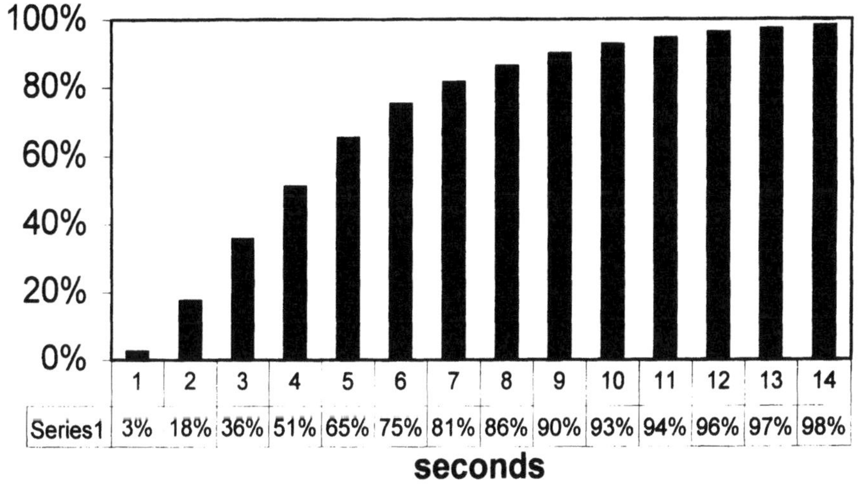

Fig. 18.5. Cumulative percentage of patients with reflux times and saphenofemoral incompetence that is severe (≤ 3 s), intermediate (4–5 s) and trivial (≥ 6 s) ($n = 1925$).

out-patient consultation, the results being explained in a standard advice leaflet accompanied by the appropriate information. Interrogating a large database of patients examined in this manner the criterion for surgical treatment as proposed would be fulfilled in no more than 36% at presentation. This approach would therefore largely achieve the aim of reducing cost to the NHS while at the same time minimising the build-up of patients with advanced venous disease requiring expensive treatment later.

References

1. Miriam Healthcare Ltd., Fundholding Price Check, 1997.
2. Freak L, Simon D, Kinsella A, McCollum C, Walsh J, Lane C. Leg ulcer care: an audit of cost effectiveness. Health Trends 1995;27:133N136.
3. Nicholls JP, Beeby NR, Williams BT. Role of the private sector in elective surgery in England and Wales 1986. BMJ 1989;298:243–247.
4. Franks PJ, Wright DDI, McCollum CN. Epidemiology of venous disease: a review. Phlebology 1989;4:143–151.
5. Brand FN, Danneberg AL, Abbot RD, Kannel WB. The epidemiology of varicose veins: the Framingham Study. Am J Prev Med 1988;4:96–101.
6. Young E, Wright DDI, Rose KR, McCollum C. Surgical outcome and patient satisfaction following varicose vein surgery. Phlebology 1996;11:169.
7. Wright DDI, McCollum CN, Greenhalgh RM. The use of non-invasive and functional tests in the identification and surgical management of venous disorders. In: Veith J, editor. Current clinical problems in vascular surgery. St Louis: Quality Medical Publishing, 115–118.
8. McIrvine AJ, Corbett CRR, Aston NO, Sheriff EA, Wiseman PA, Jamieson CW. The demonstration of saphenofemoral incompetence: Doppler ultrasound compared with standard clinical tests. Br J Surg 1984;71:509–510.
9. Lees TA, Holdsworth JD. Assessment and treatment of varicose veins in the Northern Region. Phlebology 1995;10:56–61.
10. Savin S, Sommerville K, Farrah J, Scurr JH, Coleridge Smith PD. Duplex ultrasonography for assessment of venous valvular function of the lower limb. Br J Surg 1994;81:1591–1595.
11. Wright DDI, Meek AC, McCollum CN, Greenhalgh RM. Functional tests of venous insufficiency. J Cardiovasc Surg 1987;28:97.

19 How Can Evidence on Treating Venous Disease Be Rationalised?

Gillian C. Leng, Elizabeth M. Royle and F.G.R. Fowkes

> ... it is necessary, while formulating the problems of which in our further advance we are to find the solutions, to call into council the views of those of our predecessors who have declared an opinion on the subject, in order that we may profit by whatever is sound in this suggestions and avoid their errors.
>
> Aristotle, *De Anima*

Introduction

In the current era of health care, the expectations of both the public and governments are that clinical practice should be based on the best available medical evidence. Physicians and surgeons are expected to know which treatment is best in a particular clinical situation, often despite a huge and bewildering array of available evidence. Many treatments have been rigorously tested, but the results of such evaluations often remain scattered among many medical journals and are drawn together only occasionally. The first controlled trials in the treatment of venous disease were published in the 1950s, followed by a rapid expansion in available evidence, so that by the beginning of 1998 there were over 1000 references to trials in venous disease (Fig. 19.1). Reviewing this evidence and making it easily accessible is therefore an increasingly important task. It is essential that it is properly assessed and summarised to ensure that clear evidence is available for clinical practice and also to highlight important areas for future research.

Assessing the Evidence

The best and most scientific way of demonstrating the benefits of a treatment regimen is a randomised controlled trial. Ideally, clinical practice should be based solely on evidence from good-quality trials, but lower grades of evidence may be acceptable if this evidence is lacking. There are three key criteria generally used to define a high-quality clinical trial [1]:

Randomisation using a method which cannot be broken, e.g. computer allocation scheme.
Masking of the patient, doctor and outcome assessor.
Analysis on an intention-to-treat basis.

In some situations, however, it is impossible for a trial to fulfil all these criteria. In a trial of exercise therapy, for example, it is impossible to mask either doctor or patients,

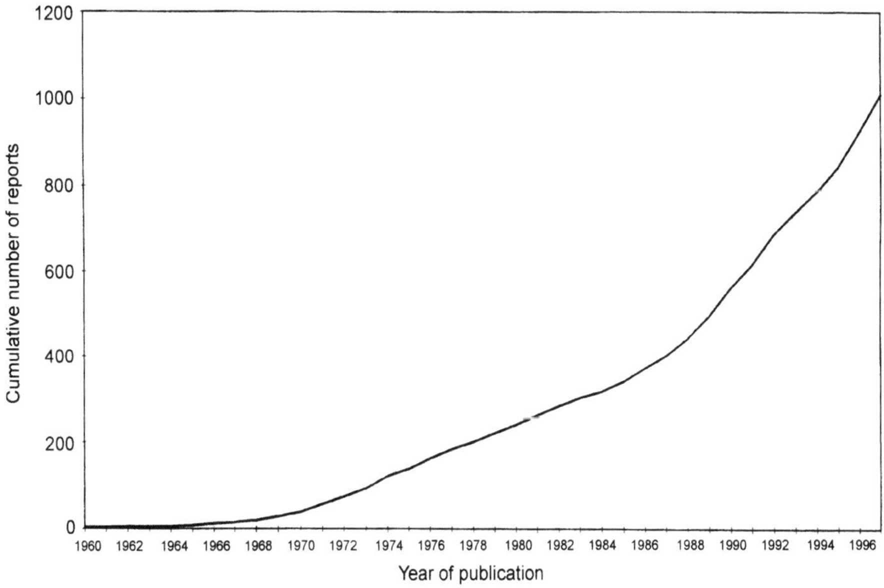

Fig. 19.1. Published evidence on treatment of venous disease, by year of publication. Data from the *Cochrane Library* (Oxford: Update Software), January 1998.

although those performing the outcome assessment can be unaware of the treatment allocation. In other cases it is neither possible nor appropriate to perform a randomised controlled trial, and in these circumstances other research strategies are required. For example, the long-term cardiovascular effects of taking oral contraceptives cannot be assessed using a randomised controlled trial. In the vast majority of cases, however, a randomised controlled trial is the best starting point for demonstrating the benefits or adverse effects of care.

Systematic Reviews and Meta-analysis

A *systematic review* differs from a more traditional literature review by following a more structured approach using pre-defined criteria. An important first step is therefore to formulate a well-focused question relevant to patient care, which will allow selection criteria for the inclusion of primary studies to be drawn up [2]. To avoid bias, it is important that these criteria are stipulated at the outset: for example, the types of participants involved, treatment, control group, outcomes, and study design.

A *meta-analysis* is a systematic review that uses quantitative statistical methods to evaluate information from the studies included for review [3]. A meta-analysis is especially useful when results from several studies lack statistical significance but appear to have effects in the same direction. The aims of performing a meta-analysis are therefore:

To estimate quantitatively the current state of knowledge concerning a treatment effect.

To improve the precision of an estimated measure of treatment effect.

To obtain sufficient power to test the statistical significance of a treatment effect.

To resolve controversy when studies appear to disagree.

To answer new questions that have not been posed in individual studies, and which the existing studies individually may not have sufficient precision or power to answer.

The benefits of combining several small studies in a statistical meta-analysis were clearly demonstrated in a recent review on compression bandages and stockings in the treatment of venous leg ulcers published on the *Cochrane Library* [4]. Three studies comparing elastic compression three-layer bandaging with inelastic compression were pooled, and the results showed a statistically significant increase in the odds of healing at 3 months with elastic compression bandaging (OR 2.26; 95% CI 1.4, 3.65) that was present in only one of the individual trials (Fig. 19.2).

Potential Problems with Systematic Reviewing

Publication bias

A systematic review can be as good only as the evidence on which it is based, and one potential pitfall is lack of evidence due to publication bias. This is particularly likely to affect trials with inconclusive or negative findings, which are less likely to be published than trials with positive benefits. This is thought to be predominantly due to the unwillingness of journal editors to publish, rather than of trialists to submit inconclusive findings [5]. To counteract this, journal editors recently agreed to a moratorium of unpublished trials, providing the opportunity for previously unpublished work to be submitted.

To reduce the effect of publication bias in a review, it is therefore important to search for trials as widely as possible. This should include scouring grey literature such as conference proceedings and theses, writing to trialists and drug companies, and searching electronic databases such as MEDLINE, EMBASE and LILACS. It is also important to hand-search journals, as up to 30% of trials may be incorrectly indexed on electronic databases [6].

Publication bias may be detected by identifying a lack of negative results using a funnel plot [7]. This is usually a plot of sample size (on the x-axis) against outcome (on the y-axis) e.g. odds ratio. With increasing sample size, the outcome measure should converge on the summary statistic in a funnel shape, but if points are missing from one side of the "funnel", publication bias should be considered.

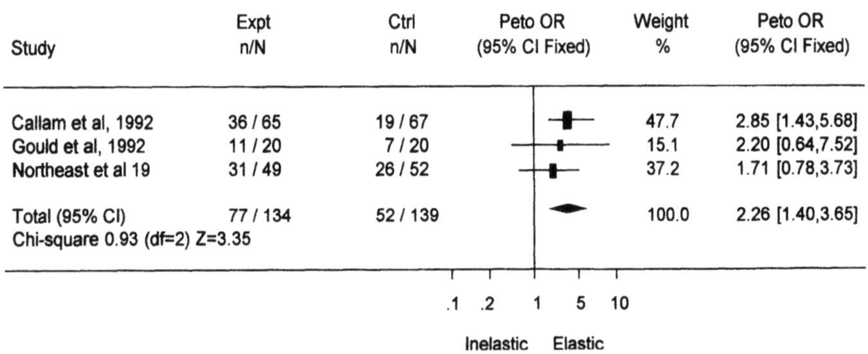

Fig. 19.2. Meta-analysis of compression for venous leg ulcers: elastic high compression (*Expt*) compared with inelastic compression (*Ctrl*). Outcome was assessed as complete healing.

Heterogeneity Between Trials

Another potential problem in statistical meta-analysis is heterogeneity between trials, often described as summing "apples and oranges". Meta-analysis is only properly applicable if the data summarised are similar or at least comparable, including treatment, patients and outcome measures [8]. Heterogeneity between trials should therefore be assessed both subjectively by clinical judgement, and by a statistical assessment prior to performing a meta-analysis.

Trial Size

It has been suggested that a meta-analysis of numerous small trials introduces so much variation that the conclusions will not be consistent with a single large trial [9]. To address this, the outcomes of large clinical trials in pregnancy and childbirth were compared with the pooled results of small trials from a comprehensive register of trials in this field (the Cochrane Pregnancy and Childbirth Database). This evaluation concluded that results were usually compatible, but discrepancies occurred even when the diversity among both large and small studies was taken into account [10]. In the absence of a mega-trial, however, a well-conducted meta-analysis represents the best available evidence. It remains unclear whether this is sufficient or whether a large trial will ultimately be required.

Trial Quality

Assessment of trial quality is an important step in performing a systematic review and the criteria used to assess quality should be stipulated in the criteria for including trials in a review. If left relatively broad, there is a danger that significant heterogeneity will be introduced and the quality of the finished review will be reduced, whereas very narrow criteria may exclude important evidence [2]. It is therefore important that trial quality is rigorously assessed prior to inclusion in a systematic review. Scales such as the one developed by Chalmers et al. [1] are now widely used (Table 19.1), although major drawbacks are lack of systematic development and evaluation [11]. In future, scales are likely to be focused on trial characteristics directly related to bias in estimating treatment effects and on the reporting of trials [12].

The Cochrane Collaboration

The Cochrane Collaboration was established in 1992 with the broad aims of "preparing, maintaining and disseminating systematic reviews of the effects of health care". The Collaboration is named after the British epidemiologist, Professor Archie Cochrane, who had the unusual distinction of conducting his first clinical trial while a prisoner of war. His wartime experiences demonstrated to Cochrane the relative unimportance of medical therapy compared with the recuperative power of the human body. This inspired him to ensure that all forms of health care would be critically evaluated, thus enabling really effective treatments to be distinguished from those which are of no benefit. In a book published by the Office of Health Economics in 1979 [13], Archie Cochrane reminded the medical profession of the need to obtain reliable evidence about the effects of the treatment it was offering: "It is surely a great criticism of our

Table 19.1. Assessing methodological quality: method of assessing quality of clinical trials, described by Chalmers et al. [1]

	3 points	2 points	1 point	0 points
Method of treatment assignment	Truly randomised, e.g. telephone or computer system, and investigator unlikely to have been able to predict (or identify) assigned treatment prior to trial entry	Randomisation involved, but method of assignment not described, or assignment made by envelope or other method that made it unlikely (but still possible) that assignment could be known or suspected by the investigators	Randomisation involved, but method of assignment not described and investigator not masked at treatment assignment	Randomisation not mentioned explicitly, or investigators could have predicted or influenced treatment assignment
Control of selection bias after treatment assignment	All patients entered into the trial and assigned treatments were included in the analysis, or any withdrawals listed and results analysed both by original treatment assigned and by treatment received	Withdrawls listed, and results analysed by original treatment assignment and by treatment received	No mention of withdrawals, or results analysed only by treatment received	Withdrawals occurred but were not described, and results analysed only by treatment received; or withdrawals accounted for >15% of the randomised patients
Masking of participants and investigators	Triple masked, so that (1) patients, (2) care givers and (3) investigators assessing outcome were unaware of treatment assignment	Outcome assessor masked to treatment assignment, or two of previous three categories were masked	Masking impossible, or impossible to judge if it had been attempted	Could have been conducted as a double-masked study but was not

profession that we have not organised a critical summary, by speciality or subspecialty, adapted periodically, of all relevant randomised controlled trials".

One of the main functions of the Cochrane Collaboration is to establish and maintain a database of all randomised controlled trials conducted to date. Electronic databases provide rapid access to information and are therefore a useful starting point, but unfortunately the low sensitivity of systems such as MEDLINE means that many of the trials on the database cannot be identified because of poor indexing [14]. It is therefore necessary to employ other search strategies, including hand-searching specialist journals, reviewing a wide range of electronic databases, registers of trials and other "grey literature" such as conference proceedings and theses. Foreign databases and journals must also be searched to ensure information is obtained on an international level. Reviewers are also encouraged to contact researchers and manufacturers to enquire about studies in progress and the availability of data from unpublished studies.

The Cochrane Collaboration is also committed to ensuring that systematic reviews are performed in all areas of health care. The Collaboration now supports many international Review Groups, dedicated to conducting reviews in a variety of specialities using standard criteria and specialist software. The first systematic reviews to be included in the Cochrane Collaboration were in the field of Pregnancy and Childbirth [15], and Cochrane Review Groups now exist in almost all areas of health care. Reviews produced for the Cochrane Collaboration all follow a similar format and are completed to high standards. They are written and published in two stages: an initial protocol, outlining plans for the review and methods to be used, and a final review which includes a description of all relevant trials and a statistical meta-analysis if appropriate. The advantage of publishing a protocol is to permit wide readership and allow comments to be made prior to completion of the finished review. There are eight main stages identified in the preparation of a systematic review prior to inclusion on the *Cochrane Library* (Fig. 19.3).

To ensure Cochrane reviews are up to date, reviewers make a commitment to maintain their reviews for the foreseeable future. The reviews are published in the Cochrane Database of Systematic Reviews (CDSR), part of the *Cochrane Library*, a quarterly electronic publication available on CD, disk and via the Internet. Publication via an electronic medium allows reviews to be updated as fresh evidence and errors are identified, thus improving their validity. In addition to the CDSR, the *Cochrane Library* contains the Database of Abstracts of Reviews of Effectiveness (DARE), the Cochrane Review Methodology Database, the Cochrane Controlled Trials Register (a database of over 150 000 controlled trials), and current information about the structure, aims and progress of the groups within the Collaboration and the Collaboration as a whole. The *Cochrane Library* also includes edited post-publication comments from users of the

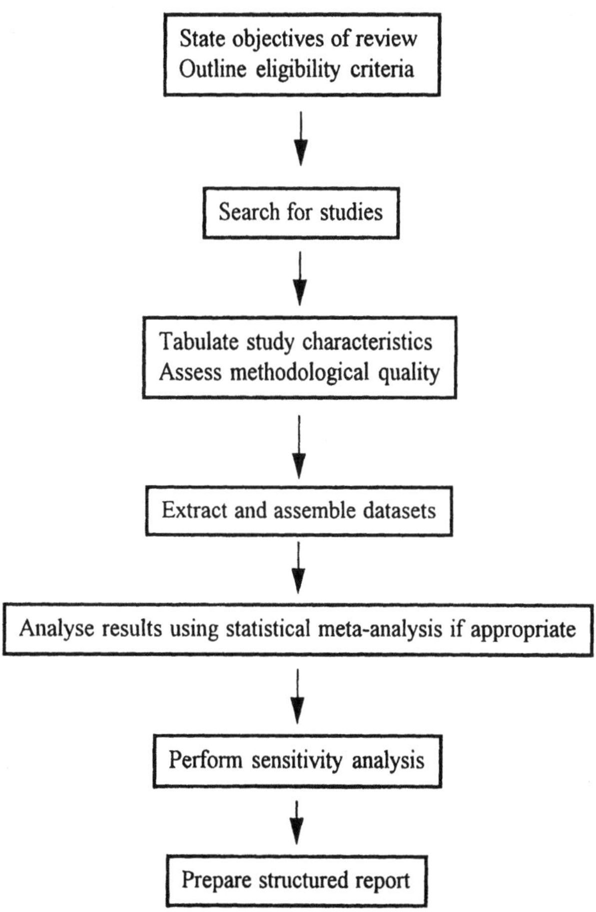

Fig. 19.3. Stages in preparing a systematic review, as outlined by the Cochrane Collaboration.

reviews and is now held in most medical libraries. Principal authors of up-to-date Cochrane reviews receive a subscription free of charge.

Cochrane Review Group on Peripheral Vascular Diseases

To evaluate the treatment of peripheral venous and arterial disorders, a Cochrane Collaborative Review Group on Peripheral Vascular Diseases was established in January 1995, based in Edinburgh. The Group has around 80 active members in 20 countries, largely comprising medical and surgical specialists but also including hospital administrators and policy makers. Its scope includes varicose veins, chronic venous insufficiency and thromboembolism, plus lower limb arterial disease and abdominal aortic aneurysm. Venous ulcers are managed by the Cochrane Review Group on Wound Healing.

Membership of the Review Group on Peripheral Vascular Diseases is available at different levels of commitment and members are not pressurised to make a greater contribution than they choose. Minimal membership, for those who do not wish to be actively involved in the Group, allows members to be kept in touch with progress and development of the Group through the quarterly Group newsletter. Other members might indicate that they are interested in acting as peer reviewers, or hand-searching journals for the Group, in which case they will be sent appropriate information and support for their work. Those interested in writing reviews inform the editorial base of the area they wish to review once they are ready to start work and are expected to deliver a draft review within 15 months of registering a title.

Establishing a database of all relevant trials is one of the main tasks of the Review Group. As a result of hand- and electronic-searching the Review Group on Peripheral Vascular Diseases has identified more than 2400 relevant articles on trials, meta-analyses and reviews. Consequently, its Specialised Register of Trials is now one of the best sources of information in the peripheral vascular field and is used by the Review Group as a primary source of trial evidence for reviewers. The majority of venous trials on the Register relate to the management of thromboembolism (Fig. 19.4), although treatment of varicose veins, chronic venous insufficiency and venous ulcers are also important areas.

The Review Group on Peripheral Vascular Diseases also works with reviewers to produce systematic reviews for publication on the *Cochrane Library*. The Group has already initiated several reviews, but many more are required. The task of reviewing all randomised controlled trials in the field of peripheral vascular diseases is enormous and anyone prepared to contribute both time and intellectual effort is welcome to contribute. This international endeavour will ensure that in future patients receive the most appropriate treatment and that any further unnecessary deaths or disability are prevented.

Acting on the Evidence

Preparing systematic reviews of treatments is only the first step in the evidence-based process. The next stage is to ensure that the results are widely disseminated, including not only evidence of efficacy but also the need for any further research. The electronic publication of the *Cochrane Library* contributes greatly to the dissemination process, but other publications such as *Evidence-Based Medicine* and the *ACP Journal Club* are

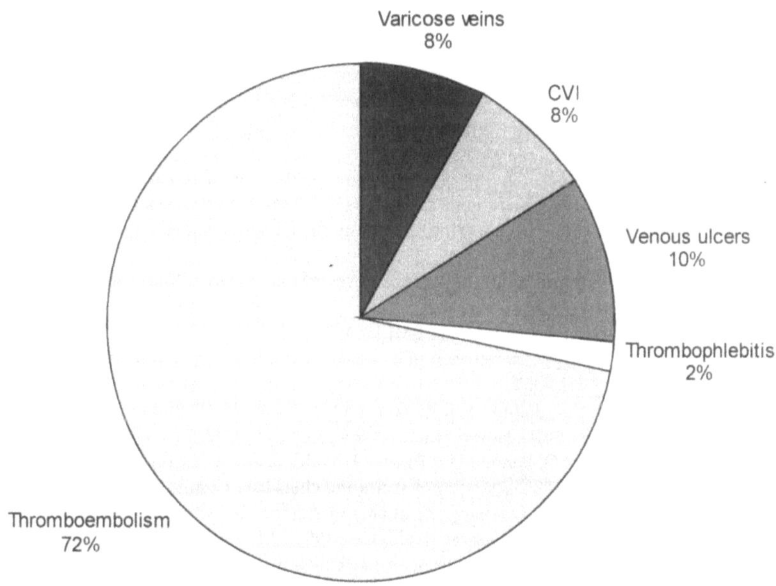

Fig. 19.4. Trials in venous disease: breakdown by disease category. CVI, chronic venous insufficiency.

also important. Despite this, the volume of information about effectiveness can be difficult to handle. An NHS Centre for Reviews and Dissemination has therefore been established in York, with the aim of making information easier to find. Provision of clear information on effectiveness for patients is also important, to help them participate in decisions about their care.

The final stage, changing clinical practice, is the most difficult. It can be facilitated by the production of clinical guidelines and audit procedures, but relies on the close co-operation between clinicians and policy makers. Any changes must be closely monitored to demonstrate real improvements in the quality, effectiveness and cost-effectiveness of health care.

Conclusions

A huge array of evidence has been published on the treatment of venous disorders, but very few systematic reviews have been prepared. It is therefore essential that more good-quality reviews are written and made readily available to all concerned. Vascular surgeons and policy makers need to work together to ensure the available evidence is used to promote clinical effectiveness, and that any change in practice is closely monitored.

References

1. Chalmers I, Adams M, Dickersin K, Hetherington J, Tarnow-Mordi W, Meinert C, et al. A cohort of summary reports of controlled trials. JAMA 1990;263:1401–1405.

2. Counsell C. Formulating questions and locating primary studies for inclusion in systematic reviews. Ann Intern Med 1997;127:380–387.
3. D'Agostino RB, Weintraub M. Meta-analysis: a method for synthesizing research. Clin Pharmacol Ther 1995;58:605–616.
4. Cullum N, Fletcher AW, Nelson EA, Sheldon TA. Compression bandages and stockings in the treatment of venous leg ulcers. In: The Cochrane database of systematic reviews. London: BMJ Publishing Group, 1997.
5. Dickersin K, Min Y-I, Meinhart CL. Factors influencing publication of research results: follow-up of applications submitted to two institutional review boards. JAMA 1992;267:374–378.
6. Dickersin K, Scheer R, Lefebvre C. Identifying relevant studies for systematic reviews. BMJ 1994;309:1286–1291.
7. Light RJ, Pillemer DB. Summing up: the science of reviewing research. Cambridge, Mass: Harvard University Press, 1984:63–72.
8. Eysenck HJ. Meta-analysis and its problems. BMJ 1994;309:789–792.
9. Borzak S, Ridker PM. Discordance between meta-analyses and large scale randomised control trials. Ann Intern Med 1995;123:873–877.
10. Cappelleri JC, Ioannidis, JPA, Schmid CH, de Ferranti SD, Aubert M, Chalmers TC, et al. Large trials vs meta-analysis of smaller trials. How do their results compare? JAMA 1996;276:1332–1338.
11. Moher D, Jadad AR, Nichol G, Penman M, Tugwell P, Walsh S. Assessing the quality of randomised controlled trials: an annotated bibliography of scales and checklists. Control Clin Trials 1995;16:62–73.
12. Moher D, Jadad AR, Tugwell P. Assessing the quality of randomised controlled trials: current issues and future directions. Int J Technol Assess Health Care 1996;12:195–208.
13. Cochrane AL. 1931–1971: a critical review, with particular reference to the medical profession. In: Medicines for the year 2000. London: Office of Health Economics, 1979:1–11.
14. Dickersin K, Schreer R, Lefebvre C. Identifying relevant studies for systematic reviews. BMJ 1994;309:1286–1291.
15. Chalmers I, Enkin M, Keirse MJNC, editors. Effective care in pregnancy and childbirth. Oxford: Oxford University Press, 1989.

Section V
Delivery of Care

20 Should Every Patient with Chronic Venous Disease Have a Duplex Scan?

D.C. Berridge and M.J. Weston

Importance of Accurate Pre-treatment Investigation and Diagnosis

"without an accurate diagnosis, there can be no reliable surgery"

It is an essential prerequisite of any intervention that an accurate diagnosis is made prior to that procedure. Traditionally, the surgery for venous disease has been largely focused on the management of varicose veins, with minimal or no investigation, and was associated with recurrence rates of up to 65% [1]. Whilst the aetiology of recurrent varicose veins is multifactorial, two main factors are undoubtedly linked: the accuracy of the original diagnosis and the quality of the subsequent surgery performed. Inadequate dissection by surgeons in training has also been cited. Persisting incompetence in 41% of patients following varicose vein surgery suggests that trainees perform surgery less effectively than consultants [2]. It is not too surprising that as many as 20–30% of new referrals to venous clinics are patients with recurrent varicose veins.

Clinical examination of patients with varicose veins looking for sites of superficial venous incompetence is notoriously unreliable [3]. This is especially so in those patients with widespread varicosities which do not conform with either the long saphenous vein or short saphenous vein distributions. Similarly, patients with recurrent varicose veins cannot be examined, and their precise venous incompetence diagnosed, with any certainty on clinical grounds alone.

The interval between the various stages of clinical examination, hand-held Doppler (HHD), duplex scanning and surgery is important as clinical deterioration occurs over time. Sarin et al. [4] found new sites of reflux in 18% of patients over a median interval of 20 months sufficient to alter the intended surgical plan. Forty patients were found to have sapheno-femoral incompetence at the initial duplex examination, which increased to 45 (a 12.5% increase) over the 20 months. Similarly, detection of sapheno-popliteal incompetence increased from 11 to 20 limbs (an increase of 81.8%).

The uncertainty of clinical diagnosis is demonstrated in Dixon's study [5]. Duplex, and subsequent surgical operative, findings in 91 legs were compared with a clinical classification of "clinically incompetent", "clinically doubtful" and "clinically competent" (Table 20.1). It can be seen that even in sapheno-femoral incompetence, considerable uncertainty exists on clinical grounds alone (11/59, 19%). For popliteal fossa incompetence, this was more exaggerated (11/27, 41%). The surgical approach was

Table 20.1. Correlation of duplex findings with surgical findings, categorised by clinical status

	Clinically incompetent	Clinically doubtful	Clinically competent	Total
Sapheno-femoral incompetence				
TP	47	11	1	59
FP		1		1
TN	1	12	17	30
FN	1			1
	49	24	18	
Popliteal fossa incompetence				
TP	11	11	5	27
FP		3		3
TN		14	47	61
FN				0
	11	28	52	
Calf perforators				
TP	9	30	8	47
FP		3		3
TN	1	9	31	41
FN				0
	10	42	39	
Other perforators				
TP	1	7	1	9
FP				0
TN		8	74	82
FN				0
	1	15	75	

After Dixon [9]. TP, true positive; FP, false positive; TN, true negative; FN, false negative.

altered by duplex scanning in 13 of 67 patients (19.4%), including removing the indication for surgery in some patients with no sapheno-femoral or sapheno-popliteal junction incompetence.

The use of HHD in clinic, using both 8 MHz and 4–5 MHz probes, can considerably aid the clinical examination. It is used to advise the patient of the likely surgery required pending full duplex scanning, as a means of selection to reduce the number of patients undergoing duplex imaging, or even as the sole investigation of these patients. Although many authorities advocate the HHD as a more reliable means than clinical examination for detecting sites of reflux, especially in primary varicose veins, the technique has its limitations [6]. The use of tourniquets has also been shown to be unreliable. The pressure required to compress superficial varicosities varies from 40 to 300 mmHg, and hence it is difficult to ensure that superficial venous reflux is prevented without causing deep venous obstruction [7].

Darke et al. [8] have reported a series of 100 limbs in 73 consecutive patients with primary and uncomplicated varicose veins. A single observer performed HHD followed by "blinded" duplex imaging. Patients with reflux of less than 0.5 s and those with "minor reflux", defined as where the duration and peak velocity of the reflux signal was less than that of the augmented signal, were excluded from analysis. Of 87 limbs with long saphenous incompetence HHD missed 4 (4.6%). Short saphenous incompetence proved more difficult, with HHD missing 2 of 21 (9.5%). Of greater concern was that HHD erroneously diagnosed sapheno-popliteal junction incompetence in a further 5 limbs. Thus potentially inadequate surgery may have been performed in 6 cases (4 long saphenous vein, 2 short saphenous vein), and inappropriate surgery in 5 (all short saphenous vein). Mercer et al. [9] compared HHD with duplex imaging in 89 limbs of 61 patients. False positive results on HHD were infrequent and good specificities were achieved: 93.3% (sapheno-femoral junction, SFJ), 93.7% (sapheno-popliteal junction, SPJ) and 85.2% (thigh perforators, TP). In contrast, the sensitivity of HHD was disappointing: 72.9% (SFJ), 76.9% (SPJ) and 51.4% (TP). Critics have argued that few patients' surgery would have been altered, but it is in the determination of what constitutes an acceptably small error that centres differ. The results of Mercer et al. [9] show that, in 5 limbs (6%) HHD suggested surgery to an entirely competent system and would have left intact an incompetent system in 19 limbs (21%). In 2 limbs (2%) both inappropriate and inadequate surgery would have been performed on HHD assessment alone. The authors maintain that this is more than "a few" and is unacceptable.

The limitations of HHD mainly arise because it is not possible to be confident which vessel is being insonated. Is it reflux at the junction, in the deep vein or in a venous tributary or cross-groin collaterals? Multilevel superficial venous incompetence can also be difficult to differentiate with either clinical examination alone or in conjunction with HHD. This is illustrated by the complexity shown by duplex scanning in a primary varicose vein cohort reported by Quigley et al. [10]. Sapheno-femoral incompetence was found in 76 (55%) of 137 limbs with primary varicose veins examined with duplex for sapheno-femoral junction incompetence. Of these, 9 (12%) had associated sapheno-popliteal junction incompetence, 19 (25%) had perforator vein incompetence, 4 (5%) had sapheno-popliteal and calf perforator incompetence, and 3 (4%) had evidence of deep venous incompetence as well. Similarly of 30 limbs with sapheno-popliteal incompetence, 13 (43%) also had sapheno-femoral incompetence, 5 (17%) had perforator vein incompetence and 1 (3%) had deep venous reflux. There were also important anatomical variations found: in 14 limbs the short saphenous vein did not join the popliteal vein, and in 4 cases it joined more than 10 cm proximal to the knee joint. There were notably more sapheno-popliteal and perforator vein incompetent segments than were found with clinical examination or HHD. In other words, the complexity of the patterns of reflux can be too great for clinical and HHD examination to unravel.

There is a third option, other than to use or not use duplex examination. Dunning et al. [11] have suggested that a selective duplex scanning policy can be used without any adverse effect on management. They studied 74 limbs of 51 patients. Of these patients, 40 had primary varicose veins, of whom 10 would have been selected to have duplex scanning performed. Their findings are impressive, with no failure of detection of significant sites of reflux despite a 30% reduction in their use of duplex scanning. However, they may be at risk of a type II error due to small numbers, such that one extra case could theoretically create a 3% error. Furthermore, other workers have been much less successful with HHD and selective duplex scanning in similar cases [6, 8, 9, 12].

The use of duplex scanning can certainly facilitate venous surgery and can lead to lower recurrence rates by allowing a more detailed anatomical map of the incompetent perforator sites [10]. This, together with the known limitations of HHD described above, suggests that it is unreasonable to restrict duplex scanning by using a selective scanning policy. Combining accurate pre-operative diagnosis and marking with careful, meticulous surgery means that inadequate and inappropriate surgery can be avoided, and recurrence rates reduced to a minimum [13]. Other workers have shown that with accurate pre-operative diagnosis utilising clinical examination, HHD and duplex scanning, the trainee surgeon can also achieve excellent results with no sites of perforator vein incompetence missed [14].

Duplex imaging can also give valuable information with regard to the patency and presence of reflux in the deep venous system. It is not infrequent that deep venous reflux is found, even in the absence of a history of deep venous thrombosis. Correction of the superficial incompetence may help to reduce or eliminate the deep venous reflux by reducing the "overload" of the deep system caused by the superficial venous incompetence. These factors will influence the prognostic advice given to the patient.

In summary, duplex scanning performs better than clinical examination or HHD in the accurate mapping of venous incompetence. The rate of varicose vein recurrence following surgery will be reduced by such improved mapping, provided that the interval between the duplex scanning and surgery is short.

Potential Impact on Quality and Outcome

There are no randomised trials that have addressed the influence of pre-operative investigations on subsequent clinical (functional and cosmetic) outcome and recurrence following varicose vein surgery. One of the main criticisms of venous surgery in the past has been the disappointment of the patient with either the initial result (especially cosmetic), the number of residual veins, or the frequency of and relatively early recurrence of varicosities. Whilst some of these factors were undoubtedly due to inadequate surgical technique, the role of inappropriate or incomplete surgery in spite of otherwise technically competent surgery cannot be ignored. If the wrong or excessive surgery is performed on primary veins in 6–9% of patients when only clinical or HHD examination has been used, then this needs to be discussed as a prognostic factor with the patient. This is in addition to the "natural recurrence" due to incompetence developing at previously competent sites, and the occurrence of neovascularisation. Clinical examination will allow correct marking of all visible or palpable veins for removal; however, as discussed earlier, it is unreliable at accurately defining the actual sites of superficial venous incompetence. The achievement of optimum quality requires the employment of the best available method of investigation; duplex scanning fulfils this role. However, there is another argument, that of cost effectiveness. This will be discussed later in this chapter.

Which Patients Should Have Duplex Scanning?

"everyone if you have the staff and resources; selective if not"

In an ideal world all patients should undergo the most detailed, least invasive imaging procedure prior to their intervention [15]. However, in an increasingly cash-limited service, it is obligatory to look at the potential cost-benefit of such a policy. It is also recognised that many radiology departments or vascular laboratories would be overwhelmed at the prospect of performing duplex scans on all patients potentially undergoing venous intervention.

Most authorities would agree that duplex investigation of recurrent varicose veins, and those arising in the popliteal fossa, should be considered as routine. Residual varicose veins following long saphenous vein ligation have been demonstrated to be due to the long saphenous vein in 68.9% of cases, short saphenous incompetence in 25.8% and deep venous incompetence in 23.8% [16]. In addition, 12 refluxing regions detected with HHD were found to be false positive when using duplex ultrasound. The same authors have also investigated recurrent varicose veins following short saphenous surgery. Most cases were due to reflux in the short saphenous vein (67%). Incompetent gastrocnemius veins (34%) and popliteal vein incompetence (20%) accounted for the majority of the rest of the recurrent varicose veins.

Whilst recurrent varicose veins may be due to inadequate dissection of the sapheno-femoral junction with incomplete ligation of all tributaries, it is becoming recognised that provided accurate surgery is performed initially, the principal cause of recurrence may be neovascularisation at the sapheno-femoral junction with vessels of less than 3 mm diameter. Jones et al. [1] demonstrated that neovascularisation was detected in up to 52% of limbs at 2 years. Nevertheless, it is equally recognised in an increasingly litigious society that inappropriate or inadequate surgery based upon inadequate pre-operative investigation might be difficult to defend. For recurrent varicose veins, duplex scanning should be considered mandatory as it is impossible to be accurate with clinical examination and HHD alone [5, 6, 23].

Bradbury et al. [3] examined 202 patients with recurrent varicose veins (267 limbs) with duplex scanning. The most frequent pattern of reflux (44.6%) was due to an intact and incompetent long sapheno-femoral junction and long saphenous vein. Less frequent but still significant causes of recurrence were an incompetent thigh perforator with long saphenous vein reflux but no sapheno-femoral junction incompetence (10.5%); and an incompetent sapheno-popliteal junction (9.7%). It is unjustified and potentially hazardous to perform "re-do" groin surgery without pre-operative duplex scanning especially in a patient with neovascularisation, deep femoral reflux or cross-groin collaterals. Patients with lipodermatosclerosis or post-ulceration are more likely to have deep reflux, combined deep and superficial reflux, short sapheno-popliteal reflux and posterior tibial vein reflux [17]. All these patients should be included if a selective policy of requesting duplex scans is used.

Sapheno-popliteal incompetence can also be difficult to differentiate from reflux either within the calf veins themselves or indeed in the popliteal vein in the presence of an otherwise competent junction. The anatomy of the sapheno-popliteal junction is so variable that accurate pre-operative marking with duplex (or intra-operative venography) is essential to allow correct positioning of the surgical incision. Vasdekis et al. [18] found that accuracy of localisation of the sapheno-popiliteal junction to within 2 cm was 56% for clinical examination, 64% for HHD and 96% for duplex scanning. Whilst the use of duplex scanning is obviously invaluable in differentiating the true pattern of recurrent reflux, using the most accurate method to determine the correct procedure in primary varicose veins will undoubtedly help both short- and long-term success and help to minimise recurrence.

For the majority of patients with uncomplicated primary varicose veins confined to the long saphenous territory, clinical examination combined with HHD is likely to be associated with a correct procedure being performed in approximately 90–95% of cases. One could argue that this is a perfectly satisfactory situation with no need for the extra expense of duplex scanning [12, 19, 20]. Kent and Weston [19] demonstrated a sensitivity at the sapheno-femoral junction of 0.93 and a specificity of 0.91 when HHD was performed immediately before duplex scanning. Nevertheless, it would still have resulted in excessive surgery in 5% and inappropriate surgery in a further 1%; that is, an overall incorrect surgery rate of 6%. Campbell et al. [20] performed clinical assessment, and HHD followed by duplex scanning in 85 patients with 122 symptomatic legs. Whilst 91% of cases were correctly identified by HHD, 9 (9%) cases of long saphenous reflux were missed. HHD assessment of the short sapheno-popliteal junction revealed correct detection of reflux in 28 of 39 cases (72%), i.e. 28% incorrect. Even allowing for low velocity reflux, 6% of patients, to quote the authors, "escaped diagnosis". This has important implications in informed consent.

The cost implication of adopting an "all-comers", "selective", or "no-duplex" standpoint will be discussed later. However, there cannot be many other instances where the surgeon would be prepared to operate knowing that he or she could be doing inaccurate or inappropriate surgery in up to 10% of cases. Some papers have shown even worse potential rates of inaccurately planned surgery. Mercer et al. [9] found that the sensitivity of HHD was 72.9% at the sapheno-femoral junction and 76.9% at the sapheno-popliteal junction. The sensitivity for thigh perforators was even less impressive at 51.4%. Sites of reflux might have been left following surgery in up to 23% of cases (Table 20.2). A confounding factor that might have made these figures worse than in other studies is the large time interval between HHD and duplex scanning. This is important because of clinical deterioration, as discussed earlier [4].

Therefore if a selective approach to the use of duplex scanning is adopted it should include all patients with recurrent varicose veins, all patients with suspected sapheno-popliteal junction incompetence, and all others with equivocal long saphenous vein/sapheno-femoral junction incompetence. Clinical examination should be augmented with the use of HHD in all cases of chronic venous disease, and in an ideal world also supplemented with colour duplex imaging.

What are the Cost Implications?

"Duplex is cheap in the overall context of the operation"

The cost implications of performing duplex scanning largely depend on the personnel running the service – whether they are technologists, surgeons or radiologists. Clearly a technologist (radiographer, trained nurse, scientist) will be less expensive than a consultant surgeon or radiologist in the same role. In addition to the actual technique of scanning, it may be important to have the clinical interpretation and experience offered by the medical personnel. There are no data available to suggest that the increased cost of the medical personnel is offset by a greater throughput. There is no evidence available that would help to determine who is the most cost-effective person to do the imaging. Indeed, in some centres the technologist may well be the most experienced and efficient person in this context. The initial outlay for the colour duplex equipment can be offset if there is spare capacity on existing machines, or by several units

Table 20.2. Implications of using hand-held Doppler (HHD) for surgical planning

	Operation based on duplex scanning			
Operation based on HHD	Stab avulsions only	SFJ ligation and LSV strip	SPJ ligation	SPJ and SFJ ligation and LSV strip
Stab avulsions only	1	8	3	0
SFJ ligation and LSV strip	2	47	1	3
SPJ ligation	0	1	9	3
SPJ and SFJ ligation and LSV strip	0	4	0	8

From Mercer et al. [15].
SFJ, sapheno-femoral junction; SPJ, sapheno-politeal junction; LSV, long saphenous vein.

potentially utilising the services of a more "central" or "common" vascular laboratory facility.

Using lease-cost figures and the salary for a laboratory technician, the cost per scan can be as little as £65. Employing a radiologist or surgeon in such a position would increase this to £85 per scan.

Who Should Provide the Service: Surgeon, Technician or Radiologist?

"the best trained person with enough time"

Who should provide the service will largely depend upon local expertise and availability. Some centres have trained vascular laboratory technologists who undertake the majority of the scanning. These individuals tend to be in demand and in short supply. Other centres employ medical physicists to provide the service. In most institutions it falls to the radiologists. Surgeons have been relatively slow to undertake training in the use of duplex scanning, although this would be a useful ability, especially in the context of outpatient assessment.

If a policy of offering a duplex scan to all patients attending with venous disease is adopted, then the large number of scans required is best provided by specialised technicians. This enables the surgeon or radiologist to fulfil their more clinically orientated role rather than using their expensive time to provide a venous scanning service. Conversely, in a selective duplex scanning service it may be more practicable because of the lower workload for the surgeon or radiologist to do their own duplex scans. A third option is for all the routine duplex scans to be done by technicians but for there to be a skilled clinician available (either a surgeon or a radiologist) who can scan problem or complex cases. The difficulty with this option lies in how the clinician maintains their expertise when dealing with only a relatively small number of venous duplex scans. These problems can only be resolved within a context of teamwork and "skill-mix".

A further major factor is the access to good-quality ultrasound equipment that is regularly updated. Only large institutions will be able to justify sole use of high-quality machines for varicose vein scanning. It may therefore be a shared device residing in radiology or the vascular laboratory, but also used for other specialities and venous thrombosis surveillance. The siting of a machine will affect which staff are best able to provide the varicose vein duplex service.

Is There a Role for Post-operative Quality Control by Duplex Scanning?

It is important for all surgeons to adopt a healthy attitude towards quality assurance. Part of this assurance is the confirmation that the intended operation has been performed properly with no residual incompetence. It is especially valuable in documenting the training quality of junior staff [17]. It is equally important that the duplex findings are always correlated with the clinical and HHD findings. Any major discrepancy should be re-checked with a second duplex examination, if necessary, prior to intervention.

The size of the workload precludes most centres from doing post-operative duplex scans on all those who have had venous surgery. Nevertheless, it should be possible for all centres periodically to scan a cohort of post-operative patients, whether as an exercise in quality assurance, audit or research. Post-operative duplex scans should be considered whenever there is a change in pre-operative protocols, different or new surgical techniques are used, or possibly as feedback for training purposes.

Conclusion

In an ideal, non-cash-limited world, everyone with primary or secondary varicose veins would have pre-operative duplex scanning, venography as required, and regular audits with post-operative duplex scanning. In reality, however, it has to be recognised that it is probably a logistical impossibility to achieve this in all hospitals. Nevertheless, patients with recurrent varicose veins, those with healed or active ulceration or lipodermatosclerosis, and those with popliteal fossa reflux should all be subject to investigation with duplex ultrasound scan. Other patients with uncomplicated primary varicose veins should be carefully examined with hand-held Doppler as a minimum.

References

1. Jones L, Braithwaite BD, Selwyn D, Cooke S, Earnshaw JJ. Neovascularisation is the principal cause of varicose vein recurrence: results of a randomised trial of stripping of the long saphenous vein. Eur J Vasc Endovasc Surg 1996;12:442–445.
2. Lees T, Sing S, Beard J, Spencer P, Rigby C. Prospective audit of surgery for varicose veins. Br J Surg 1997;84:44–46.
3. Bradbury AW, Stonebridge PA, Ruckley CV, Beggs I. Recurrent varicose veins: correlation between preoperative clinical and hand-held Doppler ultrasonographic examination, and anatomical findings at surgery. Br J Surg 1993;80:849–851.
4. Sarin S, Shields DA, Farrah J, Scurr JH, Coleridge-Smith PD. Does venous function deteriorate in patients waiting for varicose vein surgery? J R Soc Med 1993;86:21–3.
5. Dixon PM. Duplex ultrasound in the pre-operative assessment of varicose veins. Australas Radio 1996;40:416–421.
6. Salaman RA, Fligelstone LJ, Wright, Pugh N, Harding KG, Lane IF. Hand-held bi-directional Doppler versus colour duplex scanning in the preoperative assessment of varicose veins. J Vasc Invest 1995;1:183–186.
7. McMullin GM, Coleridge-Smith PD, Scurr JH. A study of tourniquets in the investigation of venous insufficiency. Phlebology 1991;6:133–139.
8. Darke SG, Vetrivel S, Foy DMA, Smith S, Baker S. A comparison of duplex scanning and continuous wave Doppler in the assessment of primary and uncomplicated varicose veins. Eur J Vasc Endovasc Surg 1997;14:457–61.
9. Mercer KG, Scott DJA, Berridge DC. Is pre-operative duplex required in all cases of primary varicose veins? Presented at the Venous Forum of the Royal Society of Medicine, London, 1997.
10. Quigley FG, Raptis S, Cashman M, Faris IB. Duplex ultrasound mapping of sites of deep to superficial incompetence in primary varicose veins. Aust NZ J Surg 1992;62:276–278.
11. Dunning PG, Payne SPK, Banerjee B, Lees TA, Lambert D. Do all patients with varicose veins need a duplex ultrasound? Presented at the Venous Forum, Royal Society of Medicine, London, October 1997.
12. Campbell WB, Halim AS, Aertson A, Ridler BMF, Thompson JF, Niblett PG. The place of duplex scanning for varicose veins and common venous problems. Ann R Coll Surg Eng 1996;78:490–493.
13. Hoare MC, Royle JP. Doppler ultrasound detection of sapheno-femoral and sapheno-popliteal incompetence and operative venography to ensure precise sapheno-popliteal ligation. Aust NZ J Surg 1984;54:49–52.
14. Turton EPL, McKenzie S, Weston MJ, Berridge DC, Scott DJS. Optimising a varicose vein service to reduce recurrence. Ann R Coll Surg Engl 1997;79:451–454.

15. DePalma R, Hart M, Zarin L, Massarin E. Physical examination, Doppler ultrasound and colour flow duplex scanning: guides to therapy of primary varicose veins. Phlebology 1993;8:7–11.
16. Tong Y, Royle J. Recurrent varicose veins following high ligation of long saphenous vein: a duplex ultrasound study. Cardiovasc Surg 1995;3:485–487.
17. Myers KA, Ziegerhein RW, Zeng GH, et al. Duplex ultrasonography scanning for chronic venous disease: patterns of reflux J Vasc Surg 1995;21:605–612.
18. Vasdekis SN, Clarke GH, Hobbs JT, Nicolaides AN. Evaluation of non-invasive and invasive methods in the assessment of short saphenous vein termination. Br J Surg 1989;76:929–32.
19. Kent PJ, Weston MJ. Duplex scanning is unnecessary in all patients presenting with primary, non-recurrent varicose veins. Personal communication.
20. Campbell WB, Niblett PG, Ridler BMF, Peters AS, Thompson JF. Hand-held Doppler as a screening test in primary varicose veins. Br Surg 1997;84:1541–1543.

21 How To Run an Efficient Venous Service?

N.J.M. London, M. Bello and M. Scriven

Introduction

This chapter describes and discusses how to provide an efficient venous service for the patient with venous ulceration. In particular, it will discuss the pros and cons of a one-stop clinic, the best way to organise such a clinic, and how the clinic might efficiently communicate and collaborate with those managing venous ulceration in the community. We will not debate whether all patients with venous ulceration should be seen in such a clinic because this will be discussed in Chapter 23.

A specialist venous ulcer assessment clinic offers a number of potential benefits for the patient with venous ulceration. First, the clinic can confirm or refute the presence of arterial disease. Although in many areas of the United Kingdom, District Nurses or Practice Nurses are trained in the measurement of the ankle:brachial pressure index (ABPI), this can be difficult if the patient has calcified distal vessels or if the ulcer is too painful to allow a pneumatic cuff to be inflated over it. Moreover, if the patient is found to have a low ABPI or poor pedal arterial signals, then an arterial duplex scan [1] can immediately be performed in the clinic and, if appropriate, the patient referred for angioplasty or surgery.

The second advantage offered by a specialist venous ulcer assessment clinic is that patients can undergo colour duplex scanning of the lower limb venous system. This is important for a number of reasons. First, it will allow the detection of the 55–60% of patients with isolated superficial venous disease who may benefit from superficial venous surgery [2,3]. Although it remains to be proven definitively, it is to be hoped that surgery in such patients will reduce ulcer recurrence rates compared with those who are treated by compression bandaging. Second, there are a small number of patients (4%) with venous ulcers who have deep venous obstruction and whose superficial veins are acting as important venous collaterals. Compression bandaging in such patients can potentially be disastrous because it further impairs venous return from the limb. Third, there would appear to be a subset of patients with superficial venous reflux and segmental deep venous reflux (reflux in a segment of the deep venous system rather than the entire deep venous system) who may benefit from superficial venous surgery [4,5]. Such patients can only be identified by duplex scanning. A final advantage of hospital attendance is that patients with leg ulcers and normal arterial and venous investigations, and who have no systemic disease that is recognised to cause leg ulceration, can have a local anaesthetic biopsy of their ulcer performed. This is important because malignancy in such ulcers needs to be excluded.

The Advantages of a One-Stop Clinic

If it is accepted that patients with venous ulceration should be assessed in a specialist hospital clinic, then the next question is whether a one-stop clinic [2] confers significant advantages over the conventional "three-visit approach" (i.e. initial attendance, followed by return for investigations, followed by return to discuss the results of investigations). The first advantage of a single-visit approach is that patients with venous ulcers tend to be elderly and often require transfer to the hospital clinic by ambulance. It therefore undoubtedly reduces costs considerably reduces cost if patients can attend on a single-visit basis rather than on three occasions. A further advantage, particularly in an elderly group of patients, is that if they know they will only have to make a single visit, they are more likely to be compliant. Understandably, many elderly patients do not relish trips to and from the hospital and if they foresee only a single visit they may be more likely to attend.

There is little doubt that it is advantageous to both physician and patient if investigations can be performed at a one-stop clinic because the aetiology of the ulcer can be explained to the patient there and then and a plan of treatment described and initiated. Finally, with MRSA being such a problem in most hospitals throughout the world, it is undoubtedly advantageous if leg ulcer patients attend on as few occasions as possible. This reduces the risk not only of MRSA being acquired by the patient during their hospital visit but also of an MRSA-infected patient bringing the organism into the hospital.

Organisation of a One-Stop Clinic

Experience has taught us that there are a number of pitfalls with respect to the organisation of a one-stop venous ulcer assessment clinic, and these will now be discussed. The first issue is where the clinic should be situated. In order for a venous ulcer patient to undergo a complete and thorough examination it is mandatory that all dressings are removed. Most vascular studies units do not have nurses attached to them and, if venous ulcer patients are seen in a vascular studies unit, there is a high chance that the vascular technologist performing the examination will not remove the dressings. This is partly because vascular technologists are not trained to remove dressings but also, if they do remove them, they are not trained or equipped to replace them. Also, the malodour left in the unit after a patient with a badly infected or colonised venous ulcer has attended can be a source of distress to both vascular technologists and subsequent patients. For all these reasons we see our single-visit venous ulcer patients in our outpatient clinic, with a dedicated mobile colour duplex scanner and an experienced vascular technologist in attendance.

The next question is how many patients can be seen in such a clinic. We have found that to remove the dressings from an ulcerated limb, perform the necessary investigations on that limb and then re-dress the ulcer takes a minimum of half-an-hour. We suggest, therefore, that no more than two patients can be seen per colour duplex scanner per hour. We would thus normally see six patients in a 3-hour clinic. Attempts to see more patients than this can result in frustration for patients, nurses and vascular technologists, and we would strongly recommend that it is preferable to run the clinic in such a way that nurses and vascular technologists have time to do their job properly!

After arrival in the clinic, patients are seen by a doctor who takes a thorough history and performs a complete physical examination. If it is thought necessary, blood tests can be performed and in our own clinic the results of such tests are available within half-an-hour. We do not routinely, however, perform full blood counts, or test levels of urea, electrolytes and albumin, because we have found that the yield of abnormalities is low. The colour duplex scanner and a vascular technologist then enter the room, "Cling Film" is wrapped around the patient's ulcer and the ABPI is measured. If it is not possible because of pain to measure the ABPI accurately, or if the distal arteries are calcified, then the technologist listens to the pedal signals using continuous wave Doppler. If the ABPI is < 0.80 or if the pedal signals are damped, a colour duplex scan is then performed of the arterial tree. It is our experience that roughly 15% of patients in a single-visit venous ulcer clinic have an arterial contribution to their problem and that the majority of these can be dealt with by angioplasty.

The venous system is then scanned in a standard manner. The results of the venous scan are reported diagrammatically on a proforma and the technologist can then discuss the results with the surgeon before taking the scanner to a patient in an adjacent room. It is logical and reasonable to ask the vascular technologist to first scan the below-knee popliteal vein, for if this demonstrates significant reflux, then superficial surgery is unlikely to be of any value and a complete venous scan is of academic interest rather than practical value. It is thus possible to reduce time and cost by having vascular technologist firstly scan the below-knee popliteal vein and, if there is significant reflux at that site, to proceed no further with the venous scan.

Communication and Interaction with Care in the Community

At the conclusion of the arterial and venous assessment, the surgeon is in a position to discuss with the patient the nature of their problem. Although, inevitably, there will be differences of opinion amongst surgeons regarding the precise indications for venous surgery, some generalisations can be made. On cases of isolated superficial venous insufficiency the pros and cons of surgery can be discussed with the patient. including the possibility that if they are very elderly or frail local anaesthetic sapheno-femoral disconnection is possible. In the patient with extensive deep venous reflux, superficial surgery has no role and the mainstay of treatment is therefore compression bandaging.

In Leicester our Health Authority has agreed to fund four-layer or short-stretch compression bandaging in the community. Patients with deep venous reflux are therefore referred back to the community for compression bandaging. The referral pathway is that the Senior District Nurse receives a copy of the letter sent to the patient's General Practitioner which clearly states the results of the arterial and venous assessment, including the ABPI. The Senior District Nurse then contacts the Specialist Leg Ulcer Nurse who covers the area in which the patient lives and within 2 or 3 weeks compression bandaging is commenced. We suggest that the patients return to our venous clinic only if there are specific problems. Patients who have had superficial venous surgery have simple occlusive dressings applied until healing occurs.

Logistic and Cost Implications

The logistic implications of a one-stop venous ulcer assessment clinic for the surgeon and hospital in which he or she works are that the outpatient clinic has to be available for half a day per week, specialist Leg Ulcer Nurses need to be available for that half-day and a mobile colour duplex scanner and vascular technologist also need to be available. It is unrealistic to expect to see more than six patients in a 3-hour clinic and a weekly clinic will generate between 10 and 12 patients each month who require superficial venous surgery.

It is possible to discuss the cost implications from the point of view of both the nation and the Hospital Trust. With respect to the Hospital Trust, it is important that such a clinic is costed appropriately and in Leicester we charge General Practitioners £140 per patient. We believe that this price is realistic and in this respect the clinic is "cost neutral". With respect to the national budget, the crucial question is whether the benefits of such a clinic, such as identifying the relatively small percentage of patients with significant arterial disease and identifying the 60% of patients who will benefit from superficial surgery, will result in improved ulcer healing and reduced recurrence rates.

Research Issues

Research is needed to determine whether patients with isolated superficial venous insufficiency who undergo corrective surgery do indeed have a lower ulcer recurrence rate at 5 years compared with those treated by compression bandaging alone. If this proves to be the case, then a prospective randomised study is required to determine whether specialist hospital-based leg ulcer assessment clinics are cost effective. The principle behind such a trial would be to randomise patients with new episodes of leg ulceration to either management entirely in the community or referral to a leg ulcer assessment clinic. Patients in the latter group who are not suitable for superficial surgery would return to the community for compression bandaging. Both approaches need to be fully costed and after 5 years the question to be addressed would be whether, allowing for recurrence rate, the cost per healed ulcer is cheaper in those who are assessed in a single-visit venous ulcer clinic. This is undoubtedly a long-term project, but only a study of this nature will determine the role of hospital-based one-stop venous ulcer assessment clinics in the management of the ulcerated lower limb.

References

1. Sensier Y, Hartshorne T, Thrush A, Nydahl S, Bolia A, London NJM. A prospective comparison of lower limb colour-coded duplex scanning with arteriography. Eur J Vasc Endovasc Surg 1996;11:170–175.
2. Scriven JM, Hartshorne T, Bell PRF, Naylor AR, London NJM. Single-visit venous ulcer assessment clinic: the first year. Br J Surg 1997;84:334–336.
3. Grabs AJ, Wakely MC, Nyamekye I, Ghauri ASK, Poskitt KR. Colour duplex ultrasonography in the rational management of chronic venous leg ulcers. Br J Surg 1996;83:1380–1382.
4. Walsh JC, Bergan JJ, Beeman S, Comer TP. Femoral vein reflux abolished by greater saphenous vein stripping. Ann Vasc Surg 1994;8:566–570.
5. Sales CM, Bilof ML, Petrillo KA, Luka NL. Correction of lower extremity deep venous incompetence by ablation of superficial venous reflux. Ann Vasc Surg 1996;10:186–189.

22 What Is the Scope of Day Care for Venous Surgery?

Ian F. Lane and Nicholas E. Bourantas

Introduction

Day care surgery was initially proposed by healthcare economists on financial grounds and rapidly advanced by the health insurance industry in the United States. Whilst in the United Kingdom there has been some resistance to this change by the medical profession and patients, it does carry advantages which lead to clinical and financial efficiency. Varicose vein surgery is ideal for day care as patients are usually young without co-morbidity, the surgical technique is predictable and ambulant patients have few complications. The incidence of varicose veins is increasing in developed countries, with the prevalence in the United Kingdom estimated to be 10–17% of the population [1]. In 1987–88 almost 50 000 patients were admitted for treatment [2,3]. Priority for treatment is assessed as low by healthcare ecomomists, based upon a perception that there is little morbidity in a disease thought to be largely cosmetic. Treatment produces a relatively small increase in quality adjusted life years compared with herniorrhaphy and surgery for other intermediate conditions. Nevertheless, strong public demand for treatment coupled with the accepted morbidity of pain and ulceration has provided an impetus to investigate cost-effective treatment other than inpatient care. A number of purchasing agencies are now refusing to fund minimally symptomatic varicose vein surgery as the disease has little priority compared with cancer surgery or major arterial reconstruction for critical ischaemia.

Traditionally, correction of valvular incompetence by ligation together with avulsion of varicosities is considered to be the optimal surgical treatment. Lengths of stay vary, particularly with cultural factors, but three nights would not have been unusual in the past. In 1966 the United Kingdom bed occupancy figures for patients undergoing varicose vein surgery exceeded the provision required for appendicectomy [4]. In an attempt to lower the cost of the procedure, length of stay has been reduced progressively and now many units are performing surgery without an overnight stay. Although initially reported in 1972, controversy has been generated by this development, particularly concerning adequacy of analgesia, incidence of deep vein thrombosis, surgical technique (with the need to strip the long saphenous vein) and patient satisfaction [5].

Pre-operative Venous Assessment

The precise surgical procedure must be planned whether a patient is scheduled for day care or overnight stay. The minimum procedure commensurate with a successful outcome is particularly important in day case surgery although this must not compromise post-operative results. Clinical examination alone is inadequate to assess lower limb varicose veins, but diagnostic ability can be considerably enhanced by the use of continuous wave Doppler ultrasound and duplex scanning [6]. Investigation of venous incompetence is addressed elsewhere in this book and is identical with that required for inpatient surgery.

Patient Assessment and Counselling

As patients are admitted only a short time before surgery, it is important that their suitability for day case procedures has been previously determined. Professional bodies and the Royal College of Surgeons of England guidelines on day case surgery state that patients for general anaesthesia should be under 70 years old, of physical status ASA group I or II and that the procedure duration must less than 60 min, this relating to recovery time [7]. This time scale limits the application for venous surgery and normally excludes bilateral procedures unless two surgeons are operating together. The new short-acting general anaesthetic agents such as sevroflurane are likely to extend operating time as well as reducing the incidence of post-operative nausea. Although patients up to 94 years of age have reportedly undergone day care surgery, often only avulsions under local anaesthetic are performed [8]. Extensive varicosities with high anticipated blood loss may preclude day care surgery. Patients needing open calf perforator surgery or post-operative bed rest for venous ulcers usually require inpatient stay although sub-fascial endoscopic perforator ligation may further expand the indications for day care. Patients require a general assessment in order to exclude pre-existing medical conditions such as diabetes mellitus, obesity, uncontrolled hypertension and cardio-respiratory disease. Other criteria required for day care selection include residence within a reasonable distance from hospital, presence of a telephone at home and a companion for the first post-operative night.

The assessment can be performed by a postal questionnaire or be nurse-led, thus saving medical personnel time compared with inpatient procedures. Personal interview is preferable and conveniently takes place at the time of the initial consultation. Routine haematology, radiology and electrocardiology is required according to local protocol. Patients ofter have concerns, particularly related to post-operative care and convalescence. The possibility of minor bleeding must be explained, as what may be considered trivial in a hospital ward can be distressing during the night at home. An information sheet is essential, giving contact telephone numbers for advice. Patients also need to be advised about mobilisation, driving and alcohol intake [9]. The experience of the University Hospital of Wales is that it is exceptional for patients to contact the on call medical staff for advice, preferring to consult their own General Practitioner (GP).

Deep Vein Thrombosis Prophylaxis

Deep vein thrombosis is associated with varicose veins, but a causal relationship has not been demonstrated [10]. Anecdotal case reports of deep vein thrombosis following bilateral varicose vein surgery have been published but there is no evidence to suggest that only unilateral surgery should be performed on a day care basis. The role of deep vein thrombosis prophylaxis is unclear as it cannot be prolonged after discharge although it is used by many vascular surgeons [11,12]. Assuming that mobilisation occurs after discharge, a single pre-operative subcutaneous dose of low-molecular-weight heparin may provide prophylaxis for the peri-operative period, with little risk of increased bleeding, although there are no clinical trials to confirm its efficacy in this situation [13]. Patients at high risk of deep vein thrombosis require inpatient surgery at present. The influence of the oral contraceptive pill or hormone replacement therapy on the incidence of post-operative deep vein thrombosis is uncertain. In the absence of scientific data, practice is likely to be determined by medico-legal factors.

Anaesthesia and Analgesia

No premedication is given for day care surgery and opiates are avoided due to their long duration of action. Laryngeal rather than endotracheal intubation is more satisfactory if spontaneous breathing with a mask is not appropriate. Endotracheal intubation, necessary if the patient is turned prone, leads to unpleasant respiratory symptoms which may distress a patient at home. Although choice of anaesthetic drug can influence recovery time, the incidence of anorexia, fatigue and headache remains high even with modern drugs [14]. Only 24% of patients would be prepared to have repeat day case surgery due to these complications. Infiltration of the wounds with 0.5% bupivacaine will provide post-operative analgesia for the period of travelling. Femoral nerve blocks have proved disappointing as the distribution of anaesthesia is limited, and they have not become popular. The use of spinal or epidural anaesthesia is limited by the compromise of post-operative mobility. It is possible to perform sapheno-femoral ligation and a limited number of stab phlebotomies under local anaesthetic infiltration. Stripping of the long saphenous vein under local anaesthetic is popular in Scandinavia but is not routinely performed in the United Kingdom.

Post-operative analgesia needs to be mild and non-opiate. Patients are provided with 5 days' supply of analgesics which can be nurse- or protocol-prescribable. A requirement for stronger analgesia is an indication for post-operative review.

Surgical Technique

It is recommended that fully accredited surgeons perform day surgery in order to minimise unnecessary tissue dissection and length of procedure. This is particularly pertinent to sapheno-popliteal ligation, where nerve damage can occur. Nevertheless surgery provides an opportunity for learning experience by trainees under supervision. Adequacy of the venous ligation can be confirmed whilst the presence of two operators reduces the duration of surgery.

Within time constraints there is no absolute contraindication to both sapheno-femoral and sapheno-popliteal ligation, although if this is performed bilaterally, immediate mobility may be compromised. Stripping of the long saphenous vein carries higher morbidity due to post-operative pain but is tolerated well. It should progress in a retrograde direction no further than the knee, thus avoiding saphenous nerve damage [15]. Serial avulsions of the long saphenous vein may provide a less traumatic alternative but are likely to be more time-consuming. Inversion stripping will leave a smaller-diameter track but the passage of the stripper may be hindered in tortuous veins. Peri-operative and post-operative pain is comparable to that of phlebectomy and it can be performed under local anaesthesia. It requires only a small exit incision which does not need suturing and is more cosmetically acceptable to patients [16]. Due to the perceived morbidity of stripping, sapheno-femoral ligation and stab avulsions alone have been advocated. This procedure may leave a long saphenous vein in situ being fed by incompetent perforators with the ultimate development of stem incompetence and recurrent varicosities. Avulsion sites do not normally require sutures and trauma can be minimised by the use of Oesch phlebectomy hooks to remove varicosities. Retrograde removal of the stripper through the groin wound will reduce incision length at the knee. Sapheno-femoral ligation and subsequent sclerotherapy to the long saphenous vein is limited by the intense thrombophlebitis that can ensue and the need for prolonged limb compression. Day surgery is not suitable for formal sub-fascial perforator exploration due to the need for bed rest post-operatively and the risk of wound breakdown although extrafascial ligation is possible. The development of sub-fascial endoscopic perforator ligation has not yet been assessed on a day care basis but early results indicate that it is fast and effective with little patient discomfort [17].

Excess blood loss will lead to unacceptable admission rates after surgery. Patients will benefit by intravenous crystalloid infusions during surgery and blood loss can be minimised by the use of a thigh tourniquet.

In a series of 157 patients (mean age 44 years; range 16–69 years) treated on the Day Unit at the University Hospital of Wales, bilateral procedures were performed in 63 (40%) with recurrent varicose vein surgery in 21 of 220 (9.5%) legs. The long saphenous vein was stripped in 30 legs and a short saphenous ligation performed in 31 limbs. Due to the unacceptable recurrence rate associated with avulsions only, the majority of patients now have the long saphenous vein stripped to the knee. Bilateral recurrent varicose vein surgery is now routinely performed by appropriately experienced surgeons.

Post-operative Care and Results

Patients are nursed with the limb elevated for 3 h in a padded firm bandage. The day following the procedure they are visited by a nurse who replaces the bandages with a lightweight anti-embolic support, providing a pressure gradient of 18–8 mmHg from ankle to knee, which is worn for 10 days. Patients are encouraged to take frequent walks and elevate their legs but no formal medical reassessment is performed unless requested by the patient themselves. This has the disadvantage that trainees cannot assess the results of their surgery. Patients usually require a community nurse visit in the immediate post-operative period. All sutures used are absorbable. The incidence of post-operative admission is low, with only 4 of 157 (2.5%) patients treated on the Day Unit at the University Hospital of Wales requiring an overnight bed. The reasons for admission were hypotension and pain control.

The outcome in 40 patients undergoing day case surgery was compared with that in 45 treated as inpatients. Post-operative analgesia was considered adequate, with no difference between the two groups. Early medical review was required by 13% of day cases compared with 6% of inpatients, although nurses may have performed an unrecorded review in the latter group. Although similar to previously published figures, post-operative GP consultation rates of up to 33% have been quoted [18]. Although there was concern by GPs that day care surgery would increase their emergency

Table 22.1. Advantages of day case varicose vein surgery

Efficient organisation with planned patient care
Minimal disruption to patients' working or domestic life
Less risk of cancelled operation
More experienced surgeons and anaesthetists
Lower infection rate than for inpatients
No "hotel" charges
Staff recruitment for normal working hours easy
Reduced cost

workload, there are no data to support this view. There was no difference in patients' symptomatic relief between the inpatient and day care groups at 1 year post-operatively.

A comparison of costs between day care and inpatient surgery must take into consideration that, whilst the surgical procedure is identical, the anaesthetic resources may be more expensive in the former. Managerial costs will be higher, particularly with patient pre-assessment, and there is a shift of costs from hospital to the community with involvement of District Nurses and GPs [19,20]. The extra costs of inpatient treatment generally relate solely to the provision of overnight nursed accommodation, which is only a small proportion of the total costs of the procedure.

Conclusions

There is no doubt that day case varicose vein surgery is clinically effective and often favoured for social reasons, particularly by women with young families (Table 22.1). Although it is less expensive than inpatient treatment the cost benefit is lower than anticipated and offset by expense in other areas. It is not possible to quantify precisely the proportion of patients suitable for day care surgery as this will depend upon referral practice and social factors. Improved post-operative analgesia, endoscopic perforator ligation and the ability to provide domiciliary deep vein thrombosis prophylaxis and wound care will further extend the indications to those with chronic ulceration. The use of 24 h stay units will enable surgery to be performed even on those with co-morbidity who would previously have required admission. Patient hotels will avoid admission for those without help at home or living an unacceptable distance from the hospital. The future expansion of short and day care surgery may be influenced by patient preference and action groups.

References

1. Burkitt DP. Varicose veins, deep vein thrombosis, and haemorrhoids: epidemiology and suggested aetiology. BMJ 1972;II:556–561.
2. Campbell WB. Varicose veins. BMJ 1990;300:763–764.
3. Department of Health and Social Security. Hospital episode statistics 1987–88. London: DHSS, 1988.
4. Anonymous. Economics of varicose veins. BMJ 1973;I:626–627.
5. Nabatoff RA, Stark DCC. Complete stripping of varicose veins with the patient on an ambulatory basis. Am J Surg 1972;124:634–636.
6. Salaman RA, Fligelstone LJ, Wright IA, Pugh N, Harding KG, Lane IF. Hand held bi-directional Doppler versus colour duplex scanning in the pre-operative assessment of varicose veins. J Vasc Surg 1995;4:183–186.
7. Guidelines for day case surgery. London: Royal College of Surgeons of England, 1992.

8. Olivencia JA. Ambulatory phlebectomy in the elderly: review of 100 consecutive cases. Phlebology 1997;12:78–80.
9. Anonymous. Follow-up day case anaesthesia in general practice. Drugs Ther Bull 1990;28:81–82.
10. Campbell B. Thrombosis, platelets and varicose veins. BMJ 1996;312:198–199.
11. Kakkar VV, Howe CT, Nicolaides AN, Renney JTG, Clark MB. Deep vein thrombosis of the leg. Is there a high risk group? Am J Surg 1970;120:527–530.
12. Campbell WB, Ridler BMF. Varicose vein surgery and deep vein thrombosis. Br J Surg 1995;82:1494–1497.
13. Andaz S, Shields DA, Scurr JH, Coleridge Smith PD. Role of low molecular weight heparin in the prevention and treatment of venous thromboembolism after surgery. Phlebology 1994;9:2–7.
14. Millar JM, Jewkes CF. Recovery and morbidity after day case anaesthesia. A comparison of propofol with thiopentone-enflurane with and without alfentanil. Anaesthesia 1988;43:738–743.
15. Cox SJ, Wellwood JM, Martin A. Saphenous nerve injury caused by stripping of the long saphenous vein. BMJ 1974;I:415–417.
16. Wilson S, Pryke S, Scott R, Walsh M, Barker SGE. "Inversion" stripping of the long saphenous vein. Phlebology 1997;12:91–95.
17. Pierik EGJM, Wittens CHA, van Urk H. Subfascial endoscopic ligation in the treatment of incompetant perforating veins. Eur J Vasc Surg 1995;9:38–41.
18. Mackaey DC, Summerton DJ, Walker AJ. The early morbidity after varicose vein surgery. J R Nav Med Ser 1995;81:42–46.
19. Ruckley CV, Garraway WM, Cuthbertson C, Fenwick N, Prescott RJ. The community nurse and day surgery. Nursing Times 1980;255–256.
20. Stott NCH. Day case surgery generates no increased workload for community based staff. True or false? BMJ 1992;304:825–826.

23 Hospital or Community: How Should Leg Ulcer Care be Provided?

Deborah A. Ellison and Charles N. McCollum

Introduction

Over the last decade great strides have been made in our knowledge of leg ulcers. Epidemiological studies have revealed an extraordinarily high prevalence although the aetiology remains much debated. The development of high-compression elastic bandage systems has improved prognosis for patients with leg ulceration [1–4]. Up to 80% of leg ulcer patients are cared for in the community [4]. Most of these patients are elderly with limited mobility and are reluctant to attend a hospital clinic on a regular basis [1,3].

The majority of venous ulcers will heal if patients are admitted to hospital for bed rest with their feet elevated for prolonged periods of time, but the elderly patient loses mobility as joints stiffen, and financial constraints and the shortage of hospital beds mean that bed rest is rarely justified. When the patient then starts to mobilise the ulcer soon recurs. It is therefore more cost-effective to develop systems of care that allow leg ulcer patients to be treated as outpatients, entirely avoiding long periods of immobility and the many complications of prolonged bed rest.

The Stockport and Trafford Leg Ulcer Study identified 323 patients in Stockport and 264 in Trafford with leg ulcers within populations of 290 000 and 240 000 respectively in each Health Authority. It would be an impossible task to assess and treat all such patients within one or two hospital clinics. Recent studies have shown that improvements in healing can be achieved within a community setting when a co-ordinated service is introduced using research-based protocols [3].

Since this is predominantly a community problem, the ideal model of healthcare should be in the community, with direct access to specialised hospital services as necessary. Specialised community leg ulcer clinics provide a focus for nurse training in leg ulcer management whilst offering structured patient assessment and appropriate research-based treatment. The purpose is not to remove responsibility from nurses but rather to provide them with the resources and training to deliver an appropriate and specialist service.

Developing a Community Leg Ulcer Service

Training

The recent Stockport and Trafford Leg Ulcer Study examined the cost and outcome of leg ulcer care throughout the populations of two large Health Authorities. In this study the district nurses within Stockport Health Authority received intensive training in leg ulcer management and set up five specialist community leg ulcer clinics over a period of 1 year [2,5]. This allowed all nurses to attend lectures and workshops. All level 1and 2 community nurses within the Health Authority underwent the leg ulcer training programme. Workshops were held for each locality prior to the clinic in that area opening. These covered all aspects of leg ulceration including the assessment of leg ulcers and implementation of research-based innovations in care to patients in the community. This was followed by a practical session on the use of the hand-held Doppler and compression bandaging. Two district nurses were nominated as co-ordinators, to ensure the smooth running of the clinics.

When the clinic opened the nurses working within that area attended four to six consecutive clinic sessions where they put the theory into practice. They were trained by the nurse specialists from the University Department of Surgery at SMUH. Subsequently, once they had been fully trained, the specialist nurse co-ordinators within Stockport Community Unit were able to take on training responsibilities. Trained nurses were then able provide care to housebound patients who were unable to travel to the community leg ulcer clinics. Following the initial training programme all nurses attended a community leg ulcer clinic on a rota for two sessions at a time. This ensured that the nurses' experience was constantly updated and provided good staffing levels for the clinic. When each community clinic was able to run independently the nurse specialists withdrew but continued to provide advice for the more difficult patients. During this time the current practice in Trafford was not changed.

Location

Community leg ulcer clinics need to be sited in the heart of the community for easy access. Patients do not then have to rely on ambulances for transport, which substantially reduces costs. Such locations make it easier for patients to use local buses or "dial-a-ride" services. Other issues to consider in locating clinics are the space available, equipment, health and safety, and infection control policies. The five clinics opened in Stockport were each on a different day, which gave patients access to a number of clinics for both primary care and to deal with any problems they experienced between visits.

Assessment

Accurate wound assessment is essential. Although this is traditionally the role of doctors, the specialist nurses in Stockport were fully trained to identify the relevant clinical signs and symptoms. They also become expert in the Doppler assessment of arterial disease. A simple hand-held Doppler is essential in a community ulcer clinic. Arterial insufficiency can be determined by comparing ankle arterial pressure with the systolic blood pressure in the arm (ABPI). An ABPI of less than 0.8 suggests that arterial disease may contribute to a delay in healing. The degree to which the ABPI is less than 0.8 indicates the severity of the disease and referral to a vascular surgeon is required for patients with symptomatic arterial disease and those with an ABPI < 0.6. Hand-held Doppler may also be used to detect venous incompetence of the short and long saphenous system, indicating patients who require assessment of venous function with a view to corrective venous surgery.

Colour-flow duplex Doppler is essential in determining the extent of the arterial or venous disease but is not essential for every patient. Hand-held Doppler in the community leg ulcer clinics will determine which patients may benefit from referral for more detailed evaluation.

Basic Methods of Treatment

Dressing and Cleansing Agents

The majority of leg ulcers are venous and will heal quickly using multi-layer elastic compression bandaging. Several randomised controlled studies of different contact dressings in combination with the four-layer compression bandage have found that none of the more expensive modern dressings performs significantly better than a simple and inexpensive non-adherent dressing [6,7]. Although there are a wide range of cleansing products available these are normally unnecessary since adequate graduated compression promotes the removal of necrotic tissue by autolysis and the formation of healthy granulation tissue. A simple and inexpensive low-adherent material such as Tricotex (Smith & Nephew) or NA Dressing (Johnson & Johnson) is all that is required.

Compression Bandaging

The inner most layer of a four-layer bandage system consists of orthopaedic wool which absorbs exudate and redistributes pressure away from the bony high points of the ankle. A bandage of crepe or a similar inexpensive material is then applied to compress the padding, preserving the elastic energy of the compression layers. The third layer consists of an elastic compression bandage applied at mid-stretch in a figure-of-eight technique. Finally a cohesive compression bandage applies further compression and holds the bandage in place for at least 1 week.

Multi-layer elastic compression bandages can be adapted to a wide range of ankle circumferences and leg sizes, enabling the application of safe therapeutic graduated compression (Table 23.1). A further advantage is that one of the compression layers

Table 23.1. Bandage regimes for different ankle circumferences

Ankle circumference	Bandage regime	Example product
< 18 cm	2 or more orthopaedic wool	Soffban
	1 light stretch bandage	Soffcrepe
	1 3a elastic bandage	Litepress
	1 3b cohesive bandage	Co-plus
18–25 cm	1 orthopaedic wool	Soffban
	1 light stretch bandage	Soffcrepe
	1 3a elastic bandage	Litepress
	1 3b cohesive bandage	Co-plus
25–30 cm	1 orthopaedic wool	Soffban
	1 3c elastic bandage	Tensopress
	1 3b cohesive bandage	Co-plus
> 30 cm	1 orthopaedic wool	Soffban
	1 3a elastic bandage	Litepress
	1 3c elastic bandage	Tensopress
	1 3b cohesive bandage	Co-plus

may be omitted for patients with mixed arterial/venous ulcers, so that a three-layer system giving approximately 20–25 mmHg compression may be applied to patients with an ABPI in the range of 0.6–0.8 [8].

Pinch Skin Grafting

Skin grafting accelerates re-epithelialisation of venous ulcers that are over 10 cm^2 once a healthy granulating wound has been achieved by compression. Pinch skin grafts may easily be applied in community leg ulcer clinics by appropriately trained nurses. They promote rapid healing by acting as "seeds" forming many epithelial islands from which epithelial growth may occur. This procedure, which is used with the standard four-layer compression bandaging, is cost-effective, accelerates healing and with adequate training can be performed by specialist nurses in the community [9].

Prevention of Recurrence

Recurrence of ulcers has been reported to be as high as 67% in patients managed conservatively [10]. Class II compression hosiery with regular 3-month follow-up appears to reduce the recurrence rate to approximately 25% each year. This involves large numbers of patients, who can be followed most easily in the community clinics. It also provides an opportunity to encourage patients to continue with exercise and leg elevation. Generally below-knee class II stockings are sufficient and are easier to apply than full-length hosiery. Obesity reduces mobility and can cause deep vein obstruction in the groin on sitting [11]. Overweight patients therefore need to be encouraged to exercise and lose weight. Ambulant patients who are not too unfit should be referred for venous investigation with a view to simple superficial venous surgery. Loss of ankle joint movement will result in failure of the calf muscle and the foot pump, causing sustained venous hypertension [12]. Ankle exercises should be taught to promote venous return and appropriate patients should be referred for physiotherapy.

Outcomes Expected from Community Leg Ulcer Clinics

The Stockport and Trafford Leg Ulcer Study compared the outcome and cost of care for leg ulcer patients in community leg ulcer clinics in Stockport Health Authority with Trafford Health Authority as a control. In this study detailed cost and efficacy were measured prospectively over a 3-month period in both districts both before and 1 year after the introduction of five community leg ulcer clinics in Stockport only. These specialist leg ulcer clinics were opened progressively over a 6-month period. As each half-day clinic can handle only 12–15 patients, just under half the available Stockport patients achieved access to a community leg ulcer clinic before the second audit of treatment and cost in the spring of 1994.

Number of Ulcerated Limbs

The number of ulcerated limbs in the Stockport population was reduced by 14% during the study from 363 in 1993 to 310 in 1994. In Trafford this number increased by 8% from 276 to 296 over the same period.

Healing Rates

The percentage of patients healing in Stockport improved significantly from 26% (66 of 252 patients) to 42% (99 of 233) after community clinics were opened, even though only half the patients in Stockport had achieved their first clinic visit [2]. The healing rate was 65% over the 3-month period in those patients who were treated in the specialist community leg ulcer clinics. In Trafford, there was no improvement in healing rates which had been 23% (47 of 203) in 1993 and 20% (43 of 213) in 1994.

Re-dressing Frequency

In Stockport the re-dressing frequency reduced markedly over the year of these studies from 2.55 per week in 1993 to 1.6 per week in 1994 across the whole population of ulcer patients, and only 1.01 per week for those patients attending the community ulcer clinics. In Trafford, where practice had not changed, re-dressing frequency remained the same at around 2.2 per week.

Cost-Benefit Analysis

In addition to these improved healing rates, a detailed analysis of the cost of leg ulcer care was also done during the Stockport and Trafford Leg Ulcer Study. This demonstrated that costs could be reduced by specialist community leg ulcer clinics in a number of ways, including the cost of dressing materials, staff and transport.

Dressing Materials

The mean re-dressing frequency in Stockport reduced over the year of these studies from 2.55 per week in 1993 to 1.6 per week in 1994 and only 1.01 per week for patients attending the community ulcer clinics. The redressing frequency in Trafford was unchanged at 2.2 per week. Overall from 1993 to 1994, annual expenditure on dressings, materials and bandages reduced from £84 777 to £61 127 in Stockport while costs in Trafford increased by 15.4% from £77 337 to £89 262. In total 118 different wound care products were being used. Following the opening of five community leg ulcer clinics using research-based treatment, although 74 different products were still being used across the district fewer than 10 products were used within the community leg ulcer clinics.

Staff and Transport Costs

Staff costs had the greatest influence on the total cost of leg ulcer care; a total of 3018 hours in Trafford and 2610 hours in Stockport were spent in attending to and re-dressing patients with leg ulcers during the first 3-month audit period in 1993. In 1994 there was a small increase in Trafford to 3047 hours but a highly significant reduction in

Stockport to only 1813 hours. This 31% reduction in nursing time was achieved by reducing both the number of patients with actively ulcerated limbs and the re-dressing frequency. This resulted in a fall of £77 097 (30.5%) in annual staff costs in Stockport from £252 439 to £175 342 [2]. The number of patients was relatively constant in Trafford and staff costs increased by 1% from £291 867 to £294 675 over the same period.

Before community leg ulcer clinics were opened in Stockport the cost of leg ulcer care to the Health Authority was over £409 991 each year, with only 26% of ulcers healing within 12 weeks. Following the introduction of community clinics using four-layer compression for patients with venous ulceration, 65% of all ulcerated limbs were healed in 12 weeks at a cost of only £253 371 in the first year and the potential for much greater savings once the prevalence of leg ulceration had been reduced further [2].

Criteria for Referral to the Vascular Surgical Service

A careful initial assessment allows patients requiring referral to the vascular surgical service to be identified and referred early (Fig. 23.1). The majority of patients with venous ulcers will respond quickly to sustained and graduated compression and do not need to be seen by the surgeon. Once healing has been achieved, compression hosiery is applied and patients are offered a venous assessment to determine whether superficial venous surgery may prevent recurrence. If there is little progress over 3 months or the ulcers have failed to heal, they should be referred to the vascular surgical service for non-invasive investigations.

Any patient found to have a resting ABPI of less than 0.5 should be referred for urgent assessment. These patients can be seen within 1 week following identification for non-invasive investigations. Appropriate vascular treatment can be undertaken and the patient transferred back to care in the community leg ulcer clinic if ABPI can be restored to > 0.6.

Research

In the past it was said that clinical trials in leg ulcer care were difficult to undertake. Now that several major studies have been successfully completed the excuse is that they are difficult in the community. Banks et al. [13] highlighted the advantages and disadvantages of undertaking clinical trials in the community. Data collection, travel time and continuity of care are all genuine problems [13]. The community leg ulcer clinic is an ideal environment for conducting randomised controlled clinical trials. Within the community setting socio-economic factors which may influence healing can be considered whilst at the same time patients are seen within a controlled environment by a limited number of staff. The large number of suitable patients available in a population of between 200 000 and 300 000 also assists recruitment to such studies.

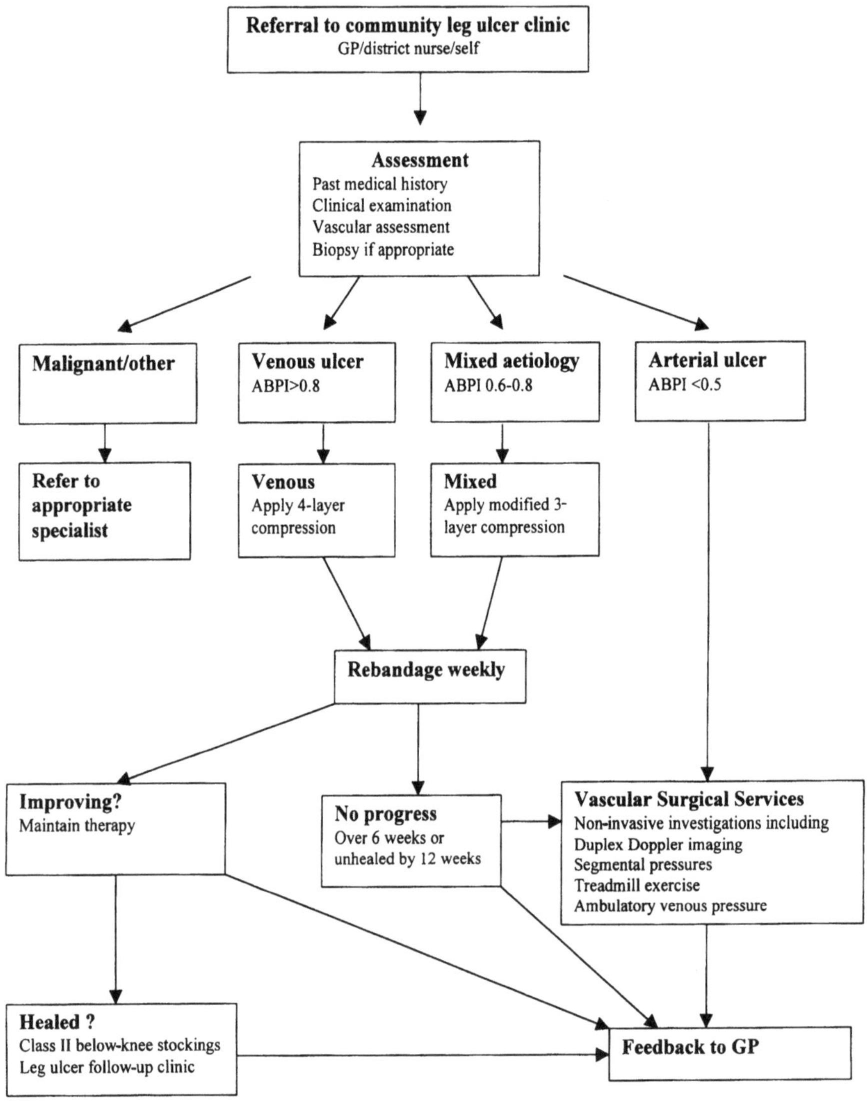

Fig. 23.1. Criteria for referral to the vascular surgical service.

Conclusion

The focus of leg ulcer therapy has moved in recent years from long-term maintenance to effective management designed to achieve early healing. The outcome of treatment for patients with active ulceration has been improved using a more scientific and research-based approach to patient assessment, adequate four-layer compression bandaging and the delivery of these innovations via patient care to the community as a whole. The introduction of community leg ulcer clinics has now been shown in three separate large clinical studies to both improve patient care and reduce costs when compared with the traditional approach. The major improvements in leg ulcer healing and cost reductions demonstrated in these studies were a direct result of training nurse specialists in leg ulcer care and introducing the four-layer bandage using a co-ordinated leg ulcer service. The reduction in prevalence of leg ulcer disease as more chronic ulcers heal leads to even greater savings in the long term.

References

1. Callum MJ, Ruckley CV, Harper DR, Dale JJ. Chronic ulceration of the leg: extent of the problem and provision of care. BMJ 1985;20:1855–1856.
2. Simon DA, Freak L, Kinsella A, Walsh J, Lane C, Groarke L, McCollum CN. Community leg ulcer clinics: a comparative study in two Health Authorities. BMJ 1996;312:1648–1651.
3. Moffatt CJ, Franks PJ, Oldroyd M, Bosanquet N, Brown P, Greenhalgh RM, McCollum CN. Community clinics for leg ulcers and impact on healing. BMJ 1992;305:1389–1392.
4. Cornwall JV, Dore CJ, Lewis JD. Leg ulcers: epidemiology and aetiology. Br J Surg. 1986;73:673–696.
5. Freak L, Simon D, Kinsella A, Lane C, Walsh J, McCollum CN. Leg ulcer care: and audit of cost-effectiveness. Health Trends 1995;207:133–136.
6. Blair SD, Backhouse CM, Wright DDI, Riddle E, McCollum CN. Do dressings influence the healing of chronic venous ulcers? Phlebology 1988;3:129–134.
7. Freak L, Simon DA, Edwards AT, McCollum CN. Comparative study of three primary dressings in the healing of chronic venous ulcers. Br J Surg 1992;79:1235.
8. Stevens J, Franks PJ, Harrington M. A community/hospital leg ulcer service. J Wound Care 1997;6:62–68.
9. Moffatt C, Oldroyd M. Pinch skin grafting: an extension of the role of the specialist nurse. Primary Health Care 1989;July:18–20.
10. Negus D. Definitive treatment: prevention of recurrence of venous ulceration. In: Negus D. Leg ulcers: a practical approach to management. Oxford: Butterworth-Heinemann, 1991:125–148.
11. Bianuie G, Kalis B. Cutaneous complications of massive obesity. Phlebologie 1993;43: 1930–1934.
12. Gaylarde PM, Dodd HJ, Sarkany I. Venous leg ulcers and arthropathy. Br J Rheumatol 1990;29:142–144.
13. Banks V, Bale SE. Practical problems of undertaking clinical trials in the community. J Wound Care 1994;3:301–304.

24 What Are The Costs of Treating Venous Disease?

Nick Bosanquet

Introduction

Since the late 1980s the availability of evidence on the costs of venous disease has much improved. The movement has been from aggregate estimates at a national level to much more firmly based local estimates on treatment costs and changes in spending as a result of different treatment regimes. There is now an evidence base from which to develop scenarios for the future.

National Costs of Venous Disease

The pioneering work at the aggregate level was that of Laing [1]. He carried out comparisons of the costs of venous disease in the United Kingdom (UK), France and Germany showing that they accounted for a comparable proportion of total treatment costs in all three countries. In the UK the proportion was highest at 2.0%, compared with 1.9% in France and 1.5% in Germany. However, the composition of spending was rather different, with more spending in the UK on community nursing and more on prescription medicines in France and Germany.

Laing also developed some estimates on the costs of long-term disability from venous disease in France and Germany. Venous disease also creates longer-term costs in disability and dependence on state-funded invalidity pensions. Here the comparisons available cover Germany and the UK. These are derived from medical certificates of invalidity processed by the social security system. They show rather greater differences in these costs than is found for expenditure on health services, invalidity costs being 1.2% of the total in Germany compared with 0.4% in the UK. Half of the total days of invalidity in Germany are accounted for by venous insufficiency: thus venous disease in Germany takes a low proportion of total treatment costs but a much higher proportion of costs of disability involving recurrent support and loss of productive capacity. In Germany 1.2% of all days of certified invalidity involved a loss of 953 million DM in 1987 and this level of loss is consistent with studies in the early 1980s.

In addition to the evidence on the monetary costs of venous disease, there was also pioneering work by Franks on the psychological costs of venous disease [2]. His work has shown that the pain, depression and anxiety suffered by patients with various types of venous disease is far greater than was previously realised. From the point of view of medical science, these conditions may not loom large: but from the patient's point of view these diseases may figure in reducing their quality of life to very low levels for years. Results for patients with leg ulcers before treatment using the Nottingham Health Profile are set out in Fig. 24.1, showing particularly strong effects on energy, pain, sleep and mobility.

Costs of Treatment Programmes

Such studies give general background; there is now a wealth of more local evidence on costs of treatment programmes which can be used by local decision-makers. One early study of this type in Riverside, UK compared the costs of treating patients with venous ulcers using traditional methods with the costs using new compression bandaging [3]. This showed that costs of treating patients with traditional methods, mainly involving the use of crepe bandages, were high. Spending in a district was £433 000 a year with only 22% of ulcers healing in each 12-week period. Much of the cost was for the time of district nurses, but there was also a significant cost for a minority of patients who had stays as inpatients. The clinics were shown to be treating an average of 18 patients a week at a cost of £17.70 per week per patient. Overall the costs of the clinics were £169 000 a year and they achieved 80% healing rates.

A later study in two districts in the North West of the UK has confirmed the earlier results from Riverside and provided a much more detailed picture of the impact of new methods on the costs of treating venous ulcers [4]. This study compares two districts with a similar population on the southern edge of the Manchester conurbation. In one district (Stockport) five leg ulcer clinics were established in convenient health centres. Patients were given an initial assessment and then treated by four-layer compression bandaging; after healing they were treated with compression stockings below the knee. In the other district (Trafford) no co-ordinated effort was made to influence the approach to the treatment of leg ulcers. After 1 year results and costs were measured in both districts. Over the period the numbers of patients achieving complete healing in 3 months rose from 26% to 42% in Stockport, while the proportions healing in Trafford remained unchanged at 20%. The numbers of ulcerated limbs was reduced by 9%

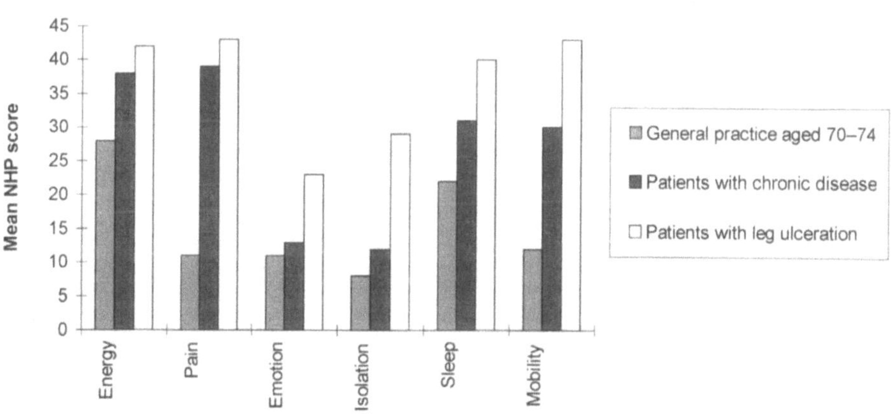

Fig. 24.1 Quality of life and leg ulceration. NHP, Nottingham Health Profile. After Frauts et al. [2].

in Stockport and the mean frequency of re-dressing was reduced from 2.5 times per week in 1993 to 1.6 times per week in 1994. In Trafford the number of ulcerated limbs rose by 5% and the frequency of re-dressing remained unchanged at 2.2 times per week.

Changes in cost followed from these changes in outcomes and in treatment methods. The cost of dressing materials and bandages rose in Trafford (Table 24.1) and fell by a third in Stockport. The numbers of hours of staff time used in leg ulcer treatment in Stockport fell by 31% from 2610 to 1813, while in Trafford the numbers of hours rose from 3018 to 3047. There were also significant changes in terms of inpatient days. The total number of days in Trafford rose from 638 to 909, while in Stockport the number of inpatient days fell from 216 to 46. The result of these changes was that total expenditure on leg ulcer treatment fell by 38% in Stockport.

This ground-breaking study was based on actual changes within a district and on audited accounts of savings actually made. It shows how new methods could be used to secure real savings. The studies do not cover all types of venous disease and even with the treatment of venous ulcers there may be some patients in whom treatment does not succeed and who have problems with recurrence. The reduction in costs of treatment for some patients may make it easier, however, to concentrate on those with intractable problems, and in whom further treatment possibly involving the use of duplex scanning and surgery might be relevant. The compression bandaging method encourages earlier detection and more rapid healing of some types of leg ulcer, and could therefore free up funding and professional time for dealing with patients who have more severe and long-term problems.

Implications of Near Treatment Programmes

Information on costs can be used for different purposes including audits about value for money. It can also provide a guide to the costs of alternative programmes. There

Table 24.1. Trafford and Stockport study: expenditure on care of leg ulcers over 13 weeks in 1993 and 1994

	Trafford		Stockport	
Item	1993	1994	1993	1994
No. of patients audited	186	194	224	205
Cost of materials	£19 334.21	£22 315.39	£21 194.14	£15 281.70
Cost of pharmaceuticals	£63.67	£24.57	£184.12	£20.15
Inpatient care:				
No. treated as inpatients	19	21	6	3
Total no. of inpatient days	638	909	216	46
Total basic hotel cost (£75.89 a day)	£48 417.82	£68 984.01	£16 392.24	£3490.94
Staff cost:				
No. of hours recorded as used in ulcer care	3017.65	3046.68	2610.00	1812.88
Total cost (£24.18/h including all overheads and travel)	£72 966.78	£73 688.80	£63 109.80	£43 835.52
Patient travel:				
No. of km by ambulance (£1.98/km)	367	1680	816	314
No. of km by car (£0.40/km)	–	19	–	230
Total travel cost	£727.32	£3336.74	£1617.33	£714.56
Total costs in 13 weeks	£141 509.80	£168 329.51	£102 497.63	£63 342.87

Source: Simon et al. [4].

is now a strong evidence base showing that the new programmes are value for money and that they compare favourably with alternatives for patients with venous ulcers. However, it would be right to stress that such gains are not always to be achieved easily. There may be a difficult transition to any new system of care, with investment in new materials and in staff training. The new system is not simply about compression bandaging but it involves communication with potential patients to persuade them to come for initial assessment and to take part in the programme through weekly visits over 12 weeks: effective bandaging to ensure pressure over the week and working with patients to prevent recurrence. Thus the new system has to be seen as an investment programme which involves considerable change for healthcare professionals: it would require management effort in establishing the credibility of the new system on the ground.

The initial study of costs in Riverside stressed that reductions in cost might appear only in the long term. Initially the management task in setting up the clinics would be considerable, involving referral, transport, assessment and sustained quality in achieving compression bandaging. Patients would need to be helped and motivated to return every week. The service required considerable training of staff and skill development. It was also thought likely that in the first year clinics would attract more referrals, thus increasing workload as patients were attracted to a more effective service. There were also concerns about possible high levels of recurrence, so that the initial gains would not be maintained in the longer term.

Later experience has shown that most of these fears were not realised in practice. The initial programmes have been shown in Stockport and other districts to be easily established. They brought more immediate gains in terms of reductions in costs so that, for example, total spending in Stockport fell by 38% over 12 months. The longer-term evidence from Riverside also showed that there was a sustained fall in prevalence, from 450 ulcers being treated in the first year to 140 ulcers in the most recent year (a reduction of 20% per year). The evidence is positive that the combination of compression bandaging followed by support stockings can lead to a permanent and not just a temporary solution.

There is still a major challenge in terms of improving information about the long-term costs of ulcers which are resistant to treatment. The Riverside study was one of the few to present costs on an annual basis. This showed (Table 24.2) average costs for all patients and for patients with long-term ulcers. Even the average costs for patients with long-term ulcers were £1334 a year: and it is likely that for some high-cost patients these costs were repeated over a number of years. More information is required both on treatment-resistant patients with leg ulcers and on costs of treating patients with other types of venous disease.

Table 24.2. Riverside study: Average annual cost (£) per patient for all patients and patients with long-term ulcers

	Patients with long-term ulcers ($N = 100$)	All patients ($N = 200$)
Inpatient days	214.60	159.30
GP consultations	26.50	18.00
District nurse visits	680.40	398.80
Bandages	119.10	77.90
Outpatient visits	293.80	213.20
Total	1334.40	867.20

Source: Bosanquet et al. [3].

Scenarios for the Future

The improved evidence base on costs allows clearer indication of how costs might change in the future. In a worst-case scenario, treatment costs will rise for recurrent ineffective treatments as changes in demography increase the numbers of patients with venous disease. There is likely to be a particular increase in numbers of patients over 75 years old with more intractable problems, leading to increases in inpatient treatment. The proportion of total healthcare spending on venous disease is likely to rise above 2%, especially in Germany where population ageing is a strong feature.

In the best-case scenario there will be rapid diffusion of the new methods to minimise long-term costs and to improve quality of treatment. The use of these new techniques will reduce the immediate costs and the longer-term prevalence of venous ulcers, and will allow greater concentration of funding and professional effort on patients who have longer-term problems. This could also provide the opportunity for investment in a new generation of programmes for helping those patients who are not helped by compression bandaging.

Changes over the past 10 years have transformed the outlook for treatment for certain types of venous disease. Eighty per cent of patients with leg ulcers can look forward to effective treatment, compared with 20% in the 1980s. These new methods are unusual in that they can lead to significant cost savings which can be achieved quite quickly. The development process now has to be extended to other groups of patients with venous disease who have not yet fully benefited from advances in treatment. A recent review by Ruckley [5] has set out an agenda which might involve more use of duplex scanning in the initial consultation, further use of simple surgery for some groups of patients and more development of targeted programmes for patients with arterial disease. There have already been significant gains for patients with leg ulcers; the next phase will be to develop targeted and co-ordinated programmes for patients with all types of venous disease. Without active planning and management, costs are likely to rise as new treatments are used piecemeal in ineffective ways. Trafford, the control district in the Stockport and Trafford study, showed a significant rise in bandage costs as professionals sought to escape from the past but without any increase in effectiveness. Doing nothing is no longer a sensible option – if it ever was.

The programme of the future would be phased and targeted so as to give appropriate care to patients at each stage. Such a programme could be designed to minimise costs and increase the effectiveness of interventions. It might have the following main elements [6]:

Early detection and treatment. There are important opportunities for patient education in identification of the early signs of leg ulcers. Treatment is likely to be much more successful, with smaller ulcers identified at an earlier stage.

Intensive treatment. Programmes have to engage patient co-operation in a programme which involves initial assessment, selection and carrying out of treatment. There has been a certain interminable and hopeless quality about leg ulcer treatment in the past which has not provided the right conditions for patient co-operation.

Prevention of relapse. It is important to ensure that the gains made in treatment are maintained so that the ulcer does not recur. It is also important to ensure that gains in social functioning are actually realised in order to prevent hospital admissions and moves towards institutional care.

The new programmes of treatment have international relevance but will have to be adapted to the particular local conditions. Thus the UK system involves much use of the time of community nurses, a resource which is not available in all countries. The use of the new techniques is likely to present a particular challenge in Germany, with its traditional heavy emphasis on support therapy for patients with venous disease. Within Germany the new more active managerial role of the Krankenkassen may supply particular opportunities to use these techniques. The social solidarity model creates a major incentive to minimise longer-term costs through effective and timely interventions. Within venous disease there is a clear division between traditional remedies often involving high-cost recurrent treatment and the new evidence base. Leg ulceration is a condition which increases with age from 1.5–3 per 1000 on average to 20 per 1000 at the age of 80 years. Unless Krankenkassen take an active role in developing the new programmes they will find themselves facing an increasing bill for traditional and ineffective remedies.

There is certainly scope for new joint programmes across Europe to reduce costs and raise quality of care for patients with venous disease; and there are also likely to be opportunities in the USA and Canada. New programmes are feasible, fundable and one of the rare areas of care where new therapies could be cost-reducing. There could be an international learning curve which would lead to mutual learning and a shared development process as programmes develop in the future. The next 10 years hold out a potential for improved quality of care for patients with venous disease, transforming a heartsink area of recurrent ineffective therapy into one where positive results could be achieved for most patients.

References

1. Laing W. Chronic venous diseases of the leg. London: Office of Health Economic's, 1992.
2. Franks PJ, et al. Community leg ulcer clinics: effect on quality of life. Phlebology 1994;9:83–86.
3. Bosanquet N, et al. Community leg ulcer clinics: cost effectiveness. Health Trends 1993;25:146–148.
4. Simon D, et al. Community leg ulcer clinics: a comparative study in two health authorities. BMJ 1996;312:1648–1651.
5. Ruckley CV. Caring for patients with chronic leg ulcer. BMJ 1998;316:407–408.
6. Bosanquet N. Venous disease: the new international challenge. Phlebology 1996;11:6–9.

Section VI
Improving Outcomes

25 How Do We Prevent Recurrence of Varicose Veins?

C. Vaughan Ruckley and Andrew W. Bradbury

The Scale of the Problem

Most surgeons in the UK, and probably elsewhere, are unaware of the long-term outcomes for their patients after varicose vein operations. Where follow-ups have been done, and published, reported rates of clinical recurrence, leading to repeat surgery, have ranged between 20% and 60% at 6–20 years of follow-up [1]. Where the intervention has been limited to high ligation combined with sclerotherapy or to sclerotherapy alone the reported recurrence rates are even higher [1]. A large part of the work of general and vascular surgeons is devoted to treating recurrent varicose veins – a disease that is more difficult to treat than the primary condition.

The shortcomings of clinical documentation and coding mean that little weight can be attached to UK national statistics. Local, data however, may be more reliable. The Lothian Surgical Audit (LSAS) [2,3] covers a population of approximately 750 000. Operations are directly coded by the operating surgeons and the databases contain > 400 000 surgical procedures. Annually over the last 15 years in Lothian 1200–1400 varicose vein operations have been performed of which 180–250 (15–20%) were performed for recurrence. In 1997 LSAS showed that 86% of primary varicose veins were treated by day care. Recurrent varicose veins are generally considered inappropriate for day care and the mean duration of stay was 3.6 days. In the UK approximately 55 000 operations are performed for varicose veins annually, of which it is estimated that 7 500 – 10 000 will be for recurrence.

Assuming an average cost of £300 per day (1997 prices in Lothian) and an average total duration of stay of 3.6 days it can be estimated that recurrence of varicose veins costs the Lothian Health service £194 400 – £270 000 per year, and by extrapolation £8.1–10.8 million for the UK annually for these operations alone. There are of course many other costs incurred by the state and by the individual arising from unsuccessful varicose vein surgery. This chapter will argue that the morbidity, the impaired quality of life and the enormous cost associated with failed varicose vein surgery are, to a considerable extent, avoidable.

Definition and Classification

When a patient with varicose veins seeks surgical treatment, the circumspect surgeon cautions that operations for varicose veins are not necessarily curative and that the condition has a natural tendency to recur. What the surgeon is less likely to disclose is that there is a close relationship between the quality of the initial care (assessment and surgical technique) and the liability to recurrence. However, the natural progression of disease may also play a part.

Varicose veins, whether simple or complex, primary or recurrent, are associated with ambulatory venous hypertension, that is the failure of the pumping mechanisms responsible for venous return to lower the venous pressure sufficiently when the patient is mobile in the erect position. Why should this defect continue to be present after varicose vein surgery? The reasons may relate either to deficiencies in the original care or to the evolution of venous disease.

Residual Varicose Veins

Varicose veins which were present before operation and which persist are more properly described as residual. They are due either to failure on the part of the surgeon to assess the varicose disease correctly or, at operation, to locate and intercept the sites of deep to superficial reflux.

Defective Surgical Technique

The surgeon may assess the varices correctly but may use a surgical technique which does not deal effectively and permanently with the sites of reflux between the deep and superficial systems, thus leading to reappearance of varices.

The Development of New Sites of Reflux

Incompetence in the valves of the veins in the legs is not a "one-off" or static process. It is known that varicose veins progress with time and that serial examinations of subjects as in the Bochum studies [4] may show new or more extensive patterns of valvular incompetence. Thus a patient who has had incompetence in the long saphenous system may subsequently develop incompetence in the short saphenous system or vice versa. Strictly speaking this category is the only one appropriately termed "recurrence" the other two being more aptly termed "residual" varicosis. However, for convenience the term recurrent will be applied in this chapter to all categories.

Most authors agree that residual varicosis and defective surgical technique, separately or in combination, are the main causes of recurrence. It follows that improvements in diagnosis and surgical technique have the potential to make an important impact on outcome and therefore to achieve substantial clinical and quality of life improvements with major savings to the health care budget.

Why Is Recurrence Important?

There are of course many additional costs other than those of "re-do"surgery arising from the unsuccessful treatment of varicose veins. Varicose veins if ineffectively treated may develop serious complications. A population survey of 600 patients with chronic leg ulcer revealed that 25% had had previous operations for varicose veins [5].

For some patients with varicose veins the problem is a cosmetic one. Symptoms frequently attributed to varicose veins include discomfort, chronic ache, heaviness, swelling, itch and cramps. Skin complications of chronic venous insufficiency, comprising pigmentation, chronic inflammation, dermatitis and ulceration (lipodermatosclerosis), affect 10–20% of the varicose vein population and 5% of the total population. The care of chronic leg ulcer has been estimated on 1991–2 prices to cost the UK National Health Service to cost up to £400 million [6], and venous diseases cost around 2% of the total health care budgets of European countries [7].

The penalty of failed care is not limited to costs. Quality of life issues have been shown to be important in venous disease [8–11].

Patterns of Recurrence

Descriptions of patterns of recurrence in the literature have been based on clinical examination, hand-held Doppler, operative findings, or imaging by duplex scanning or phlebography. These methods do not necessarily provide comparable data. Furthermore different examination techniques, descriptive terms and classifications make comparisons between series extremely difficult.

The anatomical patterns listed by authors as associated with recurrence are as follows:

Patients with Recurrent Varicose Veins in whom the Presence of a Groin Scar Indicates Intended Sapheno-Femoral Ligation (Fig. 25.1)

Type 1: Residual Connections at the Sapheno-femoral Junction

1. *Intact sapheno-femoral junction.* The surgeon has failed to identify and intercept the upper long saphenous vein and its connection with the common femoral vein.
2. *Intact tributary veins connecting the sapheno-femoral stump to thigh veins.* The dissection and clearance of the upper long saphenous vein and of its tributaries has been incomplete.
3. *Remnant of the long saphenous vein in the thigh connected to proximal long saphenous vein stump by "neovascularisation".* The surgeon either did not strip the long saphenous vein or did not adequately disconnect the divided vein from the sapheno-femoral junction.

Type 2: Residual Connections Other Than at the Sapheno-femoral Junction

1. *Intact tributary veins connecting perineal, iliac, gluteal or abdominal wall veins to thigh veins.* Residual cross-groin connections due to incomplete dissection of the tributaries of the proximal long saphenous vein.
2. *Residual incompetent long saphenous vein fed by incompetent thigh perforating veins.* The surgeon has neither removed the long saphenous vein nor disconnected it from thigh perforators.
3. *Incompetence stemming from the short saphenous system.* New or previously undetected incompetence at the sapheno-popliteal junction connecting across to the long saphenous system.

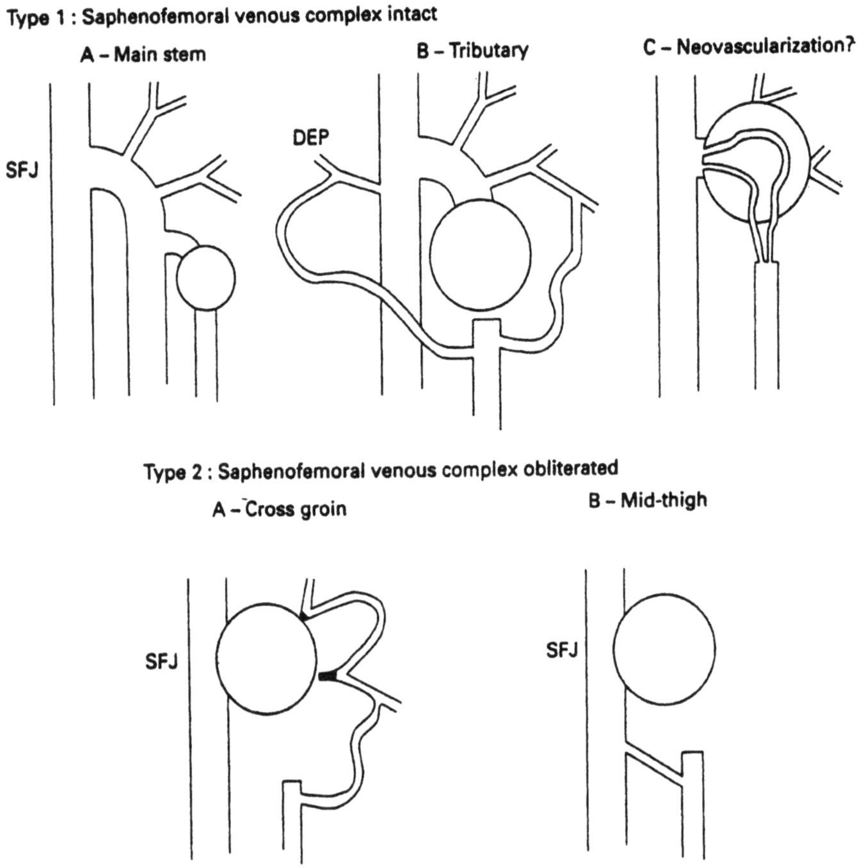

Fig 25.1. A classification of patterns of recurrence affecting the long saphenous system. SFJ, sapheno-femoral junction; DEP, deep external pudendal. Circles represent scar tissue from previous attempted sapheno-femoral ligation.

Patients with a Popliteal Scar Indicating Previous Intended Sapheno-popliteal Disconnection

1. *Intact sapheno-popliteal junction.* Failure to identify and interrupt the sapheno-popliteal junction.
2. *Residual connections.* A residual remnant of a ligated short saphenous vein connects to a tributary of the long saphenous vein, to the Giacomini vein or to the gastrocnemius veins.

Prevention of Recurrence

The causes of recurrence are implicit in the foregoing definitions and their prevention can therefore be dealt with in brief under the headings of anatomical causes, faults of assessment, imperfections of surgical technique at the primary operation and/or at "re-do" operations, and lack of follow-up care.

Anatomical Variations

The venous system in general is prone to anatomical variations. This is particularly true of the pattern of tributaries at the sapheno-femoral junction and the variety of terminations of the short saphenous vein. They are well described in standard texts [12,13]. Awareness of the common patterns should be in the surgeon's mind at all times when operating. Variations will only be detected if the exposure is adequate and the surgical dissection sufficiently thorough.

Assessment

On inspection of the leg pattern recognition is very important. Particular sites of deep to superficial reflux give rise to characteristic patterns of varices. Clinical examination therefore encompasses careful inspection with the patient standing, for sufficient time to fill the veins, on an elevated warm surface, in a good light followed by palpation and percussion. In the thin patient with a "classical" pattern of varices this may be sufficient to verify incompetence in the long saphenous system but it is often insufficient, especially for evaluation of the short saphenous sytem. The hand-held Doppler is an essential adjunct and may help the surgeon to judge when additional information is required from duplex scanning or phlebography. Many patient attributes such as obesity, oedema, lipodermatosclerosis, scarring, atypical venous patterns or a history of venous thrombosis can make simple clinical examination with or without Doppler unreliable or insufficient. An important principle is that the pre-operative assessment and marking should be carried out by the surgeon who is to perform the operation. Ideally, prior to varicose vein surgery all patients should be assessed by duplex scanning by a sonographer skilled in venous disease. Clearly this ideal is currently not universally achievable.

Surgical Technique at the First Operation.

Surgical technique, however dexterous, cannot compensate for inadequate pre-operative assessment and marking. In these days of minimally invasive and keyhole surgery the tendency to carry out sapheno-femoral or sapheno-popliteal disconnections through miniature incisions should be eschewed. It is not possible to see some of the important anatomical variants through 3 or 4 cm incisions. Small incisions carry no particular cosmetic advantage when located in the groin or popliteal creases.

By and large, varicose recurrence will be avoided, assuming accurate pre-operative marking, by the adoption of the following technical principles.

Sapheno-femoral Disconnection

The sapheno-femoral junction should be exposed through an incision at least 6 cm in length and considerably more in the fat leg. The tributaries should not be divided flush with the long saphenous vein (LSV) but should be dissected peripherally and divided at least beyond their first divisions. The sapheno-femoral junction should be fully dissected out, if necessary dividing the external pudendal artery, so that at least 2 cm of the femoral vein above and below the junction are clearly seen. The LSV should be ligated flush with the femoral vein, the site of ligation being completely separated both from the tributaries and from the divided distal stem of the LSV. The lower edge of the incision should be retracted and the knee flexed so that the upper thigh tributaries (usually the medial one) can be individually ligated.

Stripping

The benefit of stripping over high ligation alone, in terms of avoiding recurrence, has been demonstrated by a number of studies [14–17] including a number of randomised trials [18,19]. The thigh portion of the LSV should be removed down to the knee, unless the surgeon is prepared to achieve the same objective by dissecting and disconnecting every thigh perforator [20]. The validity of such a "saphenous vein preserving" approach remains to be proven, as does the reliability of the preserved vein as an arterial bypass.

Sapheno-popliteal Disconnection

A common mistake is for the surgeon to fail to find the short saphenous vein altogether. It should be marked on the skin pre-operatively with the aid of duplex scanning. Again adequate exposure is the key. The deep fascia should be divided longitudinally and the Giacomini vein located and divided. It is not the authors' policy to ligate gastrocnemius veins unless they have been shown to be incompetent and symptomatic. The deep fascia should be carefully closed.

Surgical Technique for "re-do" Varicose Vein Surgery

Many patients with recurrent varicose veins have had multiple operations. "Re-do" varicose vein operations are not easy. All too often the faults enumerated in the previous sections are repeated at subsequent operations."Re-do" operations should only be undertaken after careful evaluation including duplex scanning and/or phlebography. The sources of deep to superficial reflux must be accurately and comprehensively pinpointed and the surgery planned accordingly.

Quality Assurance and Follow-up Care

The workload involved in following up all patients after varicose vein surgery in order to monitor outcome and pre-empt recurrence is clearly more than most surgeons in state-funded practice can contemplate, yet it is an obvious way of improving outcomes which can bring recurrence rates close to zero [21]. The wearing of graduated compression hosiery for several weeks or even months after vein surgery is believed to reduce the likelihood of recurrence. Post-operative duplex scanning can identify those patients with residual reflux thereby highlighting previous defects in assessment or surgical technique and, it is hoped, leading to improvements in the service. Those patients who should continue to wear compression hosiery in the long term, for example those with deep venous reflux, can be identified, as can those who might benefit from follow-up sclerotherapy.

Who Should Do the Surgery?

It is perhaps easier to say who should not do varicose vein surgery. It should not be performed by the unsupervised inexperienced surgeon. Nor should it be done by the surgeon who is not willing or able to allocate the time or care required. The surgeon must be fully conversant with the range of anatomical variants that may be encountered and be able to call upon diagnostic techniques such as duplex scanning and/or phlebography whenever required. Some degree of recurrence of varicose veins, in some patients, may be unavoidable. Recurrence on the scale that it currently exists will not be acceptable in the future.

References

1. Eklof B, Juhan C. Recurrence of primary varicose veins In: Eklof B, Gores JE, Thulesius O, Bergqvist D, editors. Controversies in the management of venous disorders. London: Butterworth, 1989:220–233.
2. Gruer R, Gordon DS, Gunn AA, Ruckley CV. Audit of surgical audit. Lancet 1986;i:23–25.
3. Aitken RJ, Nixon SJ, Ruckley CV. Lothian Surgical Audit: a fifteen year experience of improvement in surgical practice through regional computerised audit. Lancet 1997;350:800–804.
4. Schultz-Ehrenberg U, Weindorf N, Von Uslar D, Hirche H. Prospective epidemiological investigations on early and pre-clinical stages of varicosis. In: Davy A, Stemmer R, editors. Phlebology '89. London: John Libbey, 1989:163–165.
5. Callam MJ, Harper DR, Dale JJ, Ruckley CV. Chronic ulcer of the leg: clinical history. BMJ 1987;i:1389–1391.
6. Bosanquet N. Cost of venous ulcers: from maintenance therapy to investment programmes. Phlebology 1992;Suppl 1:44–46.
7. Laing W. Chronic diseases of the leg. London: Office of Health Economics, 1992:24–33.
8. Philips T, Stanton B, Provan A, Lew R. A study of the impact of leg ulcers on the quality of life: financial, social and psychological implications. J Am Acad Dermatol 1994;31:49–53.
9. Franks PJ, Moffatt CJ, Connolly M, Bosanquet N, Oldroyd M, Greenhalgh RM, McCollom CN. Community leg ulcer clinics: effect on quality of life. Phlebology 1994;9:83–86.
10. Garratt AM, Ruta DA, Abdalla MI, Russell IT. SF 36 health survey questionaire. II. Responsiveness to changes in health status in four common clinical conditions. Qual Health Care 1994;3:186–192.
11. Baker DM, Turnbull NB, Pearson JCG, Makin GS. How successful is varicose vein surgery? A patient outcome study following varicose vein surgery using the SF 36 health assessment questionnaire. Eur J Vasc Endovasc Surg 1995;9:299–304.
12. Browse NL, Burnand KG, Lea Thomas M. Diseases of the veins: pathology, diagnosis and treatment. London: Edward Arnold, 1988:23–51.
13. Ruckley CV. Surgical management of venous disease. London: Wolfe, 1988:7–17.
14. Redwood NFW, Lambert D. Patterns of reflux in recurrent varicose veins assessed by duplex scanning. Br J Surg 1994;81:1148–1150.
15. Quigley FG, Raptis S. Cashman M. Duplex ultrasonography of recurrent varicose veins. Cardiovasc Surg 1994;2:775–777.
16. Bradbury AW, Stonebridge PA, Callam MJ, et al. Recurrent varicose veins: assessment of the saphenofemoral junction. Br J Surg 1994;81:373–375.
17. Stonebridge PA, Chalmers N, Beggs I, Bradbury AW, Ruckley CV. Recurrent varicose veins: a varicographic analysis leading to a new practical classification. Br J Surg 1995;82:60–62.
18. Sarin S, Scurr JH, Coleridge Smith PD. Assessment of stripping the long saphenous vein in the treatment of primary varicose veins. Br J Surg 1992;79:889–893.
19. Jones L, Braithwaite BD, Selwyn D, Cooke S, Earnshaw JJ. Neovascularisation is the principal cause of recurrence: results of randomised trial of stripping the long saphenous vein. Eur J Vasc Endovasc Surg 1996;12:442–445.
20. Campanello M, Hammarsten J, Forsberg C, et al. Standard stripping versus long saphenous vein saving surgery with patients as their own control. Phebology 1996;11:45–49.
21. Lofgren EP. Treatment of long saphenous varicosities and their recurrence: a long term follow up. In: Bergan JJ, Yas JST, editors. Surgery of the veins. Orlando: Grune and Stratton, 1985:285–299.

26 How Can We Improve Outcomes for Leg Ulcer Patients?

Olle Nelzén

Introduction

During the nineteeth century and until a few decades ago leg ulcer patients constituted a considerable part of the hospital inpatient population and a large proportion of leg ulcer outpatients received care from hospital-based clinics. Since the begining of the 1970s, in conjunction with the expansion of primary care, most of the care of leg ulcer patients has been tranferred to community health care. Nowadays only a few receive hospital care. Treatment was, during the same period, delegated from doctors to district and community nurses and then further to auxiliary nurses. This development has, unfortunately, resulted in a neglect of diagnostics and has focused treatment on topical wound care. Treatment to cure the true underlying causes of ulceration seems largely to have been forgotten, which explains why defective wound healing and frequent recurrences have been common. There is, however, great potential to improve the long-term outcome for leg ulcer patients and this concerns four major areas (Table 26.1.).

Leg Ulcer Healing and Recurrence

Data from Epidemiological Studies

From epidemiological studies it is known that between 60% and 70% of ulcers encountered are already recurrent [1,2]. Recurrent ulcers are even more common in the subgroup of patients with venous ulcers, where more than 70% have ulcers that have relapsed [1,3]. It is known that only about 1 in 10 ulcers is a first-time ulcer with a duration of less than a year [1,4]. The patients (n=382) in the Skaraborg study [1,5] were prospectively followed for 5 years to assess the natural history of chronic leg ulcer [6]. The overall long-term healing was poor, with only about half of surviving patients

Table 26.1. Areas where improvements are likely to result in improved outcome for leg ulcer patients

Doppler-aided diagnosis
Tailored individual treatment
Improved follow-up
Organised care pathways

being free from ulceration and without a history of recurrence at the end of follow-up (54 months). An additional 7% had experienced a recurrence which had healed at follow-up but the remaining 42% still had open ulcers or had undergone amputation. There are no other similar epidemiological series for comparison. Based on a follow-up of 186 patients healed at a dermatology clinic, in Sweden, Hansson et al. found that 52% were healed after 3 years, but only 24% had remained healed throughout the 3-year period. From a hospital-based wound healing research unit in Cardiff, Salaman and Harding [8] reported retrospective data on 490 patients treated during a 2-year period. They found an overall healing rate of 74% after 12 months but recurrences were not studied. These data concerned leg ulcers of all causes.

Venous ulcers, the largest aetiological subgroup in the Skaraborg study, had the worst prognosis. After nearly 5 years only 44% had healed without history of recurrent ulceration during follow-up [6]. The long-term outcome for patients with venous ulcers and deep venous insufficiency (DVI) appears to be worse than that for patients with ulcers caused by superficial venous insufficiency (SVI) and/or perforating vein incompetence (PVI) alone [1,6]. It is especially healing the of ulcers that is more difficult to achieve in legs with DVI, whereas recurrences appear to be more equally distributed between both groups. A total of 76% of patients with venous ulcers were eventually healed, during the 5-year period, but 42% of these subsequently experienced a recurrence. No further data are available based on unselected patients and there are only data from hospital series for comparison. In the study from Cardiff the 12-month healing rate was 72% [8]. From USA Erickson et al. [9] gave retrospective data on 99 venous ulcers of which 91% had healed after 2 years following graduated compression treatment. Over a period of 3 years 57% experienced recurrent ulceration. Mayberry et al. [10] treated 113 patients with compression and noted, retrospectively, a total healing of 93% after more than 3 years. The 5-year recurrence rate was 29% among patients compliant with compression and a similar result (30%) was recorded by others [11].

Evidence from Clinical Trials

There are certain problems using data from clinical trials to estimate leg ulcer healing: firstly patients in trials are generally heavily selected and not necessarily representative of the average patient seen in the community, secondly the authors usually give only short-term healing results, thirdly they almost never provide any data on recurrence and fourthly the trials generally have poor methodology. The results reported from randomised trials comparing different compression bandage systems show a varied picture with 12-week healing rates ranging from 0 to 100%, the majority being between 40% and 70% [12].

That short term healing can be improved in the community, by setting up community leg ulcer clinics providing treatment using a four-layer compression bandage system, has been shown in two well conducted studies [13,14]. In the Riverside study [13] the 12-week healing results were claimed to have improved from 22% prior to clinics to 69% after clinics. At 6 months 83% of venous ulcers were healed. In a similar study in Manchester [14] leg ulcer healing was assessed in two district health authorities before and after establishing leg ulcer clinics in one of them. The four-layer bandage system [13] was used in the clinics. Before the clinics both areas had 12-week healing rates around 25%. Healing then improved to 42% in the health authority in which clinics had been set up but remained unchanged in the other. Within the clinics the healing rate was even better, being up to 65%. This is in line with the Riverside study result, where obviously patients taken care of outside the clinics were not all included. The drawback of these studies is that we do not know the long-term results. It is notable that problems with recurrences, in approximately one-third of healed patients, appeared within as little as 1 year in Riverside [13].

Diagnosis

The aetiological background to leg ulcers is not always considered and there has been a tendency simply to equate a leg ulcer with a venous ulcer, although it is well known that leg ulcers can have a variety of causes. It is important to stress that a chronic ulcer is not a disease but a symptom of disease [4] and that leg ulcer is, thus, not a diagnosis! The most common background disease is venous insufficiency. On the basis of epidemiological data from Australia [15] and Sweden [5] it can be concluded that venous ulcers comprise about 55% of all leg ulcers and that about 70% of all ulcers located above the foot have a predominant venous cause [4]. Leg ulcer diagnosis is often complicated since more than a third of ulcers have a mixed, arterio-venous or multifactorial background [4,5,15]. Leg ulcers need to be classified, and an example of a leg ulcer classification for clinical use is shown in Table 26.2. [4–6]. It is essential to have an accurate diagnosis to enable the choice of the most appropriate treatment [4]. It is a reasonable demand that leg ulcers should not be treated without a prior diagnosis, preferably made by a qualified doctor at the time of the patient's first visit to the health care system [4,5,16].

The diagnosis should be reached with the aid of, at least, hand-held Doppler [1,4,5,16]. It is mandatory to use this to detect arterial insufficiency and to screen for venous

Table 26.2. Leg ulcer classification according to Nelzén et al. [4–6]

Aetiological group	Definition
1. Venous [a]	Ulcers caused by venous insufficiency or obstruction without any other causative factor present
2. Mixed venous and arterial [a]	Ulcers of predominantly venous cause combined with detectable arterial impairment. ABPI generally 0.7–0.9
3. Mixed arterial and venous [a,b]	Ulcers of predominantly venous cause combined with a minor venous insufficiency – usually superficial. ABPI generally 0.7 or lower
4. Arterial [b]	Ulcers associated with arterial insufficiency only. ABPI generally 0.7 or lower
5. Arterial and diabetes [b]	Ulcers caused by a combination of arterial insufficiency and diabetic neuropathy – "neuro-ischaemic ulcers". Any sign of arterial insufficiency (non-compressible arteries included) + neuropathy
6. Diabetes	Ulcers caused by neuropathy or diabetes-related skin disorders such as necrobiosis lipoidica diabeticorum
7. Traumatic	Pure trauma-induced ulcers with no other predisposing factor present
8. Pressure	Pure pressure-induced ulcers without any other predisposing factor present
9. Multifactorial arterial + venous + diabetic	Combinations of arterial, venous and diabetic causes, without any of the factors obviously dominating
10. Other multifactorial	Other combinations of aetiological factors with no obvioulsly dominating factor
11. Other single cause	Other single causes of leg ulcers such as vasculitis, skin tumours

ABPI, ankle – brachial pressure index.
[a] Can for clinical purposes be divided into ulcers caused by (a) DVI and (b) isolated SVI/PVI.
[b] Can be divided into ulcers caused by critical ischaemia (ABPI < 0.5) and ulcers of possible arterial cause.

insufficiency. If Doppler is not used 1 in 4 patients will receive a false diagnosis [1]. In venous ulcer patients the use of hand-held Doppler or preferably duplex Doppler is essential for the early detection of patients with isolated SVI/PVI [1,4,5]. This enables early indentification of patients likely to benefit from varicose vein surgery. In Sweden and Norway the recommended minimum requirements for leg ulcer diagnosis in primary care include an ankle-brachial pressure measurement and popliteal vein screeening with hand-held Doppler [16].

Tailored Treatment

Compression treatment has been used since the days of Hippocrates, some 2400 years ago, and has not yet solved the problem of leg ulcers. There are several reasons for this: firstly not all ulcers are pure venous ulcers, secondly it is difficult to apply compression bandages and thirdly patient compliance is far from 100% especially where prophylactic compression is concerned. Patient compliance with compression is inversely related to the recurrence rate [9–11]. From a recent review of published randomised controlled trials comparing different compression regimens it was concluded that compression improves the healing of venous ulcers but that no system had been proven superior [12]. They found that "increased use of *any correctly* applied high compression treatment should be promoted". It is very unlikely that compression treatment, in the future, will substantially improve the long-term prognosis for venous ulcer patients unless it is combined with a definite treatment to cure the underlying venous dysfunction.

What definite treatment can we offer? We know that some 90% of all ulcers are associated with a detectable circulatory deficiency, venous and/or arterial [3,5,14]. On the basis of the nature of this deficiency it has been calculated that approximately 40% of all ulcerated legs show potentially surgically curable circulatory abnormalities [5]. The potential for venous surgery has been underestimated and surgery has not been frequently used [4–6]. It has been confirmed that up to half of all venous ulcers are caused by varicose veins (SVI/PVI) alone [1,5]. Surgery is the generally accepted way of curing patients with symptomatic varicose veins and a leg ulcer is no exception. It is in fact the most severe symptom of varicose disease [4]. Results from uncontrolled surgical series all show low recurrence rates (below 10%) for "varicose" ulcers after varicose vein surgery [17]. In the absence of randomised controlled trials comparing surgery with conservative compression, there is still enough evidence to support the contention that surgery is superior to compression where leg ulcer recurrence is concerned [4]. A wider and earlier use of surgery in patients with "varicose" ulcers is likely to reduce dramatically the number of patients suffering from chronic leg ulcers. There is no evidence to support a conservative attitude in these patients although their ulcers initially may heal readily on compression therapy. On the contrary there are indications that a long-standing SVI and/or PVI, if left untreated, may progress to involve the deep venous system [18], and at that point curative surgery may no longer be possible to perform. Surgery is probably the most powerful and underused therapeutic tool for leg ulcers currently available.

Immediate arterial intervention is indicated in cases with critical ischaemia and may also be used more often in patients with less than critical ischaemia if the ulcer does not heal on conventional therapy [5]. Patients who have mixed ulcers with combined arterial and venous aetiology comprise another group with proven poor long-term outcome. In Australia mixed ulcers showed a significantly lower healing after 2.5 years than pure venous ulcers [19]. Five-year results from Sweden, based on patients from the Skaraborg study[5,6], revealed that only 29% were healed without history of recurrence compared with 46% for pure venous ulcers (Nelzén, unpublished data). Patients with mixed ulcers definitely deserve further attention. If compression does not work angiography should precede any attempts to perform superficial or perforating vein surgery, to avoid premature destruction of possible arterial conduits. In some cases it is possible to perform a simultaneous correction of both the arterial and venous deficiency by using an insufficient saphenous vein as arterial substitute. Thus, it is necessary and possible to tailor treatment for each individual patient to be able to improve the outcome. Table 26.3 shows patients suitable for referral for arterial and venous surgery.

Follow-up

Most efforts thus far have concentrated on evaluating patients and trying to improve healing. The problem of recurrent ulceration seems largely to have been forgotten [4]. On the basis of the results from the Skaraborg study [1,6] it deserves to be emphasised that prevention of recurrence is as important as the achievement of healing [4,6]. Little benefit is gained if a newly healed venous ulcer soon recurs – as is not uncommon even in trials evaluating conservative regimens [9–11,13]. In the Riverside study about one-third of healed venous ulcers recurred early, despite regular visits for compression hosiery, constituting a major problem [13]. Unless curative surgery for isolated SVI/PVI has been performed follow-up is mandatory to prevent avoidable recurrences. Patients with DVI and patients with uncorrected SVI/PVI need life-long compression prophylaxis [16].

Compliance with compression seems to vary considerably and non-compliant patients will almost invariably suffer from recurrent ulceration [9–11]. Compliance is dependent on several factors: patient information and education, type of compression device used, age of the patient and incurred costs. A major problem is that compression stockings and bandages are not generally covered by the health insurance. Patients may, therefore, often have to pay the full cost for these devices. In Sweden compression stockings may be prescribed in a few counties but not others and generally bandages have to be paid for by the patient. Unless compression devices are covered by health insurance patient compliance is not likely to rise, thus negatively affecting the long-term outcome for leg ulcer patients. A political decision is necessary to change this. In the meantime dedicated and trained personnel are essential to give patients adequate information and education. Community leg ulcer clinics may be a way of achieving this.

Table 26.3. Patients suitable for referral to vascular surgeons

All patients with venous ulcers caused by isolated SVI/PVI without signs of DVI or deep venous obstruction
Patients with mixed venous and arterial insufficiency where the patient does not tolerate graduated compression, or where the ulcer deteriorates with compression
All patients with ulcers and signs of critical ischaemia
All diabetic patients with non-healing ulcers or gangrene with noncompressible arteries or pathological ABPI
Patients with non-healing arterial ulcers despite less severe ischaemia

Organisation of Leg Ulcer Care

There is a tendency, especially in the UK, to rely on nurse-led community leg ulcer clinics to solve the problem of leg ulcers [13,14]. It is, however, unlikely that four-layer bandages will solve the problem in the long run despite obvious short-term success in healing. There is a risk that patients will be managed within the clinics without using the services of specialists. The fact that no patient in the Manchester study [14] was referred for vascular surgical services during the study period is alarming in view of the known good results of performing superficial venous surgery on patients with "varicose" ulcers. The cost savings claimed in that study are truly short term. In the Riverside study, on the other hand, it was acknowledged that a wider use of venous surgery might improve long-term outcome [13], which is more likely to be true.

It is important that doctors take charge of leg ulcer diagnosis, choice of treatment and decisions regarding referrals to specialist services. General practitioners are, at least in Sweden, encouraged to take that responsibility [16]. Nurses at leg ulcer clinics and nurses in the community are, however, also encouraged to learn basic differential diagnosis with the aid of hand-held Doppler. This is done in order to improve early detection of vascular abnormalities "out in the field" where most patients are treated. The diagnosis and treatment for a specific patient is preferably decided through a dialogue between the nurse and the responsible GP. Leg ulcer clinics seem otherwise to be an excellent way of dealing with the everyday care of leg ulcer patients.

Leg ulcer management is truly multidisciplinary. This requires establishing a collaborative network to be able to tailor the best treatment for each individual patient. Neither specialists nor nurses and GPs at community leg ulcer clinics can give the best care for their patients by acting on their own. It is important that there are established pathways for dialogue and consultation between all professionals involved. Access to vascular laboratories with duplex Doppler facilities is essential to ascertain appropriate management. Whether that is done through vascular surgeons or other departments may vary locally. An example of organised leg ulcer care pathways, from Skaraborg county Sweden, is shown in Fig. 26.1. At present one of the most important tasks seems to be to bring surgeons, vascular surgeons and GPs into these networks, which they have previously tried to avoid.

Future Implications

One problems remains unsolved, namely the fact that about half of all people with leg ulcers are self-caring [4,20]. Is this perhaps a reflection of the poor results achieved through, mainly, conservative management over the past decades within the health care system? It is a problem of great concern since most of the self-carers are young individuals who often have ulcers caused by curable disease such as varicose veins [4,20]. As their long-term prognosis is poor without professional treatment they will, eventually, seek help from public health care. Thus, there seems to be a considerable patient delay involved in leg ulcers. To this delay is added the delay often caused by health carers neglecting to perform a proper diagnosis that enables the most appropriate treatment to be chosen (Fig. 26.2). Educating not only health care professionals but also the general population seems to be one of the most important tasks for the future. Who knows, perhaps TV commercials and/or the Internet would be ways of attacking this problem?

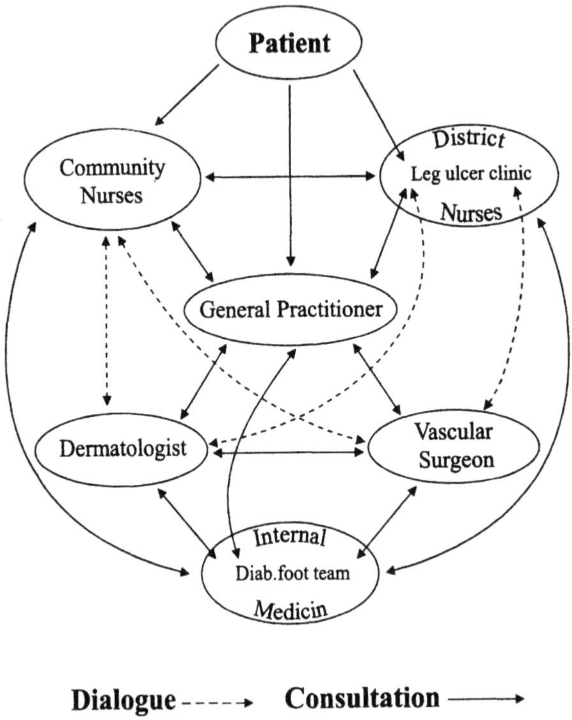

Fig. 26.1. Example of organised care pathways for the management of patients with leg ulcer. The example shows the present situation in Skaraborg county, Sweden.

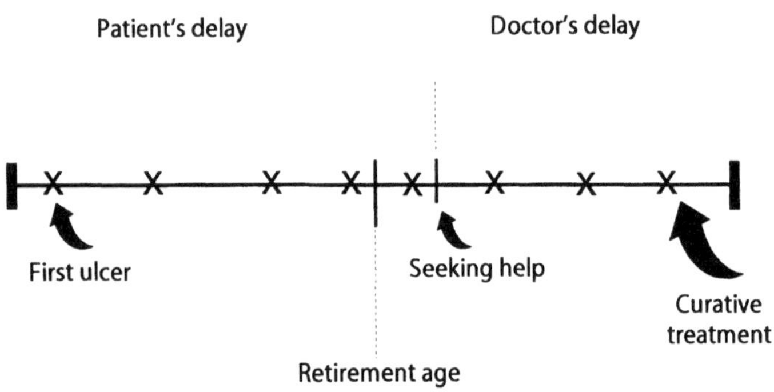

Fig. 26.2. The typical patient history for a patient with venous ulcer. *Crosses*, ulcer episode

Conclusions

By means of a wider use of Doppler-aided diagnosis, tailored individual treatment and improved follow-up, as well as by organising care in a multidisciplinary network, the long-term outcome for leg ulcer patients is likely to improve. The increased interest in leg ulcer care and treatment has, it is hoped, lifted this problem from the backyard of medicine. I believe that the establishment of community clinics in combination with venous surgery that is initiated early and performed accurately will have the most profound positive effect on the prognosis for patients with chronic ulcers. In fact a large number of those are in reality not "chronic" at all. There is real potential to reduce the leg ulcer population substantially, probably by one half, within a decade from now.

References

1. Nelzén O, Bergqvist D, Lindhagen A. Venous and non-venous leg ulcers: clinical history and appearance in a population study. Br J Surg 1994;81:182–187.
2. Callam MJ, Harper DR, Dale JJ, Ruckley CV. Chronic ulcer of the leg: clinical history. BMJ 1987;294:1389–1391.
3. Baker SR, Stacey MC, Jopp McKay AG, Hoskin SE, Thompson PJ. Epidemiology of chronic venous ulcers. Br J Surg 1991;78:864–867.
4. Nelzén O. Patients with chronic leg ulcer: aspects on epidemiology, aetiology, clinical history, prognosis and choice of treatment. Comprehensive Summaries of Uppsala Dissertations from the Faculty of Medicine 664. Uppsala: Acta Universitatis Upsaliensis, 1997:1–88.
5. Nelzén O, Bergqvist D, Lindhagen A. Leg ulcer etiology: a cross sectional population study. J Vasc Surg 1991;14:557–564.
6. Nelzén O, Bergqvist D, Lindhagen A. Long-term prognosis for patients with chronic leg ulcers: a prospective cohort study. Eur J Vasc Endovasc Surg 1997;13:500–508.
7. Hansson C, Andersson E, Swanbeck G. A follow-up study of leg and foot ulcer patients. Acta Derm Venereol (Stockh) 1987;67:496–500.
8. Salaman RA, Harding KG. The aetiology and healing rates of chronic leg ulcers. J Wound Care 1995;4:320–323.
9. Erickson CA, Lanza DJ, Karp DL, Edwards JW, Seabrook GR, Cambria RA, et al. Healing of venous ulcers in an ambulatory care program: the roles of chronic venous insufficiency and patient compliance. J Vasc Surg 1995;22:629–636.
10. Mayberry JC, Moneta GL, Taylor LM Jr, Porter JM. Fifteen-year results of ambulatory compression therapy for chronic venous ulcers. Surgery 1991;109:575–581.
11. Dinn E, Henry M. Treatment of venous ulceration by injection sclerotherapy and compression hoisery: a 5-year study. Phlebology 1992;7:23–26.
12. Fletcher A, Cullum N, Sheldon TA. A systematic review of compression treatment for venous leg ulcers. BMJ 1997;315:576–580.
13. Moffatt CJ, Franks PJ, Oldroyd M, Bosanquet N, Brown P, Greenhalgh RM, et al. Community clinics for leg ulcers and impact on healing. BMJ 1992;305:1389–1392.
14. Simon DA, Freak L, Kinsella A, Walsh J, Lane C, Groarke L, et al. Community leg ulcer clinics: a comparative study in two health authorities. BMJ 1996;312:1648–1651.
15. Baker SR, Stacey MC, Singh G, Hoskin SE, Thompson PJ. Aetiology of chronic leg ulcers. Eur J Vasc Surg 1992;6:245–251.
16. NMCA and MPA. Treatment of venous leg ulcers. In: Waersted A, Westbye O, Beermann B, Strandberg K, editors. Recommendations of a workshop on treatment of venous ulcers. Oslo: The Norwegian Medicines Control Authority and Swedish Medical Products Agency, 1995:9–32.
17. Walsh JC, Bergan JJ, Beeman S, Comer TP. Femoral venous reflux abolished by greater saphenous vein stripping. Ann Vasc Surg 1994;8:566–570.
18. Darke SG, Penfold C. Venous ulceration and saphenous ligation. Eur J Vasc Surg 1992;6:4–9.
19. Stacey MC, Baker SR, Rashid P, Hoskin SE, Thompson P. The influence of arterial disease, diabetes and rheumatoid arthritis on the healing of chronic venous ulcers. Proceedings of the 4th European conference on advances in wound management, Copenhagen. London: Macmillan Magazines, 1995:153–156.
20. Nelzén O, Bergqvist D, Lindhagen A. The prevalence of chronic lower-limb ulceration has been underestimated: results of a validated population questionnaire. Br J Surg 1996;83:255–258.

27 Quality of Life for Leg Ulcer Patients

Peter J. Franks

Introduction

Few clinicians or patients would disagree with the proposition that the presence of leg ulceration plays an important part in patients' lives. However, there is relatively little objective evidence to support this, and little is known of its precise impact in those who suffer from this affliction. Ulcer patients are frequently elderly and suffer from many health-related problems, most particularly poor mobility and numerous other pathologies common in this age group. The problem that we have in examining quality of life in these patients is that health issues may not reflect problems of the leg ulceration per se, but may be a consequence of and part of the patients' overall health. This chapter will attempt to draw together some of the concepts behind quality of life measurement and some of the evidence available from published studies in patients with leg ulceration and will then examine how this area may develop in the future.

What Is Meant by Quality of Life?

Quality of life, health-related quality of life, functional status and health status are terms often used interchangeably to describe a patient's state of well being. Whilst quality of life may encompass areas of life such as financial security and freedom of expression, most investigators wish to examine the impact of a disease (on the individual or on populations) which relates most closely to their state of health. Health-related quality of life (HRQL) is an easier concept to describe, with general consensus on the areas of life to be measured – most frequently physical, mental, social functioning and general health [1].

Why Measure Quality of Life?

Traditionally medicine has considered survival as the primary end-point for life threatening diseases. However, early trials of cancer therapies demonstrated that the use of these toxic agents led to extreme side-effects, often with little benefit in terms of survival. From these studies it became clear that not only was *quantity* of life important, but that *quality* of life could be equally, if not more important. Moreover, whilst some feel that health is merely the absence of disease, the World Health Organisation has enlarged this definition to "a state of complete physical, mental and social well being and not merely the absence of disease" [2].

HRQL fits well into the concept of this broader sense of health, since patients may "feel" ill without any clinical evidence of disease. This concept is important since it gives the patients' views of their own health, rather than clinical judgements made by a doctor. Moreover, whilst clinicians have chosen to rely on clinical measurements as outcomes of care, there is a growing recognition that these may be inadequate in describing the impact of a disease process on a patient. In leg ulceration the severity of the disease is often described in terms of the area of ulceration, yet it is recognised that small ulcers may cause as much discomfort and pain as larger areas of ulceration. For the individual patient the size of an ulcer may be irrelevant to its impact on his or her life. Moreover, although leg ulceration is largely a problem in the elderly, there is evidence that a substantial proportion of patients have their first ulceration before the age of 60 years. The impact of ulceration is likely to be different in these younger patients, particularly in relation to time lost from work and job loss [3], whilst the elderly may have lower expectations of health, and consider their ulceration as an inevitable part of their gradual decline with old age. Hence, ulceration may have a different impact according to the individual being assessed. Thus, we must consider that patients may differ in their expectations in terms of both clinical outcome and its impact on HRQL. Whilst it is expected that healing will be the outcome of choice in all patients, in certain situations this may not be either feasible or desirable. It must be acknowledged that even though treatment techniques have advanced over the last 10–15 years, to enable healing in the majority, there may be a significant minority in whom either these techniques are either inappropriate or fail to produce the desired outcome. We must look for outcome measures to evaluate success of treatment other than simple healing.

How Health Related Quality of Life Is Measured

There is no correct way to measure HRQL and different techniques may be employed according to the different requirements of individual studies for example, qualitative interviews with patients [4], carers or families or a more structured approach using standard validated questionnaires. Whichever tool is chosen, to be of value it must conform to a number of requirements:

Appropriateness. The tool must be appropriate for the patient group being studied.
Reliability. It must be stable under conditions of repeated measurement, particularly in relation to intra- and inter-observer differences.
Validity. The tool must measure what it purports to measure.
Sensitivity to change. It must be capable of detecting change when there is a real difference in the patient's status.

Generic and Disease-specific Tools

There is considerable debate over the relative values of generic and disease-specific tools. Generic tools were developed to measure HRQL over a wide variety of diseases and disease states. They have the advantage of having been frequently validated among a number of diseases, often within different cultures, and translated into a variety of languages. The generic tools are frequently favoured because they require no development work to use and are well validated. In addition, they may be of great value in assessing the relative impact of different diseases. The principal disadvantage of such tools is that they may not ask questions of relevance to the particular patient group being investigated. The tool may thus fail to detect changes in health which may be important to the patient. The most popular generic tools used in the study of leg ulceration have been the Nottingham Health Profile (NHP; 38 questions) [5] and the Short Form 36 (SF-36; 36 questions) [6]. Whilst there may be others which provide similar information, these have not been evaluated in ulcer patients.

Disease-specific tools have the advantage of being relevant to the disease being investigated and are more likely to be sensitive to changes in state experienced by the patient. Their principal disadvantage is the time and effort required to validate such tools for each disease and the inability to compare patients across disease classifications. Studies so far have concentrated on the use of generic tools, although recently there has been a general appreciation of the need for disease-specific tools. Preliminary studies have started to develop tools specifically for patients with leg ulceration and venous disease. The following sections will examine the evidence collected using both types of tool.

Leg Ulcer Disease and Quality of Life

Much of our understanding of the impact of leg ulceration on patients with leg ulceration has come from the administration of the NHP. In a study in the Wirral, Cullum et al. [7,8] identified 88 patients with chronic leg ulceration, and compared them with 60 control subjects of a similar mean age. Perceived bodily pain using the NHP was significantly higher in the ulcer patients versus the controls. Energy loss was significantly greater in the patients with ulceration, but there was no significant difference between groups in respect of emotional reactions. Results from the other scores of the NHP were not discussed.

In a Lothian and Forth Valley clinical trial of 200 patients suffering from leg ulceration there were significantly worse scores on the NHP for patients suffering from venous ulceration than age/sex/social class norms for pain, social isolation and physical mobility [9]. These results were in a agreement with a study reported from Cardiff, where there were significantly poorer scores for 54 patients with chronic leg ulcers compared with age/sex norms in all domains of the SF-36 except for mental health [10].

Factors that Affect Quality of Life in Leg Ulceration

Age and Gender

This area of study has raised a number of issues, not least how HRQL assessments need to be interpreted in the light of population gender differences. The first study to investigate gender in patients suffering from leg ulceration was performed in Sweden, and examined differences between 51 men and 74 women using the NHP [11]. To adjust for the effects of gender and age, a score for each patient was derived relative to the percentage of their expected value from population normal values. Thus, a percentage score of 100 meant that the patient had a score equal to their age/sex norm, a higher score meant that the patient had a poorer HRQL than expected, whilst a score of less than 100 meant the patient had a better quality of life than expected. This method of analysis demonstrated significantly poorer HRQL in men than women for pain and physical mobility. More recently, Price and Harding [10] disputed this, finding poorer HRQL in women in respect of physical functioning, vitality and social functioning, with a poorer, though non-significant difference in general health.

Recently we have investigated this apparent paradox using information collected from a number of audits of leg ulcer care throughout the UK. In an examination of 758 patients with leg ulceration we have shown that indeed the scores are poorer in women for all domains of the NHP (Fig. 27.1a). However, this is due to women having higher normal scores than men in the general population [12]. When adjusted for age and sex normal values, the excess scores show significantly poorer quality of life for men associated with their ulcer in the domains of energy, pain, sleep and social isolation (Fig. 27.1b). A similar pattern is noted for age. Whilst using crude scores gives consistently poorer HRQL for the more elderly patients (Fig. 27.2a), following adjustment for age and sex the excess score attributable to the presence

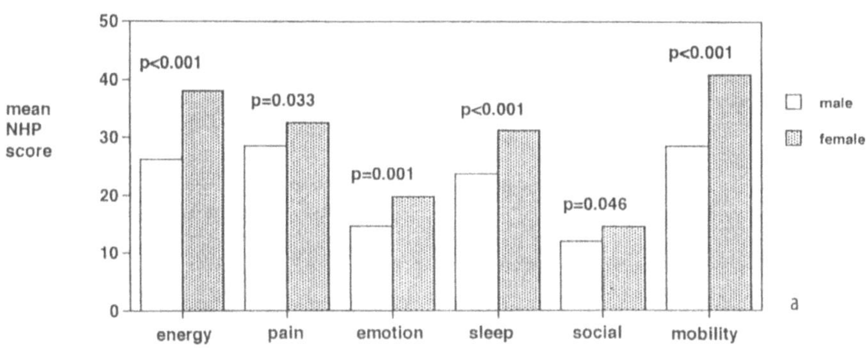

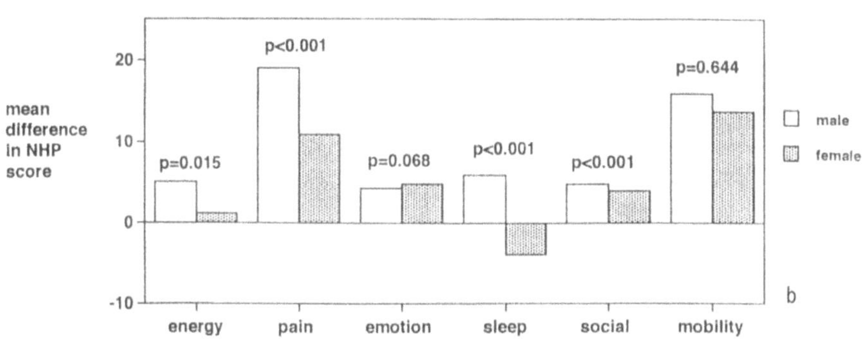

Fig. 27.1a,b. Differences in scores on the Nottingham Health Profile (NHP) in men and women compared using the Mann Whitney test. **a** Raw scores indicate that women appear to suffer to a greater extent than men. **b** After adjustment for age and sex, the excess scores were significantly greater in men, indicating that they appear to suffer to a greater extent than women.

of leg ulceration appears to be greatest in the youngest age group (<65 years) (Fig.27.2b). In these analyses it also appeared that the lowest impact was in the 75–84 year age group, with an increased impact in the most elderly group (>85 years).

Ulcer Duration and Size

Whilst it might be considered that increased ulcer size and duration may have a deleterious affect on the patient's HRQL, there is little evidence to substantiate this. The Swedish study found no evidence of longer duration of ulceration impacting on their patients [11], whilst in Cardiff increased bodily pain and poorer general health were found in the patients with longer duration of ulceration [10]. However, this observation may have been confounded by the longer-duration ulcers being present in the more elderly patients. In our analysis of 758 patients we were unable to find any differences in quality of life scores in relation to ulcer duration. Moreover, the only outcome parameter was only significantly related to ulcer size >10 cm2 was increased bodily pain, confirming evidence from the Wirral [7,8].

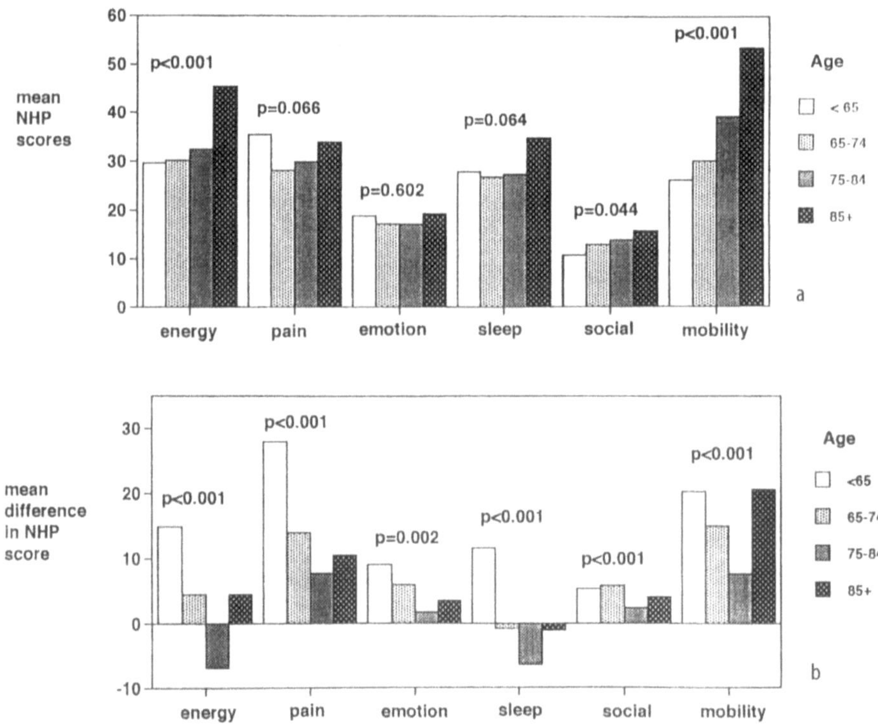

Fig. 27.2a,b. Differences in scores on the Nottingham Health Profile (NHP) by age compared using the Kruskal Wallis test. **a** differences in mean scores appear to indicate that the more elderly suffer to a greater extent than the younger patients. **b** After adjustment, the greatest impact of the ulceration appears to be in the youngest age group, with lowest impact in those aged 75–84 years.

Other Factors

Whilst there has been some evidence to show an association between low social class and poor HRQL, analyses of our data provided no evidence to substantiate this after adjusting for age and sex. However, employment status was associated with differences in excess pain scores, being greatest in patients who had retired from work due to illness, and lowest in those patients who were either retired or who were currently employed. Perceived pain was lowest in the patients receiving district nurse care at home and poorest in those receiving practice nurse care, whilst sleep was best in those who attended outpatient departments for treatment and again worst in those who received practice nurse care.

The Impact of Therapy on Quality of Life

The first attempt to use a generic tool to examine outcomes in patients suffering from leg ulceration appeared in the Riverside project in London during the early 1990s [13]. This project was designed to evaluate the impact of delivering care to patients in the community using largely existing resources, but with the re-organisation of care around community leg ulcer clinics, staffed by community nurses overseen by a clinical nurse specialist liaising with the acute hospital service. The principal treatment for patients with venous ulceration was the four-layer bandage (4LB), which had been devised in a hospital outpatient setting but appeared to offer benefits to the majority of patients who were being treated in the community [14]. The Symptom Rating Test (SRT) [15] was used to detect changes in psychiatric morbidity in patients during the clinic audit cycle. After 12 weeks of treatment there were significant reductions in anxiety, depression and hostility, and improvements in cognition. Both patients whose ulcers had healed and those whose ulcers remained unhealed after 12 weeks experienced benefits in terms of reduction in SRT scores. However, those patients whose ulcers had healed experienced significantly greater improvements in terms of depression and hostility than those who remained unhealed. Thus, healing the ulcer appeared to offer significant psychiatric benefits in these patients.

Recently, the NHP has been used as an outcome measure in a Lothian and Forth Valley randomised trial of therapy in 200 patients suffering from venous ulceration [9]. During the 24 weeks of follow-up patients significantly improved in terms of energy, pain reduction, emotional reactions, sleep and physical mobility. Again, healing the ulceration had a significantly greater effect on patients in terms of energy, pain, emotional reactions, sleep and mobility. There were also significantly greater improvements in energy and physical mobility when using the 4LB compared with the Granuflex bandage.

Disease-Specific Tools

The first attempt to develop a disease-specific tool was described by Hyland et al. in 1994 [16]. They used focus groups to discuss problems associated with leg ulceration, and from these developed a tool. The first section of the final questionnaire examines the impact of leg ulceration in terms of pain, sleep, time self-treating and time thinking about the ulceration. The second section consists of 29 questions which examine the patient's lifestyle and mechanisms used to avoid further injury. At present, the repeatability and sensitivity to change are being evaluated.

A further tool has been developed in France to examine patients suffering from all forms of chronic lower limb venous insufficiency; this consists of 20 questions [17]. Again, whilst information has been provided on the development of the tool, including reliability measurements and some evidence on sensitivity to change, there is still a need to check the external validity by comparing the results of this tool with those of a standard generic tool such as the NHP or SF-36.

Although both tools offer promise in assessing HRQL in patients with leg ulceration, it remains to be seen whether they are sufficienty user-friendly and fulfil the requirements of investigators in this area.

Conclusion

Whilst most clinicians and researchers acknowledge the impact that leg ulceration has on patients, there is still little evidence on its importance in terms of quality of life and how its impact may be modified by effective treatment. Whilst complete healing will always be the principal therapeutic aim in these patients, it must be acknowledged that in some cases this may not be possible and alternative outcome measures such as HRQL must be employed.

To date the evidence suggests that whilst the presence of leg ulceration appears to affect most patients, there is poorer HRQL in men, particularly in the areas of perceived pain, sleep quality and social isolation. Moreover the impact is related to age, with younger patients suffering from more acute lack of energy, increasing bodily pain, poorer sleep and mobility. Whilst effective treatment almost certainly improves the patients' HRQL, particularly in the areas of perceived pain and mobility, it remains to be seen whether successful treatment can return a patient to expected levels of functioning and psychological well being.

Clearly, there is much work to be done before we can understand some of the issues in quality of life in these patients. Although it might be expected that pain is important, leg ulceration also appears to have a major impact on the patient's social life, mobility and sleep quality. The generic tools which have been used can only offer crude indications of the impact of the problem on the patient's lifestyle. In the future it is likely that these will be used in combination with questions which address issues related directly to ulceration. It is clear that clinical outcomes such as complete ulcer healing are limited in assessing the value to the patient of health care programmes and treatment regimens. Whilst these outcomes will remain as key evidence of success, other methods must be employed to evaluate therapeutic benefits in patients in whom complete healing may not be possible.

References

1. Fallowfield L. The quality of life: the missing dimension in health care. London. Souvenir, 1990.
2. World Health Organisation. The first ten years. Geneva: WHO, 1958.
3. Phillips T, Stanton B, Provan A, Lew R. A study of the impact of leg ulcers on quality of life: financial, social and psychologic implications. J Am Acad Dermatol 1994;31:49–53.

4. Walshe C. Living with a venous leg ulcer: a descriptive study of patients' experiences. J Adv Nurs 1995;22:1092–1100.
5. Hunt SM, McEwan J, McKenna SP. Measuring health status. London: Croom Helm, 1986.
6. Ware JE, Snow KK, Kosinski M, Gandek B. SF-36 Health Survey: manual and interpretation guide. Boston Health Institute, New England Medical Center, 1993.
7. Hamer C, Cullum NA, Roe BH. Patients' perceptions of chronic leg ulcers. J Wound Care 1994;3:99–101.
8. Roe B, Cullum N, Hamer C. Patients' perceptions of chronic leg ulceration. In: Cullum N, Roe B, editors. Leg ulcers: nursing management. Harrow: Scutari Press, 1995:125–134.
9. Franks PJ, Bosanquet N, Brown D, Straub J, Harper DR, Ruckley CV. Perceived health in a randomised trial of single and multi-layer bandaging. Phlebology; (Suppl) 1:17–19.
10. Price P, Harding K. Measuring health-related quality of life in patients with chronic leg ulcers. Wounds 1996;8:91–94.
11. Lindholm C, Bjellerup M, Christensen OB, Zedrfeld B. Quality of life in chronic leg ulcers. Acta Derm Venereol (Stockh) 1993;73:440–443.
12. Hunt SM, McEwan J, McKenna SP. Perceived health: age and sex comparisons in the community. J epidemiol Community Health 1984;38:156–160.
13. Franks PJ, Moffatt CJ, Connolly M, Bosanquet N, Oldroyd M, Greenhalgh RM, McCollum CN. Community leg ulcer clinics: effect on quality of life. Phlebology 1994;9:83–86.
14. Moffatt CJ, Franks PJ, Oldroyd M, Bosanquet N, Brown P, Greenhalgh RM, McCollum CN. Community clinics and impact on healing: BMJ 1992;305:1389–1392.
15. Kellner R, Sheffield BF. A self rating scale of distress. Psychol Med 1973;3:88–100.
16. Hyland ME, Ley A, Thomson B. Quality of life of leg ulcer patients: questionnaire and preliminary findings. J Wound Care 1994;3:294–298.
17. Launois R, Reboul-Marty J, Henry B. Construction and validation of a quality of life questionnaire in chronic lower limb venous insufficiency (CIVIQ). Qual Life Res 1996;5:539–554.

28 Developing and Implementing Leg Ulcer Guidelines

Tracey Gillies

Introduction

Clinical guidelines have been proposed as one method by which it may be possible to improve clinical outcome or the processes involved in the provision of care. In this chapter a brief overview of guideline methodology is given before addressing the development and implementation of leg ulcer guidelines in Scotland by the Scottish Leg Ulcer Project.

Clinical guidelines have beeen defined by the Institute of Medicine as"systematically developed statements to assist practitioner and patient decisions about appropriate health care for specific clinical circumstances" [1] A number of desirable characteristics of a clinical guideline are described, which include validity, reproducibility and reliability, representative development, clinical applicability and flexibility and clarity. Validity is influenced by the membership of the development group, the method by which evidence is identified and synthesised and the way in which the guideline is developed from this evidence [2]. A number of different methods have been described including consensus, both formal and informal, evidence-based and explicit guideline development [3]. Evidence-linked guideline development, it has been suggested, is most likely to result in a valid guideline. However, it is easier to produce a guideline than to demonstrate any health gain following production of that guideline. Dissemination and implementation are the key steps which must follow the guideline development if any change in clinical outcome is to occur, although they are frequently overlooked. It is difficult to quantify these steps although the use of various strategies known to influence both dissemination and implementation can be noted [4].

Grimshaw et al. [5] have reviewed the evaluations of such guidelines to address the question of whether clinical guidelines can change the behaviour of health care professionals. They identified 91 studies, grouping these by study design and field into clinical care, preventative care, prescribing practice or the use of investigations. In particular, they looked at the intervention made to promote the use of the guideline and the effect on process (whether the guideline was followed) and outcome (whether there was any benefit in health outcome for the patient). They found that properly developed guidelines do change clinical practice and may lead to a change in patient outcome. However, the factors influencing guideline adoption are complex. Local ownership of guidelines is important but guidelines developed only at a local level are perceived as less credible than those developed nationally. Implementation strategies were found to be most effective when they impinged on the consultation with the patient (such as patient specific reminders), active participation was needed in education programmes and the influence of local opinion leaders was shown to be prominent. Overall, successful strategies need to take effect close to the point of patient contact.

There are a number of obstacles to the successful implementation of guidelines at a personal, group and organisational level, and a behavioural framework has been drawn up to identify these and introduce strategies to overcome them [6]. It has been proposed that there are those who are "early adopters", the "middle majority" and the "late adopters", each group having different characteristics, motivation for change and needs when introduced to guidelines [7]. No one method will reach all but face-to-face instruction, assessment and feedback by respected peers combined with practical support has been found to be effective. Grol [7], working with General Practitioners, noted that too much effort is spent improving knowledge and attitudes and too little on improving skills and actual behaviour. A questionnaire carried out amongst hospital doctors of all grades in an English healthcare region found that 77% expressed welcoming attitudes towards guidelines, with most claiming to use guidelines at least once a month [8]. Lack of awareness, poor development and impracticality were cited as the commonest reasons why guidelines were not adhered to. Another survey of senior staff in 270 acute hospitals in the United Kingdom found that whilst 99% were in favour of clinical guidelines, only 19% had a hospital strategy for their implementation [9].

Scottish Leg Ulcer Project: Background

The Scottish Leg Ulcer Project (SLUP) began with the general agreement of a number of interested clinicians that there was a need to improve leg ulcer care in Scotland, and in particular to translate the healing rate of venous ulcers seen in specialist centres to the wider community. A national survey of leg ulcer care was carried out to identify the needs of those working in primary health care. A random sample of 673 General Practitioners (GPs) and 441 Community Nurses working in all 15 Health Boards were sent a questionnaire asking them what leg ulcer services were available in their area, their level of satisfaction with the current service and areas where they would like to see improvements. Community Nurses were also asked who was involved with care in their area, and whether they had access to protocols. Response rates of 76% for GPs and 82% for Community Nurses were obtained. Satisfaction with the current service was expressed by 285 (56%) of GPs, although only 155 (30%) had access to a recognised leg ulcer specialist. A diagnosis as to the aetiology of the ulcer was made by GPs and Community Nurses together in 68% and by Community Nurses alone in 21% of cases, but the choice of treatment was most often left to the nurse alone. Only 9% of Community Nurses had access to local protocols for management of leg ulcer patients, although 89% said such protocols would be helpful. Training and education was the area most frequently identified as a way in which the leg ulcer service could be improved. The deficiencies in specialist support, education and lack of clear guidelines for the management of leg ulcer patients were identified by both GPs and Community Nurses as shortcomings in the service provided.

This survey raised a number of issues about the management of leg ulcer patients in Scotland and how it could be improved. Successful treatment methods for venous ulcers based on multilayer graduated compression bandaging have been well documented in the literature [10], but these results have not been reproduced in the wider community. Furthermore, the survey gave a clear indication that a guideline on leg ulcer management would be welcomed by those providing the majority of the care for leg ulcer patients. The survey was completed at the same time as there was a certain amount of negative feeling towards clinical guidelines being expressed in the medical literature [11–13]. Many guidelines have been developed that have little or no evidence base and merely represent the opinions of a few individuals. Those who believe that valid guidelines serve a useful purpose are aware that they need an effective implementation strategy in order to improve clinical outcomes but that guidelines cannot be used as a panacea for inadequate service provision, training or resources [4,9].

A proposal was then made for the main project to study the implementation of a well-constructed guideline on leg ulcer care on a large scale across Scotland. The guideline has been produced by the Scottish Intercollegiate Guideline Network (SIGN) and has been developed in parallel with the main project by an independent group. The structure and principles behind SIGN guidelines are described below

Scottish Intercollegiate Guideline Network

SIGN was set up in 1993 by the Royal Colleges in Scotland and their Faculties in response to the report on clinical guidelines produced by the Clinical Resource and Audit Group (CRAG) [14]. This group recognised the differences between nationally developed guidelines which were more likely to be scientifically valid and those developed locally which would have a stronger sense of ownership and so be more likely to be accepted and used in everyday practice. The proposed solution was a two-tier process in which SIGN would first undertake development of evidence-based national guidelines to set out the principles of good clinical practice. Local protocols would then be developed based on these, according to specific resources and circumstances [15].

By the end of 1997, 21 guidelines had been published by SIGN covering many diverse topics in all specialties of medicine but concentrating on those areas that have been identified as priorities for the National Health Service (NHS) in Scotland. These are cardiovascular and cerebrovascular disease, mental health and cancer. Large subjects are generally unsuitable for guideline development and need to be split into more manageable topics. The St. Vincent Declaration to improve the care of diabetic patients, for example, was taken as the starting point for six different guideline development groups, each focusing on one aspect of the declaration [16]. There has been an increasing attempt by SIGN to ensure that a guideline adheres to a closely defined remit, concentrating on particular areas in which there is a wide variation in clinical practice or outcome and strong evidence for best practice [17]. New proposals now have to demonstrate the need for the guideline and that the evidence upon which it will be based is strong enough to allow clear recommendations to be made before they are adopted for development by SIGN. This is to ensure that succinct and relevant guidelines are produced.

Each guideline is developed using a standard method, although these methods are constantly evolving. Once the proposal has been accepted by SIGN, a chairman of the development group is appointed. Group membership aims to cover all key disciplines involved with the care outlined in that particular guideline and includes a member responsible for undertaking the literature search with help from the Information Officer in the SIGN Secretariat. Wherever possible a group should include at least one patient or patient representative. Members should be drawn from the whole of Scotland so that there is adequate geographical representation of all regions. This further facilitates ownership when the guideline is disseminated. Guidelines are not developed in isolation and there is strong collaboration with other groups who have worked in the field. These include groups carrying out systematic reviews within the Cochrane Collaboration and groups undertaking broader work for the NHS such as the Scottish Health Purchasing Information Centre (SHPIC).

Following a preliminary meeting to clarify the remit of the guideline and areas which are to be included or excluded, a systematic review of the literature is carried out using an explicit standard search strategy. Following initial sifting of the identified literature to identify relevant evidence, papers are then considered by the group. Depending on group size, the subject may be split for consideration by smaller subgroups. SIGN undertakes training courses in critical appraisal techniques which all group members are encouraged to attend. Critical appraisal concentrates on methodological aspects (for example, the method of randomisation used, whether all the subjects were accounted for, whether analysis was carried out on an intention-to-treat basis and clinical aspects (whether the paper answered the question it set out to, whether an appropriate method was used, whether these finding could be extrapolated to ordinary clinical practice). Papers that are used as evidence in the guideline are judged by the group to be methodologically acceptable and assigned a level of evidence. The evidence from these papers is then linked to the recommendation for practice made by the group using the grades of recommendation. The levels of evidence and grades of recommendation are based on those developed by the US Agency for Health Care Policy and Research. This explicit linkage of recommendation and supporting evidence is intended to maximise the validity of the guideline.

When a draft report has been synthesised by the group, a national open meeting is held. All interested parties are invited to attend, and the draft guideline is presented. Comments and feedback are most important and are carefully considered and incorporated if accepted. The national meeting also serves to stimulate thinking about the subsequent development of local protocols, facilitate implementation of guideline recommendations and increase involvement. A further draft is then sent for peer review and consultation before the guideline is passed to the SIGN Editorial Board for formal evaluation. The critical appraisal of the guideline carried out by the Editorial Board is set out and available to the development group [18]. Not all guidelines meet the stringent criteria set down as part of the appraisal process in their first edition. If approved, the guideline is published as a pilot edition, and all guidelines are reviewed and updated after 2 years.

At present SIGN guidelines are distributed to all GPs, Consultants and Managers. It is proposed to increase distribution to Specialist Registrars in the near future. However, distribution does not ensure that the guideline or its contents are disseminated to those whose practice it may most influence, and SIGN does not take part in the next part of the process: developing local protocols from the national guideline and implementing these.

The Care of Patients with Leg Ulcer: A SIGN Guideline

A SIGN guideline development group was set up in July 1996 to produce a guideline on the management of patients with a leg ulcer. Although all types of ulcer are included, most attention is paid to venous leg ulcers, and in particular the assessment of these ulcers and their management within primary health care services. Diabetic leg ulcers were not covered extensively as these are the subject of a separate guideline. Full consideration was taken of the NHS Management Executive guideline on the management of leg ulcers, although this was developed by a consensus method and remains at draft stage. The SHPIC guideline on leg ulcers was also available to the group.

The guideline development group was chaired by Mr Douglas Harper and comprised five hospital-based doctors, two GPs, two Community Nurses, a pharmacist, a Leg Ulcer Nurse Specialist, a public health physician, a physiotherapist and a patient.

Although overall the literature on the care of leg ulcer patients is wide, noticeably few randomised controlled trials with large numbers of subjects and good methodology were found. This influenced the grade of recommendation assigned to some points in the guideline. Similarly, there are a large number of trials addressing ulcer healing but very few of these were rigorously conducted on an adequate sample size. The delivery of care, whether by community-based specialist clinics or some other method, was not addressed by the guideline group.

The national meeting to discuss the guideline was held on 4 September 1997 and was well attended. A number of parallel workshops were held in the afternoon to discuss those aspects seen by the development group as under-supported by evidence (such as the role of surgery) or contentious to a number of participants (the role of dressings). These generated valuable feedback. The pilot edition is due to be published in May 1998.

The Scottish Leg Ulcer Project: Main Project

The project is a randomised controlled trial to evaluate the impact of the implementation of national guidelines, with and without systematic nurse training, on the outcome of care for patients with chronic leg ulcers. It has been funded jointly by the Scottish Office and CRAG and is expected to run for 2 years. The project officially began in July 1997 but was under development for 2 years from July 1995, following the results of the national survey on leg ulcer care. The background to the project has been described above.

The hypothesis upon which the trial is based is that healing rates of leg ulcers will be greater when evidence-based guidelines of care are introduced systematically, with an approach that includes nurse training, than when guidelines are simply issued. Thus the trial aims are as follows:

1. To determine baseline healing rates prior to the introduction of national (SIGN) guidelines.
2. To determine changes in healing rates following dissemination of guidelines.
3. To determine changes in healing rates following the systematic introduction of guidelines including nurses training.
4. To compare the changes in healing rates in (2) and (3).

Healing rates (as defined by the ulcer-free leg) form the main endpoint to be measured in the study, although a costing analysis will be carried out on a small subset at intervals.

The participating areas in the trial cover all parts of Scotland, both urban and rural, with an included population of approximately 2 million. Ethics approval has been obtained for all participating areas.

Following a period of baseline data collection in all areas, geographical localities have been randomised to dissemination of the guidelines alone (control: aim 2) or dissemination of the guidelines coupled with a cascade system of training of Link Nurses and subsequently Community Nurses (intervention: aim 3). Baseline data collection began in September 1997 for 6 months. Randomisation by distinct geographical locality has been carried out. The baseline data are particularly important in a study such as this where the proposed effective intervention (guidelines plus training) is being implemented in a number of geographically disparate areas. Without baseline data, results will be un-interpretable due to variation in baseline performance both within and between intervention and control areas.

Data Collection

Information about every patient with a leg ulcer being cared for by a Community Nurse within the project area is being collected every 3 months by a postal census. Simple recording forms (one to be completed per patient) were sent to all Caseload Managers as identified by participating Community Trusts in the first census carried out in September 1997. These were completed, returned and the information entered on a database. Patient names have not been entered in order to comply with the Data Protection Act, but unique codes are used to identify both the Community Nurse and the patient. The participating areas are divided into three and the census weeks staggered in order to ease administration within the central SLUP office through which all data are collected. At each subsequent census, information is sought about the patients previously identified with a leg ulcer. The Community Nurse is asked to return the form stating whether the leg is ulcer-free, or whether the patient is unavailable for assessment. Information about transfer of patient care is sought as this allows patients to be tracked between different areas. Notification of any new ulcers is requested. Ambiguities are clarified by telephone and non-responders reminded twice by telephone. Information is only sought about the site on the leg of ulceration and the duration of the current episode of ulceration. To encourage continued participation with the somewhat tedious process of repeated form completion every 3 months, a decision was made to limit the information collected so that the forms could be completed with the minimum of effort. A letter was sent to all GPs in participating areas explaining the project and asking for their co-operation. No objections were received.

Postal censuses will continue at 3 monthly intervals throughout the 2 year duration of the study. This system of data collection is entirely separate from the implementation of the guidelines and is the same for both intervention and control areas (Fig. 28.1). Although somewhat cumbersome, direct contact with each Community Nurse would seem to be the only reliable way to collect the necessary information across such a large population. The existing methods used by Community Nurses to record provision of care vary widely between Community Trusts and there is no common way to pool this information.

The method of data collection by 3 month census and the recording forms were piloted in Tayside. This area was chosen because Community Nurses enter their workload in a coded form into a computerised system. It was hoped that this would establish the completeness of response by cross-checking the completed forms against the central Tayside database. However, cross-checking was difficult because of ambiguities and lack of specificity in the codes used by the nurses.

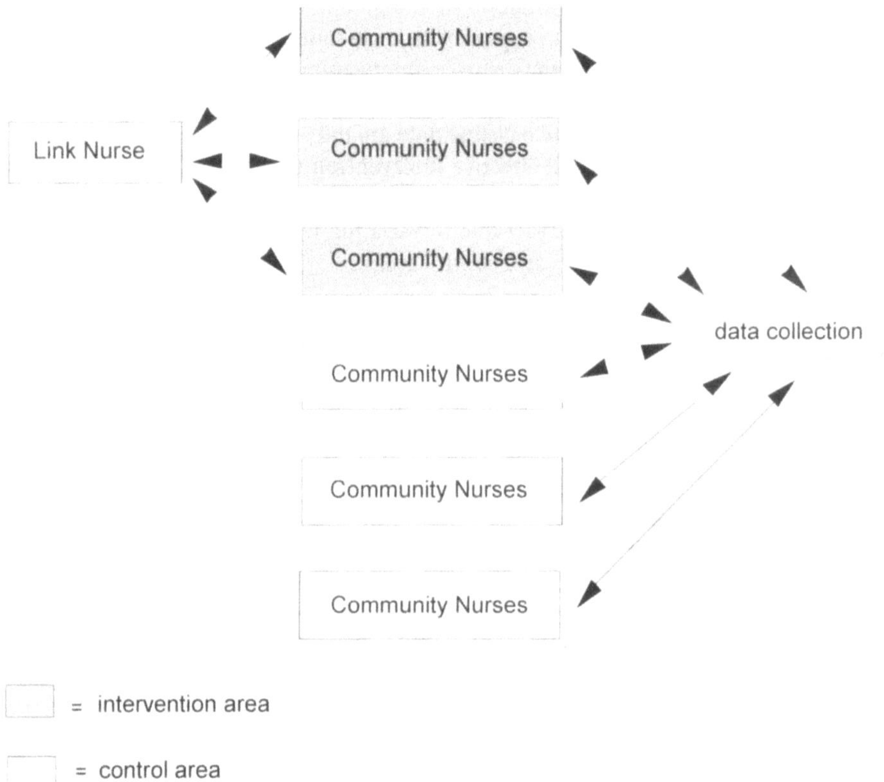

Fig. 28.1. Schematic representation of different areas in the Scottish Leg Ulcer Project showing that data collection is separate from cascade training.

A number of valuable lessons were learnt from the pilot study which have been incorporated into the main study; namely, sending census forms directly to the Caseload Manager rather than through an intermediary such as the Locality Manager, clarifying the date on which information is to be collected and asking those Caseload Managers with no patients with leg ulcers at the time of the census to return the form stating this fact. The pilot study included practice nurses but it became clear that there was no infrastructure corresponding to the Community Trusts through which these nurses could be regularly contacted, and a decision was made to limit the main study to those nurses employed by Community Trusts as either Community Nurses or Treatment Room Nurses.

Concern had been expressed about those patients who were receiving care in long stay institutions or in acute-stay wards in hospital. Therefore all wards, nursing and residential homes were surveyed once during the pilot study to determine the point prevalence of leg ulcers in these areas. The numbers were small (10 patients in total) and in the main study patients in such establishments have only been entered if they are receiving care from a Community Nurse

In the 2 months between the start of the project and the first census, members of the project team visited each area to hold a "roadshow". All Community Nurses in the area were invited and encouraged to do so by their Locality Manager. The purpose of the roadshow was to explain the aims and structure of the project, to introduce the recording forms to be used at each census and demonstrate completion of the forms, and to outline what would be involved in training. It was explained to all areas that training of the intervention areas would take place in the spring of 1998 and of the control areas at the end of the project if a beneficial effect of training by an improvement in healing rates was demonstrated. The main aims of the roadshow were to make individual nurses feel part of such a large project, thus ensuring a full and continued response rate in the censuses, and to familiarise them with the census forms.

Guideline Dissemination

The SIGN guidelines on the management of chronic leg ulcers are due to be published in May 1998 and will be distributed by SIGN in the normal way to all areas.

Control Areas

Data collection will continue throughout the duration of the project in control areas. The SIGN guidelines will be available in these areas through normal channels of distribution and no attempt will be made to influence implementation. It is likely that some areas will draw up local protocols based on the guidelines.

Intervention Areas: Training

Each intervention area has identified one or more Link Nurses and training of these nurses has taken place during the first 3 months of 1998. The role of the Link Nurse in the project is a pivotal one and Community Trusts were asked to identify committed, motivated individuals with an interest in leg ulcers. The place of the Link Nurse is twofold: to draw up local protocols with local leg ulcer specialists based on the SIGN guidelines and to provide cascade training for all nurses in each intervention area who care for leg ulcer patients. The number of Link Nurses required for each intervention area is dependent on the geographical distribution of the area and the number of nurses within that area to be trained. In total, 51 Link Nurses were identified by participating areas.

Each Link Nurse was required to attend a 1-day "core theory" study day and a 3-day practical course. Two core theory days and six practical courses at different regional centres were held. The core theory day concentrated on the contents of the SIGN guideline with an overview of the project. Workshops were held on the subject of developing local protocols and organising cascade training. The practical courses covered patient assessment techniques including Doppler assessment, bandaging skills and teaching skills. Although Link Nurses who had successfully completed a certified leg ulcer course were excused part of the practical course if necessary, they were encouraged to attend, thinking not of the acquisition of new skills but how they could best pass on those skills to others. All Link Nurses had to pass an Objective Structured Clinical Examination on the last day of the practical course to ensure that they had all achieved a minimum standard.

The responsibility of one of the SLUP trial co-ordinators has been organisation of the training and continuing support of the Link Nurses. Each Link Nurse has been given a teaching pack which includes an extensive collection of slides, handouts for duplication on assessment, bandaging, care of the skin and dressings, videos on Doppler assessment and bandaging techniques, and samples of different bandaging systems and graduated compression stockings. The amount of training each Link Nurse will need to carry out will depend on current practice in each area; some areas already have leg ulcer care protocols which can be adapted if necessary to fit in with the SIGN guidelines, but in others training and protocol development will need to begin from scratch. The trial co-ordinator will liaise with each Link Nurse, providing further resources, advice or support as necessary. It is proposed that as much of the cascade training as possible will have been completed by the summer of 1998 to coincide with publication of the SIGN guidelines. This will allow the maximum time for data collection on healing rates in the control and intervention areas. Each Link Nurse will become a local leg ulcer expert and provide training for new Community Nurses in the area as required.

Training in Control Areas

If analysis of the healing rates shows a benefit for those areas where there has been training in the use of the guideline, then similar cascade training will be offered to control areas. Obviously if no benefit of training is demonstrated, it will not be offered.

Preliminary Results

Only the results of the first two rounds of censuses giving the first baseline healing rates are available at present, and these are shown in Fig. 28.2. Ulcerated legs rather than leg ulcer patients have been noted. A total of 1508 patients were identified in the first census and 1446 in the second, with less than 1% lost to follow-up in the second

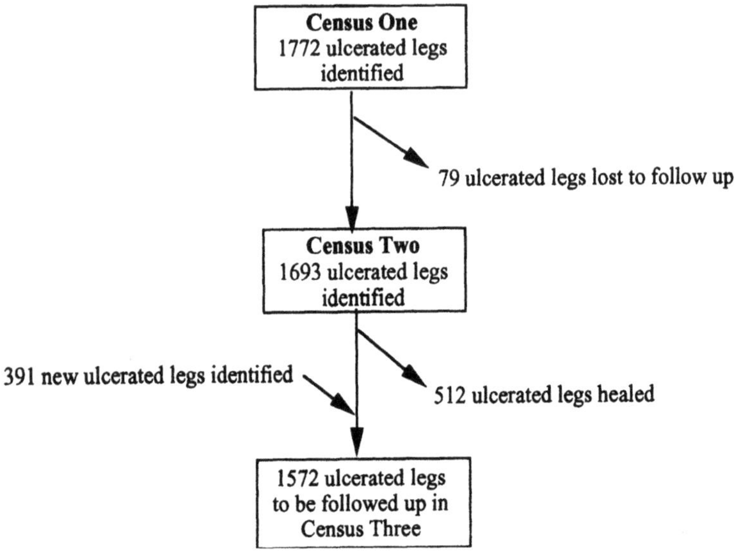

Fig. 28.2. Preliminary results of the first two censuses from the Scottish Leg Ulcer Project, given as numbers of ulcerated legs identified.

census. Of these 62 patients for whom no information was available, two are not compliant with treatment, one is away on holiday and two have entered long-term care. The remainder have died or moved to another area.

Conclusions

This is an exciting project because it has the potential to improve leg ulcer care for patients in a large part of Scotland as well as providing necessary further information about guideline implementation. Guidelines are one of a number of ways in which clinical practice can be altered in order to improve outcome, but merely developing a guideline is insufficient: there must be a clear strategy for implementation. As effective methods are labour-intensive this brings considerable short-term resource implications, although there may be longer-term cost savings if the hoped for improvement in clinical outcome is achieved.

References

1. Field MJ, Lohr KN, editor. Guidelines for clinical practice: from development to use. Washington: National Academy Press, 1992.
2. Grimshaw J, Russell I. Achieving health gain through clinical guidelines. I. Developing scientifically valid guidelines. Qual Health Care 1993;2:243–8.
3. Woolf SH. Practice guidelines, a new reality in medicine. Arch Intern Med 1992;152:946–952.
4. Grimshaw JM, Russell IT. Achieving health gain through clinical guidelines. II> Ensuring guidelines change medical practice. Qual Health Care 1994;3:45–52.
5. Grimshaw J, Freemantle N, Wallace S, et al. Developing and implementing clinical practice guidelines. Qual Health Care 1995;4:55–64.
6. Robertson N, Baker R, Hearnshaw H. Changing the clinical behaviour of doctors: a psychological framework. Qual Health Care 1996;5:51–54.
7. Grol R. Implementing guidelines in general practice care. Qual Health Care 1992;1:184–191.
8. Mansfield C. Attitudes and behaviours towards clinical guidelines: the clinician's perspective. Qual Health Care 1995;4:250–255.
9. Renvoize EB, Hampshaw SM, Pinder JM, Ayres P. What are hospitals doing about clinical guidelines? Qual Health Care 1997;6:187–191.
10. Moffat CJ, Franks PJ, Oldroyd M. Community clinics for leg ulcers: an impact on healing. BMJ 1992;305:1389–1392.
11. Feder G. Clinical guidelines in 1994. BMJ 1994;309:1457–1458.
12. Haines A, Feder G. Guidance on guidelines. BMJ 1992;305:785–786.
13. Sudlow M, Thomson R. Clinical guidelines: quantity without quality. Qual Health Care 1997;6:60–61.
14. CRAG. Clinical guidelines: a report by a working group set up by the Clinical Resource and Audit Group. Edinburgh: Scottish Office, 1993.
15. Petrie JC, Grimshaw JM, Bryson A. The Scottish Intercollegiate Guideline Network Initiative: getting validated guidelines into local practice. Health Bull 1995;53:345–348.
16. WHO (Europe) and International Diabetes Federation (Europe). Diabetes care and research in Europe: the St. Vincent Declaration. Diab Med 1990;34:655–661.
17. Petrie J, Harlen J. SIGN comes of age: but what next? Health Bull 1997;55:362–364.
18. SIGN. Clinical guidelines: criteria for appraisal for national use. Edinburgh: SIGN, 1995

Index

FSC
www.fsc.org
MIX
Papier aus verantwortungsvollen Quellen
Paper from responsible sources
FSC® C105338

If you have any concerns about our products,
you can contact us on
ProductSafety@springernature.com

In case Publisher is established outside the EU,
the EU authorized representative is:
Springer Nature Customer Service Center GmbH
Europaplatz 3, 69115 Heidelberg, Germany

Printed by Libri Plureos GmbH
in Hamburg, Germany